基础病理形态学
Basic Pathological Morphology

主编　李懿萍　卜晓东

Editors in Chief
Yiping Li　Xiaodong Bu

东南大学出版社
SOUTHEAST UNIVERSITY PRESS
·南京·

图书在版编目（CIP）数据

基础病理形态学 / 李懿萍，卜晓东主编 . —南京：
东南大学出版社，2023.2
ISBN 978 - 7 - 5766 - 0596 - 9

Ⅰ. ①基⋯　Ⅱ. ①李⋯ ②卜⋯　Ⅲ. ①病理形态学
Ⅳ. ① R361

中国版本图书馆 CIP 数据核字（2022）第 248827 号

责任编辑:陈潇潇　责任校对:李成思　封面设计:王　玥　责任印制:周荣虎

基础病理形态学
Jichu Bingli Xingtaixue

主　　编	李懿萍　卜晓东
出版发行	东南大学出版社
社　　址	南京四牌楼2号　邮编：210096　电话：025-83793330
网　　址	http://www.seupress.com
电子邮件	press@ seupress.com
经　　销	全国各地新华书店
印　　刷	南京艺中印务有限公司
开　　本	787 mm×1092 mm　1/16
印　　张	18.25
字　　数	410千字
版　　次	2023年2月第1版
印　　次	2023年2月第1次印刷
书　　号	ISBN 978 - 7 - 5766 - 0596 - 9
定　　价	68.00元

＊ 本社图书若有印装质量问题,请直接与营销部联系,电话（传真）:025-83791830。

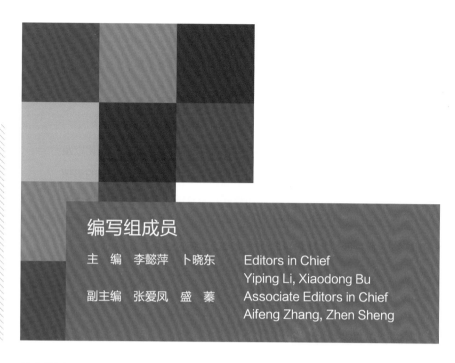

编写组成员

主 编 李懿萍 卜晓东　　Editors in Chief
　　　　　　　　　　　　Yiping Li, Xiaodong Bu
副主编 张爱凤 盛 蓁　　Associate Editors in Chief
　　　　　　　　　　　　Aifeng Zhang, Zhen Sheng

编者（按姓氏笔画为序）

卜晓东　东南大学医学院病理学系
许　纯　南京大学医学院附属鼓楼医院病理科
李懿萍　东南大学医学院病理学系
张爱凤　东南大学医学院病理学系
陈平圣　东南大学医学院病理学系
徐月霜　东南大学医学院病理学系
盛　蓁　东南大学医学院病理学系
潘　旻　东南大学医学院病理学系

Contributors

Xiaodong Bu　Department of Pathology, Medical School, Southeast University

Chun Xu　Department of Pathology, Affiliated Drum Tower Hospital, Medical School, Nanjing University

Yiping Li　Department of Pathology, Medical School, Southeast University

Aifeng Zhang　Department of Pathology, Medical School, Southeast University

Pingsheng Chen　Department of Pathology, Medical School, Southeast University

Yueshuang Xu　Department of Pathology, Medical School, Southeast University

Zhen Sheng　Department of Pathology, Medical School, Southeast University

Min Pan　Department of Pathology, Medical School, Southeast University

前言
PREFACE

病理学主要是从形态学角度来研究疾病的病因，疾病时器官、组织的病理变化以及其发生发展规律的一门医学桥梁学科。众所周知，理论来自实践，没有几百年来的病理学实践就没有今天的病理学理论。医学生在本科阶段学习病理的时间十分有限，所以为了提高学习效率，首先学习前人从实践中总结出来的一些理论，然后再通过观察标本和切片的病理形态来验证这些理论，是非常必要的。只有通过理论课和实习课的结合，才能真正理解和掌握教科书上的理论知识，为以后学习临床学科及从事临床或科研实践奠定较扎实的基础。

如果说掌握基本病理形态是病理学入门捷径，那么一本高质量实习教材就是成功指南。国内出版的用于医学生病理实习的教材不少，但由于各院校在标本切片方面的差异性，此类教材难以推广，所以几乎每个院校均有各自的病理实习指导用书。如果有一本通用性强的实习教材，则不仅扩充了学习资源，而且可以相应扩大学习自由度，有利于学生的个性化发展。

我们根据病理教学大纲，依托多年来积累的线上线下教学资源，以及借鉴国内外同类教材编写经验，推出了这本《基础病理形态学》，希望能实现上述愿景。

本教材为中英双语，内容丰富，既有学习要求、理论回顾、典型病理标本和组织图像、案例分析、习题作业等板块，还附有线上课程（病理与健康：https://www.icourse163.org/course/SEU-1001755397；病理形态实验学：https://www.icourse163.org/course/SEU-1206290801；普通病理学：https://www.icourse163.org/course/SEU-1463109174；系统病理学：https://www.icourse163.org/course/SEU-1206526803）、数字病理切片库链接，以实现资源共享。本教材附有680余幅典型病理图片，它既是病理学实习指导，也是病理学图谱，还是联系相关病理资源的平台，所以既可作为医学本科生、留学生病理实习指导书，也可作为医学研究生和低年资病理医生的基础参考书。

在本书编写过程中，得到了江苏省中西医结合医院病理科曾铮、李瑞平，南京金陵医院病理科吴楠，南京脑科医院病理科王娟，江苏省人民医院江北院区病理科史传兵，江苏省肿瘤医院病理科张晓毅，东南大学附属中大医院病理科张丽华、魏晓莹、丁粉干、徐佳佳等多位同道的大力支持，在此深表谢意！

由于编者水平有限，本教材难免存在不足之处，还望同道们不吝赐教。

陈平圣 于南京

2022年12月

Pathology is a medical bridge discipline to study the etiology, pathological changes of organs or tissues, and their development. It is known to all that theory comes from practice. Without hundreds of years of pathological practice, there would be no pathological theory as we have today. However, the time is very limited to study pathology for undergraduates. Therefore, in order to improve learning efficiency, it is very necessary to study theoretical knowledge summarized by predecessors from practice firstly. Then we can identify them by observing the pathological morphology of specimens and sections in person. Only by combining theoretical courses with experimental courses, we can really master the theoretical knowledge in textbooks and lay a solid foundation for learning clinical disciplines in clinical practice and scientific research in future.

Since mastering basic pathological changes is a shortcut to pathology study, a high-quality practice textbook is a successful guide. Many textbooks for pathology practice have being published in China. The specimens and sections described in textbooks are different due to the editors in various colleges so that almost every college has its own pathology practice guidance. Therefore, it is difficult to popularize such textbooks. If there is a universal textbook, it will expand not only learning resources, but also learning freedom, which is favorable to the personalized development of students.

To achieve the above willingness, we compile the book after consulting abundant information. The writers have collected the data including pathology syllabuses of various colleges, online and offline teaching resources accumulated over years, and related teaching materials at home and abroad.

This textbook, *Basic Pathological Morphology*, is bilingual in Chinese and English. The content is rich, and covers learning requirements, learning guidance, typical pathological specimens and histological images, clinical case analyses, exercises, as well as the shared resource links including online courses and digital pathological section library. This textbook is attached with more than 680 typical pathological pictures, so it is not only a practice guidance of pathology and a color atlas of pathology, but also an interlinkage of relevant online pathology resources(Pathology and health: https://www.icourse163.org/course/SEU−1001755397; Experimental pathology: https://www.icourse163.org/course/SEU−1206290801; General pathology: https://www.icourse163.org/course/SEU−1463109174; Systemic pathology: https://www.icourse163.org/course/SEU−1206526803). Therefore, it can be used as a practice guide for medical undergraduates and international students, as well as a basic reference book for medical postgraduates and junior pathologists.

We really appreciate selfless support from many colleagues during the process of writing this book. They are Zheng Zeng, Ruiping Li (Department of Pathology, Jiangsu Province Hospital on Integration of Chinese and Western Medicine), Nan Wu (Department of Pathology, Nanjing Jinling Hospital), Juan Wang (Department of Pathology, Nanjing Brain Hospital), Chuanbing Shi (Department of Pathology, Pukou Branch of Jiangsu Province Hospital), Xiaoyi Zhang (Department of Pathology, Jiangsu Cancer Hospital), Lihua Zhang, Xiaoying Wei, Fengan Ding, and Jiajia Xu (Department of Pathology, Zhongda Hospital, Southeast University).

Due to the limited level of editors, some mistakes and omissions may exist in this textbook. We appreciate readers' criticisms and suggestions for future revision and improvement.

Pingsheng Chen, Nanjing

December, 2022

病理与健康

病理形态实验学

General Pathology

Systemic Pathology

目录
CONTENTS

学习入门

　　解剖学和组织胚胎学是基础病理形态学学习的必备知识,掌握正常形态方可学习异常形态,同学们务必打牢基础。

　　病理实习课提倡理论联系实际。在观察标本切片时,要全面细致,自行验证所学的理论;同时又要用理论指导实践,发现病变,且分清主次。为了使实习取得预期的效果,一定要有独立思考、刻苦钻研的精神;要有实事求是的科学态度,认真观察每一个标本和每一张切片,切忌走马观花、不懂装懂。

　　通过观察标本切片、尸检示教和分析讨论尸检病案,不仅要学习病理学的基本理论,认识基本病变,还要通过观察与分析病理现象,培养自己的归纳、推理能力,以便得出正确结论。因此,观察标本切片时要认真思考,透过现象抓住本质。看到大体标本的病变,要联想此处镜下改变,反之亦然。不仅如此,还要联想病变是怎样形成的,对该器官及全身有何影响,并联系所学过的病理及其他基础学科知识,推断与形态改变有关的机能与代谢变化以及病人可能发生的临床表现,以做到理论联系实际、宏观联系微观、局部联系整体、形态联系机能代谢、基础联系临床。简言之,即用"动"的、发展的、整体的观点看待静止的、局部的标本切片及实习材料,以期对所学的疾病获得一个完整和动态的概念。

一、主要学习资源

　　病理学的实习材料,主要来自尸检和活检,包括人体病变器官制成的大体标本和病变组织制成的切片。此外,尚有线上教学视频,既有三维标本展示、组织切片和尸检示教等,也有数字切片平台。

　　1. 大体标本:是用于肉眼观察病变的器官和组织。我们所观察的大体标本,多数是用10%福尔马林(即4%甲醛溶液)固定的,与新鲜标本比较,颜色已有所改变,但并不妨碍我们对病变的观察。

　　2. 组织切片:是取自大体标本病变部分的组织。经切片染色后,封固在玻片上,需用显微镜观察形态。

　　观察大体标本可以认识病变器官或组织的全部状态,病变的性质、部位和分布等,因而能对病变进行初步诊断。观察组织切片则可以认识病变的微细结构,并能对病变加以较为精确的鉴别,以确定病变的性质和范围,做出最后诊断。但因它仅为病变的一小部分组织,所以有一定的局限性。要想对病变做出全面、正确的诊断,必须既观察组织切片又观察大体标本,把两者有机地结合起来。

二、 大体标本的观察方法与步骤

1. 先确定标本是什么器官,是器官的哪一部分。有的标本是由外科手术取下的,这种标本常常是部分器官或某种组织,且有时不易见到正常的部分,这时就要注意设法判明标本是取自什么器官、什么组织。

2. 观察器官的体积(大小)及重量,若是实质性器官(肝、肾、脾),注意是否肿大或缩小;若是有腔器官(心、胃、肠),注意其内腔是否有扩大或狭窄,腔壁有无变薄或增厚,腔内有无内容物、是什么性质的内容物,并要观察黏膜或内膜色泽,注意它们是否光滑,有无出血、溃疡和假膜形成等。

3. 观察器官的形态,注意有无变形(如肝硬化时变为结节状等),然后分别观察表面及切面的下列各种变化:

① 光滑度(光滑或粗糙)。

② 湿润度(湿润或干燥)。

③ 透明度(正常器官包膜菲薄而透明,当有病变时可变混浊而失去光泽)。

④ 颜色(暗红、淡黄、棕黄、灰白、黑色等),还得注意标本颜色是源于福尔马林固定后的变化,还是自然颜色。

⑤ 硬度(变硬、变软、坚实或松脆等)。

⑥ 切面(是否平整,边缘有无外翻,质地是否均匀,色泽及正常解剖结构有无改变等)。

4. 观察表面和切面有无病灶(即器官中或组织中病变特别明显的部分)及病灶的特征:

① 位置:在器官的哪一部分。

② 数目及分布:单个或多个,区域分布或弥漫分布。

③ 大小:体积＝长×宽×厚,并以毫米或厘米为单位。有时也可以用实物大小如芝麻大、粟米大、绿豆大、黄豆大、鸡蛋大、拳头大等形容。

④ 形状:乳头状、菜花状、息肉状、三角形、楔形等。

⑤ 颜色:红色表示病灶内含血液,黄色表示含有脂肪或类脂,绿色或黄绿色表示含有胆汁,棕黄色一般表示含有含铁血黄素,灰白色一般为纤维结缔组织等。另外,有些特殊病变常有特殊颜色改变,因此要注意比较病灶与周围组织的颜色有何不同。

⑥ 质地:如硬、软、韧、脆、致密、疏松等,并与周围组织进行对比。

⑦ 与周围组织的关系:如病灶边界明显还是模糊,有无包膜,是否充血、出血,对周围组织有无压迫、浸润、破坏等。

5. 病理诊断:根据所观察到的病理变化,结合理论知识对大体标本上的病变做出初步诊断。诊断的写法是**器官名称＋病理变化**,如肝淤血、脑出血、肾贫血性梗死等。

三、 病理组织切片的观察方法与步骤

一般采用普通光学显微镜观察。大家使用的切片大多是石蜡切片,经苏木素-伊红(H.E.)染色后,细胞浆及结缔组织呈粉红色,细胞核呈紫蓝色。有时采用特殊染色(如苏丹Ⅲ、锇酸等)。

观察病理切片必须按照下列步骤:先全面了解,再重点观察;先应用正常组织学知识判定病变部分属于什么器官、什么组织,再应用病理学知识识别病变的性质、范围和程度等。

观察步骤如下:

第一步:先用肉眼观察切片,初步了解整个切片的情况。通过这一步骤,有时能认出其为何种组织,如肺、脑等最易辨认。而切片上的组织如有显著病变部分,则可确定其位置以及与周围组织的关系,使镜下观察时不致遗漏。

一般来说,肉眼观察切片应注意三点:

1. 切片上的组织是什么形状。如为环状,则大致为有管腔器官的横切面等。

2. 组织是同质的还是有显然不同的部分。

3. 组织的边界是自然的,还是切割的。自然的边缘常为该器官的包膜或浆膜。

第二步:用低倍镜观察,这是最常见的观察步骤。观察时上下、左右移动切片,在全面细致地观察切片之后,先要确定是何种组织,然后观察病变所在及病变性质,再观察病变与正常组织的关系等。大多数病变都可能而且应该在低倍镜下观察到。

观察时注意以下几点:

1. 切片上组织如系同质的,要辨认出是什么组织;如系显然不同的组织构成,则要认出是什么器官,是否与肉眼观察所预断者相符合等。

2. 切片组织之边界如为自然的,注意是否有上皮覆盖,是哪一类上皮,是否正常,有无结缔组织包膜,包膜是否增厚等。

3. 对切片上有病理改变(不正常状态)的组织,应进一步确定其性质,可注意下列四项:

① 病变组织的分布,其结构及与周围组织的关系与正常状态有何不同;

② 病变区内细胞的大小、形状、结构、数量等是否正常;

③ 有无特殊物质,如细菌、寄生虫、色素、异物等出现,其性质、数量、部位及与周围组织的关系如何;

④ 病变是否由肿瘤性增生的细胞组成,其分化程度及与周围组织的关系如何等。

第三步:用高倍镜观察。高倍镜一般用于观察细胞水平的一些较微细的结构变化,最后确定病理变化的性质,做出病理诊断。使用时一定要先用低倍镜找到要观察的部分,固定在视野中心,再换用高倍镜观察。因高倍镜放大倍数大,所以观察的范围实际上很小,不易看到病变的全貌及与周围的关系。因此,一定要先用低倍镜观察,再有目的地进行高倍镜观察;否则无目标地在高倍镜下移动切片,不仅不易找到观察的目标,而且会浪费很多的时间和精力,事倍功半。另外,若不经过低倍镜观察,直接用高倍镜看切片,

不但不易对准焦点，且接物镜可能下降太低而撞击玻片，导致物镜和切片的损坏。

第四步：用油镜观察。一般情况用低倍镜和高倍镜观察即可做出病理诊断，不必使用油镜。油镜仅在查看组织中微生物时以及一些特殊情况下才使用。

本书所列显微图片后的括号内均备注了放大倍数，绝大多数为 H.E. 染色，所以正文将不再多做说明，若同时有特殊染色、荧光染色和电镜图片呈现时将会特别注明。

四、 绘图和描述的意义与要求

绘图和描述的意义：

1. 帮助同学深入细致地观察病变，器官和组织病变的形态经过绘图或文字描述，使实践与理论结合得更好，经过绘图或文字描述，印象较深。

2. 科学绘图及文字描述是一项基本技能训练。借助它，科学工作者可以把观察到的形象记录下来。因此，医学生必须掌握科学绘图和文字描述的技巧。这不仅可以提高对病变的分析和描述能力，而且还可以培养严谨的科学工作作风。绘图只要求对病变的形态用正确的图形来表达，应重点突出，画面整洁，不要求工笔画，但也不能潦草、敷衍。文字描述要求用词准确，条理清楚，书写整洁，使别人看后能对描述的病变有形象的概念，应避免重复累赘、杂乱无章或过于简单、马虎草率。

总之，对绘图和描述的要求就是要说明问题。如何才能说明问题呢？主要应做到以下三点：

① 正确显示或表达出病变部位，例如绘制肝淤血，必须显示肝小叶的中央静脉淤血的程度；描述大叶性肺炎时，必须说清楚是哪个肺叶等。

② 能正确地显示或表达出所观察到的病变的各种特点，这是很重要的。

③ 对每一个具体结构或病变特点的描绘，首先要抓住形象特征。例如中性粒细胞，应该画出分叶状核；淋巴细胞，应画出圆形深染的核及其外周少量胞浆。此外，各细胞间大小比例必须正确。再如，文字描述梗死区时，要写出梗死灶的大小、形状、颜色、质地等。

至于绘图时究竟画高倍好还是低倍好，采取哪个视野，应根据具体情况而定。一般说来，低倍图利于显示病变全貌，高倍图利于显示细微结构，必要时也可以在画低倍图像后佐以高倍图像以更清楚地表达出病变特征。

必须指出，在绘图时必须防止两种偏向：一种是为了说明问题，全部按照图谱描下来，这种脱离实际的作风不好；另一种是完全按照单个视野中所见依样画葫芦，这种画法的真实性是好，但如一个视野中所见并未包括全部特点，这样做就不能说明问题。此时可把两个或几个视野所见综合画出，如此，既较好地表达了病变特征，又不损害它的真实性。同样文字描述时，也要避免照抄教科书上有关病变的文字，或者对每个细节都详细描述，忽略重点，舍本逐末。

Introduction to Learning

Anatomy and histology as well as embryology are knowledge cornerstones to basic pathological morphology. Students must lay a solid foundation to learn abnormal morphology better.

It is advocated to integrate theory with practice in pathology practice courses. It is important to observe the specimens and sections comprehensively and detailedly, which contributes to verify the theoretical knowledge. Simultaneously, theoretical knowledge should be used to guide practice, which helps to find out the major and minor lesions, primary and secondary lesions. In order to achieve the expected learning effect, it is recommended not only to keep the spirit of independent thinking, diligent study, and scientific down-to-earth attitude, but also to avoid glancing over things hurriedly and pretending to know all.

By observing specimens and sections, autopsy teaching and case analyses, not only basic theory, basic lesions, but also induction and reasoning capabilities can be trained to draw accurate conclusions. Therefore, perceiving the essence through the appearance is the key point to study specimens and slices. When observing gross specimens, think of the associated microscopic changes, and vice versa. Furthermore, to cultivate clinical thinking way, after identifying the lesion, think about its developing process and the impact on the organ and the host and infer the functional and metabolic changes, and the clinical manifestations related to the morphological changes. Try to integrate theory with practice, macro with micro, parts with whole, morphology with functions, basic changes with clinical abnormalities. In short, the static and local practice materials, mainly specimens and sections, should be viewed in a "dynamic", developmental and overall approach.

1. Main learning resources

The practice materials of pathology mainly come from the working accumulation of human autopsy and biopsy, including gross specimens from diseased organs and sections from diseased tissues. In addition, there are online teaching videos, such as three-dimensional specimens, tissue sections, autopsy teaching, as well as digital section platform. It is worth mentioning that students can also browse digital sections on the website provided.

1.1　Gross specimens

They are used to observe the diseased organs and tissues with naked eyes. Most of them were fixed with 10％ formalin (i. e. 4％ formaldehyde solution). Compared with fresh specimens, the color has changed, but it has not influence on observing lesions.

1.2　Tissue sections

They are taken from the lesions of gross specimens. After being sectioned and dyed, they are sealed on the glass slides to be observed under the microscope.

By observing the gross specimens, you can recognize the diseased organs or tissues in a whole, clarify the nature, location and distribution of the lesions, and finally make preliminary pathological diagnoses. By checking tissue sections, the microstructure of the lesions can be accurately identified to determine the nature of the lesions and definite the pathological diagnoses. However, it has some limitations because the slices have been made of partial tissues. Therefore, to make a comprehensive and correct diagnosis, you must integrate the information you have observed from both tissue sections and gross specimens. Clinically, we need to further combine the morphological changes with clinical materials including clinical manifestations, radiographic and laboratory examinations to make the final pathological diagnosis.

2. Observation of gross specimens

2.1　First determine what organ the specimen is, then clarify the specific location of lesions in the organ. Some specimens removed surgically often present certain parts of organs and tissues, and sometimes it is difficult to find out normal parts. Thus, it is necessary to identify what organs and tissues the specimens have been taken from.

2.2　Observe the volume (size) and weight of the organ. If it is a parenchymal organ (liver, kidney or spleen), you should pay attention to whether its size becomes large or small. If it is a hollow/cavitary organ (heart, stomach or intestine), notice the changes: the volume of the inner cavity and thickness of the wall; the contents in the lumen: normal or abnormal, if with abnormal contents, identify their nature; the mucosa or intima: color, smoothness (smooth or rough), injured changes (bleeding, necrosis, ulcer, pseudomembrane).

2.3　Look into the shape of organs and pay attention to whether there is deformation (such as nodular appearance for liver cirrhosis). Therefore, it is very important to familiarize with the morphology of healthy organs, tissues, and cells. A good learner of pathology often reviews human anatomy and histology. The changes on the surface and cut surface are observed as follows.

(1) Smoothness (smooth or rough).

(2) Tissue moisture (wet or dry).

(3) Transparency (Generally, the capsule of normal organs is thin and transparent. Under

pathological condition, the capsule can become thick, turbid and lose original luster).

(4) Color (dark red, light yellow, brown yellow, gray, or black, etc.). Consider that color changes of the specimens were caused by fixation with formalin or the natural color of diseased organ.

(5) Hardness (hardening, softening, firmness or brittleness, etc.).

(6) Cut surface (whether the section is flat, whether the edge is everted, whether the texture is consistent, whether the color and anatomical structure are abnormal, etc.).

2.4　Note whether there are lesions on the surface and cut surface, and the characteristics of lesions.

(1) Location: involved part of the organ.

(2) Number and distribution: single or multiple, regional or diffuse.

(3) Size: Volume= length×width×thickness (unit: mm or cm). Sometimes it can also be described as the size of real objects, such as sesames, corns, mung beans, soybeans, eggs or fists.

(4) Shape: papillary, cauliflower, polypoid, triangular, or wedgy, etc.

(5) Color: red indicates hemorragic area, yellow for fat or lipids, green or yellow green for bile, brown yellow and gray white generally for hemosiderin and fibrous connective tissue, respectively. In addition, some special lesions often have specific color changes, so you should take into account the color differences between lesions and surrounding tissues.

(6) Texture: hard, soft, tough, brittle, dense, loose, and the texture difference between lesions and the surrounding tissues.

(7) Relationship with surrounding tissues: for example, the lesion border (clear or unclear), outmost tissue (with capsule or without), congestion, bleeding, and the effect on surrounding tissues (compression, infiltration, and destruction, etc.).

2.5　Pathological diagnosis: make a preliminary diagnosis of the lesions on the gross specimen according to the observed pathological changes and the corresponding theoretical knowledge. The diagnosis is defined as **organ name ＋ pathological changes.** For example, liver congestion, cerebral hemorrhage, renal anemic infarction, etc.

3.　Observation of tissue sections

It is usually observed by ordinary optical microscope. Most sections are generally paraffin sections. After stained by hematoxylin and eosin (H.E.), the cytoplasm and connective tissue are pink and the nuclei are purple blue. Sometimes special dyes are used (such as Sudan Ⅲ, osmic acid, etc.).

To observe sections better, the following steps are recommended. First get the whole impression by scanning comprehensively, and make a preliminary judgement what the observed organ and tissue, and possible pathological changes are. Then focus on the part of possible lesions to identify the nature and extent of the lesions based on the pathological knowledge.

The detailed steps are as follows.

3. 1　Step 1

To get an overall impression of the section with naked eyes.You can sometimes identify the tissue you are observing, such as lung and brain. For the tissue with a significant lesion, its location and relationship with the surrounding tissue can be determined, which makes us not to miss the lesion under the microscope.

Generally speaking, three key points should be considered when observing slices with naked eyes:

(1) The shape of the tissue on the slice. If the tissue is annular, it is mostly possible to be the cross-section of a luminal organ.

(2) The texture and color of the whole tissue is consistent or obviously different.

(3) Is the tissue edge natural or cut? The natural margin is often the capsule or serosa of the organ.

3. 2　Step 2

To observe tissue section with low-power magnification. The step is the most important part to be done for observers. When observing, carefully move the section up, down, left and right to cover the whole tissue. For most sections, tissue, lesions, the location, border, and nature of lesions can be identified at low magnification. The following points should be noticed during observation.

(1) If the tissue on the slice is homogeneous, the tissue should be recognized. If it is obviously different, the organ must be identified and consistent with the preliminary judgement by naked eyes.

(2) If the margin of the tissue is natural, to identify that it is covered by epithelium or capsule, and histological structure is normal or abnormal. For covering epithelium, it is needed to define the type of epithelium.

(3) For the tissue with pathological changes on the section, its nature should be further elucidated, and the following four items can be noted.

① The distribution of diseased tissues, difference between the lesions and normal tissues based on its microscopic structure, and their relationship with surrounding tissues.

② The size, shape, structure and quantity of cells in the lesions.

③ Abnormal substances, such as bacteria, parasites, pigments and foreign bodies, and their nature, quantity, location and relationship with neighbouring tissues.

④ Tumor cells in the lesions, and the differentiation degree and the relationship with adjacent tissues.

3. 3　Step 3

To observe with a high-power magnification. This step is generally used to determine some fine structural changes at the cell level, confirm the nature of pathological changes, and make final pathological diagnoses. To do that, you must first find the part to be particularly observed with a low-power objective, and fix the key area in center of the visual field. Due to large magnification of high-power objective, the viewing zone is too small to observe the whole slice. As we have known, moving the slice aimlessly under a high-power objective will not only make it difficult to find the target, but also waste time. In addition, if you use a high-power objective at the beginning of observation, it is hard to focus on the tissue. Simultaneously, if the objective len drops too low, both the objective lens and slice can be damaged. Therefore, you must start observing with a low-power objective, and then change for a high-power objective.

3.4 Step 4

To observe tissue slice with oil immersion lens. Generally, oil objective is not necessary to be used because pathological diagnosis can be made by detecting with low-power objective and high-power objective. The oil len is only used in observing microorganisms in the tissues and some special cases.

Most histological images are shown with magnifications stated in the parentheses by H.E. staining in this book, which is no more described in the main body. However, if the pictures are from special staining, immunofluorescence staining, and transmission electron microscopy (TEM), we will supplement the necessary explanation.

4. Significance and requirements of drawing and text description

4.1 Significance

(1) Help students to observe morphological changes deeply and carefully, and make a better integration of practice and theory.

(2) Scientific drawing and text description are basic skills for learners of pathology. Observers can record and share what they see by these skills. This can not only improve the ability to analyze and describe lesions, but also cultivate a rigorous scientific attitude.

Therefore, medical students should master the skills of scientific drawing and text description.

4.2 Requirements

In short, the drawing only requires typically graphic expression of the lesion. A neat picture is required, and scribbled and perfunctory drawing should be avoided. The text description requires well-organized and concise words, which can exhibit a vivid concept of the described lesions. Redundant, poorly-organized, too simple or careless text explanations should be prohibited.

(1) Accurately display or express the location of lesions. For example, when drawing liver congestion, it is necessary to show the congestion degree of hepatic lobules and portal areas. When describing lobar pneumonia, it is required to clarify the involved specific lobe, etc.

(2) It is important to correctly display or express the characteristics of the observed lesions.

(3) Grasp typical characteristics when describing the pathological changes of each specific structure or lesion. For example, lobulated nuclei must be drawn for neutrophils, while round and deeply stained nuclei and a small amount of cytoplasm should be presented for lymphocytes. The proportion of various cells in the same tissues should be rational. Monocytes are usually larger than erythrocytes in a picture. If describing an infarct area, the text should contain its size, shape, color, and texture. The vision is drawn based on high or low-power fields, which depends on specific cases. Generally speaking, low-power images are conducive to display a whole picture of lesions, and high-power images are powerful to reveal microscopic structure. If necessary, a combination of the high-power image and corresponding low-power image can contribute to elucidate the morphological characteristics better.

(4) Two prejudices must be prohibited in drawing. One is to copy the atlas to explain lesions better, but the observed images in the tissue are not considered thoroughly. The other is to draw pictures completely according to the observed images in a single field of vision. The authenticity of this painting method is good, but the observed picture in a vision field can not cover all the features and represent the lesion. In this case, two or more visual fields may be drawn comprehensively, which can express the morphological features of the lesion without influencing its authenticity better. Similarly, when describing a lesion, we should avoid copying the related text from textbooks or other pathology books, or describe all the abnormal changes in detail, which will neglect morphological characteristics of lesions.

陈平圣 (Pingsheng Chen)

第一章

细胞、组织的适应和损伤，损伤的修复

一、目的要求

1. 掌握不同类型萎缩的形态变化及其对机体的影响。
2. 掌握细胞水肿、脂肪变及玻璃样变的形态学特征及其对机体的影响。
3. 掌握不同类型坏死的形态学特征、鉴别点以及坏死的结局。
4. 掌握肉芽组织的构成及其功能。
5. 了解淀粉样变、黏液样变、病理性色素沉着、病理性钙化等的形态特征。

导学

细胞 组织

适应
- 萎缩
- 肥大
- 增生
- 化生

可逆性损伤
- 细胞水肿
- 脂肪变
- 玻璃样变
- 淀粉样变
- 黏液样变
- 病理性色素沉着
- 病理性钙化

不可逆性损伤
- 坏死
  凝固性坏死
  液化性坏死
  纤维素样坏死
  干酪样坏死
  脂肪坏死
  坏疽
- 凋亡

二、大体标本

1. 适应

1.1　子宫老年性萎缩（图 1-1）

标本为全切子宫及双侧附件。子宫体积缩小，重量减轻。

1.2　小腿骨骼肌萎缩（图 1-2）

标本为两小腿相应水平之横断面，粗者取自健侧，细者取自萎缩侧，显示萎缩侧肢体已明显变细，骨骼肌萎缩甚至消失，由纤维脂肪组织充填取代。

1.3　心肌褐色萎缩（图 1-3）

心脏体积缩小，心尖部变尖，心外膜下冠状动脉弯曲（蓝箭）。心肌呈褐色，是由于脂褐素在心肌纤维内聚集所致。

1.4　肾压迫性萎缩（图 1-4）

肾脏的冠状切面，可见肾体积增大，失去原有的外形，整个肾脏呈多房状，肾实质明显萎缩变薄。该病变形态多见于肾盂和输尿管结石患者导致的尿路梗阻。

1.5　子宫肥大（图 1-5）

标本为妊娠子宫，子宫体积明显增大，切面可见宫壁肌层高度增厚。子宫肥大常常伴有宫壁的平滑肌细胞增生。

1.6　肠代偿性肥大（图 1-6）

标本为一段肠管，部分区域肠管狭窄（蓝框），狭窄以上的肠腔扩张（蓝箭），肠壁肥厚。

2. 可逆性损伤

2.1　肾水肿（图 1-7）

肾脏的冠状切面，可见肾体积略增大，包膜紧张、混浊、颜色变灰。切面见实质隆起，边缘外翻，皮质增厚，皮髓质分界不清，条纹模糊。

2.2　肝水肿（图 1-8）

肝脏略增大，包膜紧张，失去光泽，似沸水煮过样外观。切面实质隆起，边缘外翻，色泽较灰白。

2.3　肝脂肪变（图 1-9）

肝组织切面实质稍隆起，色泽淡黄，有油腻感。右图显示苏丹Ⅲ染色，呈橘红色。

2.4　脾包膜玻璃样变（图 1-10）

脾脏体积增大，部分包膜明显增厚（蓝框），色灰白，呈半透明之外观。注意与正常厚度的包膜（黑框）相对比。

2.5　睾丸白膜玻璃样变（图 1-11）

睾丸切面可见白膜明显增厚，色淡灰白，呈半透明状外观（蓝箭）。该病变形态多见于慢性鞘膜积液患者。

2.6　皮肤黏液样变（图 1-12）

标本为两块皮肤及皮下组织。一块为正常皮肤（黑箭），另一块为黏液样变的皮肤，可见表皮变皱，真皮由于纤维结缔组织增生而明显增厚，呈灰白色，略有半透明黏液样背景（蓝箭）。

2.7　肺含铁血黄素沉着（图1-13）

一侧肺组织切面，可见肺质地粗糙、干燥，并有铁锈色或棕褐色的色素沉着，即含铁血黄素。

2.8　眼脉络膜恶性黑色素瘤（图1-14）

标本为眼球的矢状剖面，可见色素膜起源的恶性肿瘤细胞富含黑色素，已全部占据球内玻璃体，并累及眼球后组织。

2.9　肺炭末沉着（图1-15）

一侧肺组织，可见肺膜面布满大小不等的黑色斑点，乃大量炭末沉着所致。

2.10　皮肤文身（图1-16）

标本为皮肤，表面可见黑色图案。是将色素注射入皮肤后，被吞噬细胞吞噬，并携运于真皮层的结缔组织中所致。

2.11　肺结核钙化灶（图1-17）

一侧肺组织切面，组织内可见灰白色质硬小结节（蓝箭），形如石灰，这是因为该处组织坏死后有钙盐沉积所致。该标本属于哪一种类型的病理性钙化？

3. 不可逆性损伤

3.1　脾凝固性坏死（图1-18）

脾脏切面可见灰白色坏死区，质地致密而干燥，边界清楚，周围绕有一圈黑褐色的充血出血带。

3.2　脑液化性坏死（图1-19）

脑冠状切面，可见大脑左右侧不对称，一侧大脑半球体积缩小，基底节区可见液化性坏死灶（蓝箭），呈疏松网状结构，该侧脑组织略有塌陷。

3.3　淋巴结干酪样坏死（图1-20）

数个淋巴结增大、粘连成一个团块，切面可见大小不等的黄白色坏死区（蓝箭），质地细腻均匀，类似干酪。

3.4　皮下脂肪坏死（图1-21）

标本为皮肤组织，皮下可见一囊状空隙，是由于脂肪坏死后液化流失所形成的假性囊肿，囊壁内可见残留絮状坏死脂肪组织。

3.5　手干性坏疽（图1-22）

手远端皮肤变黑，干涸似木炭。手足坏疽的常见原因是血栓形成、栓塞和血管痉挛。

3.6　肺空洞（图1-23）

肺切面可见肺组织缺损而形成空洞（蓝圈），此乃慢性纤维空洞型肺结核，由于病灶内的干酪样坏死物质通过支气管引流排出所致。

3.7　脾凝固性坏死灶机化（图1-24）

脾脏切面可见一个小灶坏死区（蓝箭），灰白色，部分呈半透明，此乃坏死后发生机化所致。脾脏包膜面可见由于纤维组织收缩牵拉所形成的局部凹陷。

4. 损伤的修复

皮肤一期愈合（图 1-25）

皮肤表面有先前手术切口愈合的瘢痕，颜色较周围皮肤略淡，有光泽，较平坦。

三、组织切片

1. 适应

1.1　小腿骨骼肌萎缩（图 1-26）

与残留的正常骨骼肌（黑星）相比，萎缩的骨骼肌细胞（蓝箭）肌浆减少，染色不均，细胞体积明显缩小，甚至完全消失，肌束间可见大量的脂肪组织（蓝星）填充取代。

1.2　前列腺结节性增生（图 1-27）

前列腺腺体数量明显增多，腺腔大小不一，甚至扩张呈囊状，腺泡上皮细胞增生活跃，细胞层次增多（蓝箭），部分腺腔内可见增生的上皮细胞形成乳头状结构（蓝星）。

2. 可逆性损伤

2.1　肾小管上皮细胞水肿（图 1-28）

肾脏皮质内可见肾小球（蓝星）、近曲小管（蓝箭）和远曲小管（黑箭）等结构断面。近曲小管上皮细胞普遍肿大，细胞界限不清，导致近曲小管管腔变窄，形态不规则。上皮细胞胞浆内充满伊红染颗粒，部分已脱落至腔内，细胞核结构仍清楚。

2.2　肝细胞水肿（图 1-29）

肝小叶及门管区结构尚完整，小叶内可见部分肝细胞肿胀（蓝箭），胞浆疏松化，染色变淡，细胞核尚存。蓝星示中央静脉。

2.3　肝脂肪变（图 1-30）

肝小叶内肝细胞胞浆几乎全部被大小不等的圆形透亮空泡（蓝箭）所占据，胞核受压偏位，蓝星示中央静脉。其空泡原为脂滴，在制片过程中被二甲苯所溶解。

2.4　脾包膜玻璃样变（图 1-31）

淡伊红染区域为高度增厚的脾脏包膜（蓝线），其下方为脾脏实质（蓝星）。实质内脾小体明显减少，脾小梁增粗，纤维组织增生，脾窦扩张。包膜内胶原纤维肿胀，互相融合成为均匀一致的伊红染的片状或梁状结构。

2.5　睾丸白膜玻璃样变（图 1-32）

淡伊红染区域为增厚的睾丸白膜（蓝线），其下方可见不同断面的生精小管（蓝星）。白膜高度增厚，胶原纤维肿胀互相融合成为均匀一致的结构。

2.6　脾小动脉玻璃样变（图 1-33）

脾脏内的小动脉管壁增厚（蓝箭），伊红染，均质状，管腔狭窄。脾小体萎缩变小，数目也减少。

2.7　浆细胞玻璃样变（图 1-34）

浆细胞胞浆内可见大小不等的均质、红染、毛玻璃样，小球状物质蓄积，即 Russell 小体（蓝箭）。该形态为浆细胞胞浆内出现的玻璃样变，主要由变性的免疫球蛋白积聚而成。

2.8 胰岛淀粉样变（图1-35）

胰岛间质内可见不定形的淡伊红染物质蓄积（蓝星），内分泌细胞数量明显减少。该淀粉样物质主要由胰岛淀粉样多肽构成，刚果红特殊染色可呈橘红色，多见于2型糖尿病患者。

2.9 血管壁黏液样变（图1-36）

小动脉管壁中可见大量灰蓝色黏液样物质蓄积（蓝星），其中可见数量不等的星芒状成纤维细胞（蓝箭）散在分布，动脉管壁固有结构厚薄不一，血管腔明显变小。

2.10 皮内痣（图1-37）

小巢状聚集的黑色素细胞主要位于真皮上部，黑色素细胞胞浆内外可见黑褐色的色素沉积（蓝箭），真皮表皮交界处及表皮侧未见增生的黑色素细胞巢，这是与交界痣的区别所在。黑星示表皮。

2.11 肺炭末沉着（图1-38）

明显增厚的肺间质内可见大量的黑色炭末沉着（绿星），部分肺泡腔内尚可见胞浆内吞噬有炭末的巨噬细胞（蓝箭），这属于外源性色素沉着。

2.12 动脉中层钙化（图1-39）

动脉中膜内可见波浪线样或颗粒状、小团块状的嗜碱性钙化灶（蓝箭），注意与正常的动脉管壁结构相对比（蓝星）。

3. 不可逆性损伤

3.1 肾凝固性坏死（图1-40）

左侧结构不清的伊红染区域即为肾坏死区，右侧可见结构清楚的肾小球及肾小管，二者交界区域有充血出血现象，称为炎症反应带。坏死区内肾小球（蓝箭）和肾小管（蓝星）的固有细胞胞核俱消失不见，惟轮廓尚存，故呈一片伊红染色。

3.2 脑液化性坏死（图1-41）

与周围残余的伊红染神经毡结构比较，脑组织中可见灶性的淡染区域（蓝圈），即软化灶形成。该区域内神经组织坏死后液化，大量水分和溶解的脂类物质在H.E.染色中呈现疏松的筛网状形态（蓝星），可见反应性肥大和增生的星形胶质细胞（蓝箭），此为损伤后的修复性改变。

3.3 淋巴结干酪样坏死（图1-42）

细胞核较为密集的蓝色区域为残存的淋巴结结构（绿星），而伊红染区域内的淋巴结正常结构已不复存在，代之以大片呈伊红染、细颗粒状的坏死组织（蓝星），此即干酪样坏死灶。与肾凝固性坏死比较，干酪样坏死灶中坏死组织崩解较彻底，不仅细胞核消失，而且组织轮廓不复存在。

3.4 皮下脂肪坏死（图1-43）

皮下创伤性脂肪坏死的早期，可见脂肪细胞核消失，胞浆内脂滴外溢融合（蓝星），脂肪小叶间隔内可见明显的出血灶（黑星）。

3.5 血管壁纤维素样坏死（图1-44）

小血管管壁厚薄不一，部分管壁内可见条块状、深红染的无结构坏死区域（蓝箭），其染色性质类似于纤维素，因此得名。该坏死形态多见于变态反应性疾病。

4. 损伤的修复

4.1　肉芽组织（图 1-45）

组织结构疏松，内有大量新生的毛细血管（蓝星），形态大小不一，或横断，或纵切。多数毛细血管管腔内充满红细胞，并可见小灶性出血（黑星）。在毛细血管之间可见多数成纤维细胞（蓝箭），呈梭形或纺锤形，其间还有各种炎细胞浸润，主要是中性粒细胞（绿箭）和巨噬细胞（黑箭）。

4.2　皮肤一期愈合（图 1-46）

真皮层内可见大量伊红染的胶原瘢痕组织（蓝星），瘢痕组织表面覆盖有已经完全再生的表皮（黑星），表皮结构完整，未见明显增生性改变。

4.3　瘢痕疙瘩（图 1-47）

真皮层（蓝星）内伊红染的胶原带之间可见大量平行排列的成纤维细胞或肌成纤维细胞（蓝箭），增生活跃，表皮（黑星）结构尚完整。

四、 临床病理讨论

案例 **1**　患者，男，70 岁，上腹部不适伴恶心 7 天余。胃镜检查：胃窦部黏膜红白相间，以红为主，见点状糜烂；其余食管、贲门、胃底、胃体、胃角、幽门、十二指肠球部及降部等未见明显异常。胃窦部黏膜活检组织 2 块送病理检查。镜下可见图 1-48 中所示的黏膜改变。

（1）图中箭头所示的细胞为何种细胞？

（2）该患者胃黏膜中出现了哪一种适应性改变？

案例 **2**　患者，男，10 岁，左侧颈部皮下脓肿切开引流后 20 天，未能愈合，再次行扩大引流术，切除脓肿周围部分组织送病理检查。肉眼观：灰白色不规则组织 1 块，质地较硬，大小约 10 mm×5 mm×3 mm。镜下所见如图 1-49 中所示。

（1）真皮层中可见何种组织形态？

（2）该组织最后的结局如何？

五、 思考题

1. 变性的常见类型有哪些？肉眼及镜检的特点各是什么？

2. 坏死的类型有哪些？肉眼及镜检的特点各是什么？坏死的结局有哪些？

3. 何谓坏疽？坏疽的类型有哪些？

4. 何谓机化？其意义如何？

5. 肉芽组织是如何发生发展的？

6. 名词解释：萎缩，化生，坏死，脂肪变，玻璃样变，营养不良性钙化，转移性钙化，凝固性坏死，干酪样坏死，液化性坏死，坏疽，凋亡，再生，肉芽组织，一期愈合。

Chapter 1

Adaptation, Injury of Cell and Tissue, Tissue Repair

Ⅰ. Aims

1. To grasp the morphological changes of different types of atrophy and the effects of atrophy on the body.

2. To grasp the morphologic characteristics of cellular swelling, fatty change, hyaline degeneration and their clinical effects.

3. To grasp the morphological characteristics and outcome of different types of necrosis.

4. To grasp the composition and function of granulation tissue.

5. To understand the morphological characteristics of amyloid change, mucoid degeneration, pathological pigmentation and pathological calcification.

Guidance to study

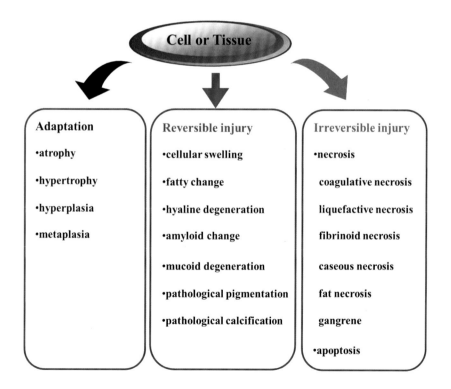

‖. Gross specimens

1. Adaptation

1.1　Senile atrophy of uterus（Fig. 1-1）

It is a uterus with two sides of oviducts and ovaries. There is a decreasing size and weight of uterus.

1.2　Skeletal muscle atrophy of shins（Fig. 1-2）

Here are the amputated shins at the same level. One is normal, and the other（slim one） shows atrophy. The skeletal muscle fibers reduce in the atrophic one. The fat and fiber tissues fill in it.

1.3　Brown atrophy of heart（Fig. 1-3）

The atrophic heart shows the decreased size, and the coronary arteries（blue arrow）on the surface are tortuous. The brown color indicates the accumulation of lipofuscin in atrophic myocardial fibers.

1.4　Atrophy of kidney due to pressure（Fig. 1-4）

The kidney lost its normal shape and became multilocular. The size of kidney increases but the cortex of kidney is thin. The atrophic change is common in patients with pelvis and ureteral calculi.

1.5　Hypertrophy of uterus（Fig. 1-5）

This is a significantly enlarged pregnant uterus. The myometrium of uterine wall is highly thickened. Uterine hypertrophy is often accompanied by smooth muscle cell proliferation.

1.6　Compensatory hypertrophy of intestine（Fig. 1-6）

This is a segment of intestine with a stricture area in the middle（blue box）. The diameter of intestine increases（blue arrow）, and the intestinal wall is thicker in left side than that in adjacent area.

2. Reversible injury

2.1　Cellular swelling of kidney（Fig. 1-7）

Both the size and weight of kidney increase. The color is pale on the section. The cortex is thick and the boundary between cortex and medulla is not clear.

2.2　Cellular swelling of liver（Fig. 1-8）

The liver increases in size and has a pale boiled appearance. On section, the liver becomes swollen with a bulged parenchyma.

2.3　Fatty change of liver（Fig. 1-9）

The fatty liver is enlarged and yellow, with a greasy appearance. Fatty liver shows orange after being stained by Sudan Ⅲ (right).

2. 4　Hyaline degeneration of spleen capsule（Fig. 1-10）

The volume of the spleen increases, and part of the capsule (blue box) is obviously thickened. The color is gray and translucent. Pay attention to the difference from the normal capsule (black box).

2. 5　Hyaline degeneration of albuginea of testis（Fig. 1-11）

Albuginea of testis is thick, grey, and has a translucent appearance (blue arrow).

2. 6　Mucoid degeneration of skin（Fig. 1-12）

Here are two pieces of skin and subcutaneous tissue. One piece is normal tissue (black arrow), but the other shows shrinkage of the epidermis, with thickened mucoid appearance of the dermis (blue arrow).

2. 7　Hemosiderosis of lung（Fig. 1-13）

Here is one side of the lungs. On the cut surface, the lung is brown or rusty in color.

2. 8　Ocular choroidal malignant melanoma（Fig. 1-14）

It is the sagittal section of the eye. The malignant tumor cells originated from the uvea are rich in melanin, and the tumor tissue has occupied the vitreous body and involved the retroocular tissue.

2. 9　Anthracosis of lung（Fig. 1-15）

There are small or big black focal aggregates throughout one side of lungs, and the aggregates are pigment deposition including coal.

2. 10　Tattoo of skin（Fig. 1-16）

A black pattern can be seen on the skin surface. When the pigment was pricked with a pin into skin, it is phagocytosed by macrophages, and subsequently deposited in the dermis.

2. 11　Calcification of pulmonary tuberculosis（Fig. 1-17）

There is a grey and hard small nodule (blue arrow) in the lung, which looks like limestone. This local deposit of calcium salt occurs in necrotic tissue of the lung.

3. Irreversible injury

3. 1　Coagulative necrosis of spleen（Fig. 1-18）

On the section of spleen, there is a gray-white necrotic area with clear boundary, which is dense and dry, and surrounded by a circle of black-brown bleeding zone.

3. 2　Liquefactive necrosis of brain（Fig. 1-19）

The left and right hemicerebrum are asymmetric. One side of hemicerebrum shrinks in size. There is a necrotic area (blue arrow) in the basal ganglia, showing a rete-liked appearance.

3. 3　Caseous necrosis of lymph nodes（Fig. 1-20）

Several lymph nodes become large and coalesce into a mass, in which yellow-white necrotic areas(blue arrow)are similar to cheese.

3. 4　Subcutaneous fat necrosis(Fig. 1-21)

A cystic cavity can be seen on the section of subcutaneous tissue, and the lining of cyst is the necrotic fat. Most of the necrotic tissue has lost.

3. 5　Gangrenous necrosis of hand(Fig. 1-22)

The distal portion of hand shows a black, dry, and shriveled appearance. This is an example of "dry" gangrene in which there is mainly coagulative necrosis. The common causes are thrombosis, embolism and vasospasm of the blood vessels.

3. 6　Lung cavitation(Fig. 1-23)

The section of lung tissue with chronic fibro-cavitary pulmonary tuberculosis shows a cavity, which is a residual cavity(blue circle)after the local caseous necrotic tissue flows into the bronchi.

3. 7　Organization of coagulative necrosis of spleen(Fig. 1-24)

A small organized area secondary to necrosis can be seen on the section of spleen, which is gray-white and partially translucent(blue arrow). Local depression formed by traction of scar tissue can be seen on the capsule of spleen.

4. Tissue repair

Healing by first intention of skin(Fig. 1-25)

It is a scar on the skin surface after the healing of previous surgical incision, with white and shining appearance.

‖. Tissue sections

1. Adaptation

1. 1　Skeletal muscle atrophy of shins(Fig. 1-26)

Compared with the residual normal skeletal muscle (black asterisk), the cytoplasm of atrophic skeletal muscle cells (blue arrows) is lightly stained and uneven, and the cells significantly reduce in both size and number. The atrophic muscle bundles are replaced by adipose tissue(blue asterisks).

1. 2　Prostatic nodular hyperplasia(Fig. 1-27)

The numbers of prostate glands increase significantly, and the sizes of them are different. The glands are dilated, even cystic. The hyperplastic epithelial cells are multilayered (blue arrows), and the papillary infoldings are common(blue asterisks).

2. Reversible injury

2. 1   Cellular swelling of renal tubule（Fig. 1-28）

Glomerulus（blue asterisks）, proximal convoluted tubule（blue arrows）and distal convoluted tubule（black arrow）can be seen in renal cortex. The proximal convoluted tubules（black arrow）present narrow and irregular lumens lined by enlarged epithelial cells with unclear boundary. The cytoplasm of epithelial cells is filled with eosin-stained granules. Some of them have collapsed and dropped off into the lumen, but the nuclei of cells are still remained.

2. 2   Cellular swelling of liver（Fig. 1-29）

The structure of hepatic lobule and portal area is still intact. Some swollen hepatocytes show small, clear vacuoles within the cytoplasm（blue arrows）, and the staining of them becomes weak, but the nuclei remain. The blue asterisk indicates the central vein.

2. 3   Fatty change of liver（Fig. 1-30）

The cytoplasm of hepatocytes is almost occupied by round vacuoles（blue arrow）of different sizes, and the nuclei are compressed and decentered. Vacuoles are originally lipid droplets, which are dissolved by xylene during H.E. staining process. The blue asterisk shows the central vein.

2. 4   Hyaline degeneration of spleen capsule（Fig. 1-31）

The light eosin-staining part of the section is the highly thickened capsule of spleen（blue line）, below which is the spleen parenchyma（blue asterisk）. Splenic corpuscles decrease significantly in number, splenic trabeculae are thickened, and splenic sinuses are dilated. In high magnification, the swollen collagen fibers fuse into a uniform eosin-stained sheet structure.

2. 5   Hyaline degeneration of albuginea of testis（Fig. 1-32）

The highly thickened albuginea（blue line）covering the testicular seminiferous tubules （blue asterisk）shows uniform eosin-staining appearance. In high magnification, the collagen fibers swell and fuse with each other.

2. 6   Hyaline degeneration of central artery in spleen（Fig. 1-33）

The homogeneous eosin stained walls of arterioles are thickened（blue arrows）with narrow lumens. The number of splenic corpuscles is decreased.

2. 7   Hyaline degeneration of plasma cells（Fig. 1-34）

Homogeneous, eosin-stained, ground glass-like globular substances of different sizes can be seen in the cytoplasm of plasma cells, namely Russell bodies（blue arrows）. It is the hyaline degeneration in the cytoplasm of plasma cells, which is mainly formed by the accumulation of degenerated immunoglobulin.

2. 8　Amyloid change of pancreatic islets（Fig. 1-35）

Amorphous, eosin-stained extracellular substance (blue asterisks) can be seen in the islet interstitium. The number of endocrine cells is significantly reduced. The amyloid substance is mainly composed of islet amyloid polypeptide, and Congo red stain gives a red color to tissue deposits. Amyloid change of pancreatic islets can be seen in patients with type 2 diabetes.

2. 9　Mucoid change of vascular wall（Fig. 1-36）

A large amount of gray-blue myxoid substances (blue asterisks) and scattered stellate fibroblasts (blue arrow) can be seen in the small artery wall. The vascular lumen becomes narrow and the thickness of wall is different.

2. 10　Intradermal nevus（Fig. 1-37）

Small nests of melanocytes are in the upper dermis. Dark-brown melanin deposition (blue arrows) can be seen inside or outside the melanocytes. There is no proliferative melanocyte nest at the epidermal side of dermoepidermal junction, which is the difference from the junctional nevus. The black asterisk shows epidermis.

2. 11　Anthracosis of lung（Fig. 1-38）

A large number of black carbon pigments (green asterisks) deposit in the thickened lung interstitium, and macrophages (blue arrow) phagocytizing carbon in the cytoplasm can be seen in some alveoli. Anthracosis of lung belongs to the exogenous pigmentation.

2. 12　Arterial medial calcification（Fig. 1-39）

Wavy, granular, and lump-like basophilic calcification (blue arrows) can be seen in the arterial media. Pay attention to the difference from the normal arterial wall (blue asterisk)

3.　Irreversible injury

3. 1　Coagulative necrosis of kidney（Fig. 1-40）

The eosin-stained area with unclear structure on the left is the area of renal necrosis, and the glomeruli and renal tubules with clear structure can be seen on the right. There is a congestion and bleeding boundary between the necrotic and non-necrotic area. At high magnification, the nuclei of glomeruli (blue arrows) and renal tubules (blue asterisks) in the necrotic area disappear, but the structure outline remains.

3. 2　Liquefactive necrosis of brain（Fig. 1-41）

Compared with the residual eosin-stained neuropil, the focal lightly stained area (blue circle) is liquefactive necrosis. In this area, the brain tissue is liquefied after necrosis, and a large amount of water and dissolved lipids display loose cribriform-like structure (blue asterisks). Hypertrophic and proliferative astrocytes (blue arrow) can be seen as a reactive repair after injury.

3. 3   Caseous necrosis of lymph node (Fig. 1-42)

The remained structure of lymph node (green asterisk) can be seen around the eosin-stained necrotic area (blue asterisks), which shows fine granular appearance. Compared with renal coagulative necrosis, the caseous necrosis in lymph node is disintegrated completely, not only the nuclei disappear, but also the tissue structure outline no longer exists.

3. 4   Subcutaneous fat necrosis (Fig. 1-43)

In the early stage of subcutaneous traumatic fat necrosis, the nuclei of adipocytes disappear and overflowed lipid droplets fuse together (blue asterisks). The obvious bleeding foci (black asterisks) are in the septa of fat lobules.

3. 5   Fibrinoid necrosis of vascular wall (Fig. 1-44)

The wall of blood vessel is varying in thickness. There are amorphous bright red necrosis areas (blue arrow) in part of the wall. The staining of this substance is similar to fibrin on H.E. preparations, so it is named as fibrin-like. Fibrinoid necrosis is often seen in allergic diseases.

4. Tissue repair

4. 1   Granulation tissue (Fig. 1-45)

It shows loose connective tissue with a large number of newborn capillaries (blue asterisks) in different shapes and sizes. Most capillary lumens are filled with red blood cells, and small focal bleeding (black asterisk) can be observed. There are fibroblasts (blue arrow) in spindle shape, neutrophils (green arrow) and macrophages (black arrow) among capillaries.

4. 2   Healing by first intention of skin (Fig. 1-46)

Eosin-stained collagen scar (blue asterisk) can be seen in the dermis. The surface of scar is covered with completely regenerated epidermis (black asterisk), without obvious proliferative changes.

4. 3   Keloid (Fig. 1-47)

A large number of fibroblasts or myofibroblasts (blue arrows) arrange in parallel between the eosin-stained collagen bands in the dermis (blue asterisk). These cells present active proliferation, and the epidermis is intact (black asterisk).

Ⅳ. Clinical pathological discussion

Case 1

A 70 years old male had upper abdominal discomfort with nausea for more than 7 days. Under endoscopy, the mucosa of gastric antrum was red and white, mainly red, with punctate erosion. No obvious abnormalities were found in esophagus, cardia, fundus, gastric body, gastric angle, pylorus, duodenal bulb and descending part. Two pieces of gastric antrum mucosa biopsy tissues were sent for pathological examination. Microscopically, part of the mucosa was shown in Figure 1-48.

(1) What kind of cell is shown by the blue arrow in the figure?

(2) What kind of adaptive changes have occurred in the patient's gastric mucosa?

Case 2

A 10 years old boy failed to be healed 20 days after incision and drainage of the subcutaneous abscess in the left neck. He underwent extended drainage again, and some tissues around the abscess were removed. The tissues were sent for pathological examination. Macroscopically, it was one piece of gray hard irregular tissue, about 10 mm×5 mm×3 mm in size. The microscopic change was shown in Figure 1-49.

(1) What kind of tissue can be seen in the dermis?

(2) What was the final outcome of this tissue?

Ⅴ. Questions

1. What are the morphologic characteristics of different types of reversible injury?

2. What are the morphologic characteristics of different types of necrosis? What are the outcomes of necrotic tissue?

3. What is gangrene? What are the types of gangrene?

4. What are organization and its significance?

5. How does granulation tissue develop?

6. Terms: Atrophy, Metaplasia, Necrosis, Fatty change, Hyaline degeneration, Dystrophic calcification, Metastatic calcification, Coagulative necrosis, Caseous necrosis, Liquefactive necrosis, Gangrene, Apoptosis, Regeneration, Granulation tissue, Healing by first intention.

Ⅵ. 附图 (Figures)

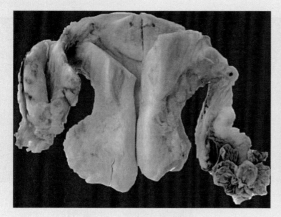

图 1-1 子宫老年性萎缩
Fig.1-1 Senile atrophy of uterus

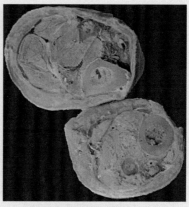

图 1-2 小腿骨骼肌萎缩
Fig.1-2 Skeletal muscle atrophy
of shins

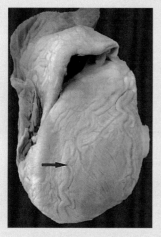

图 1-3 心肌褐色萎缩
Fig.1-3 Brown atrophy
of heart

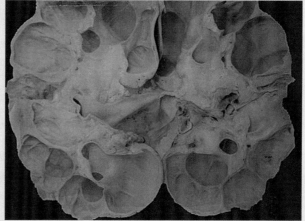

图 1-4 肾压迫性萎缩
Fig.1-4 Atrophy of kidney due to pressure

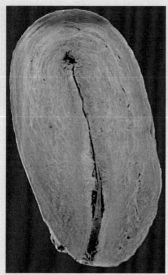

图 1-5 子宫肥大
Fig.1-5 Hypertrophy of uterus

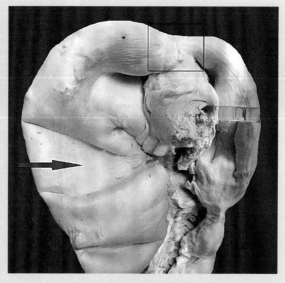

图 1-6 肠代偿性肥大
Fig.1-6 Compensatory hypertrophy of intestine

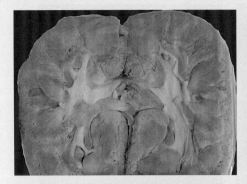

图 1-7　肾水肿
Fig.1-7　Cellular swelling of kidney

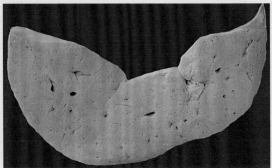

图 1-8　肝水肿
Fig.1-8　Cellular swelling of liver

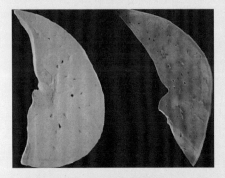

图 1-9　肝脂肪变
Fig.1-9　Fatty change of liver

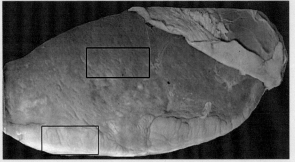

图 1-10　脾包膜玻璃样变
Fig.1-10　Hyaline degeneration of spleen capsule

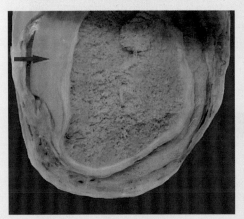

图 1-11　睾丸白膜玻璃样变
Fig.1-11　Hyaline degeneration
　　　　　of albuginea of testis

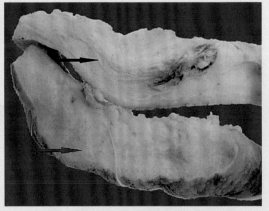

图 1-12　皮肤黏液样变
Fig.1-12　Mucoid degeneration of skin

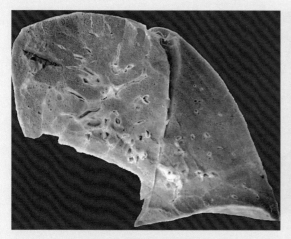

图 1-13　肺含铁血黄素沉着
Fig.1-13　Hemosiderosis of lung

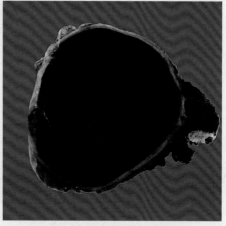

图 1-14　眼脉络膜恶性黑色素瘤
Fig.1-14　Ocular choroidal malignant melanoma

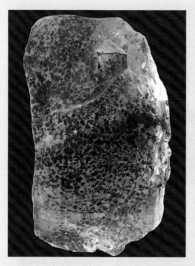

图 1-15　肺炭末沉着
Fig.1-15　Anthracosis of lung

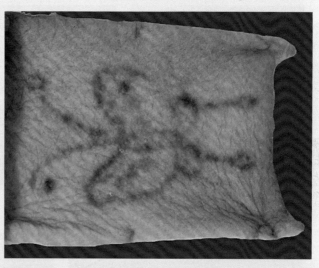

图 1-16　皮肤文身
Fig.1-16　Tattoo of skin

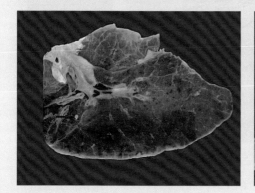

图 1-17　肺结核钙化灶
Fig.1-17　Calcification of pulmonary tuberculosis

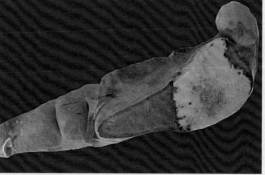

图 1-18　脾凝固性坏死
Fig.1-18　Coagulative necrosis of spleen

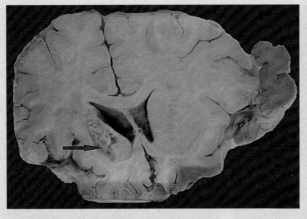

图 1-19　脑液化性坏死
Fig.1-19　Liquefactive necrosis of brain

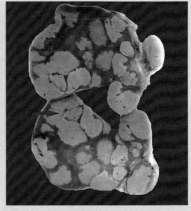

图 1-20　淋巴结干酪样坏死
Fig.1-20　Caseous necrosis
of lymph nodes

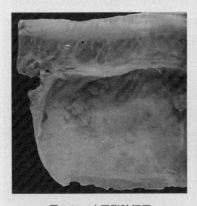

图 1-21　皮下脂肪坏死
Fig.1-21　Subcutaneous fat necrosis

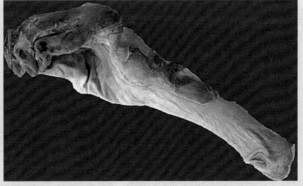

图 1-22　手干性坏疽
Fig.1-22　Gangrenous necrosis of hand

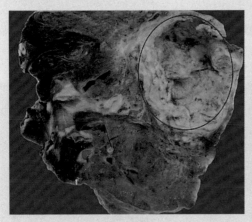

图 1-23　肺空洞
Fig.1-23　Lung cavitation

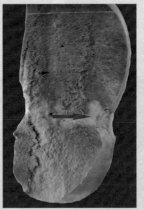

图 1-24　脾凝固性
坏死灶机化
Fig.1-24　Organization of
coagulative necrosis of spleen

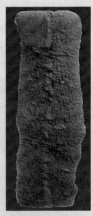

图 1-25　皮肤
一期愈合
Fig.1-25　Healing
by first intension
of skin

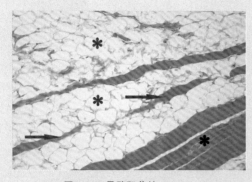
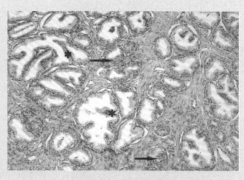

图 1-26　骨骼肌萎缩（×200）
Fig.1-26　Skeletal muscle atrophy（×200）

图 1-27　前列腺结节性增生（×100）
Fig.1-27　Prostatic nodular hyperplasia（×100）

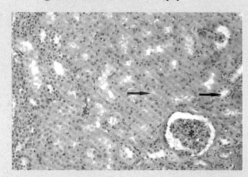

图 1-28　肾小管上皮细胞水肿（×200；×400）
Fig.1-28　Cellular swelling of renal tubule（×200；×400）

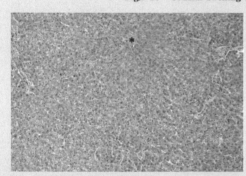
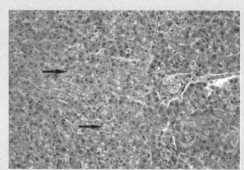

图 1-29　肝细胞水肿（×100；×200）
Fig.1-29　Cellular swelling of liver（×100；×200）

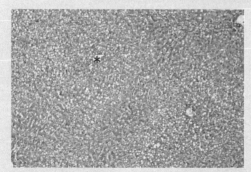
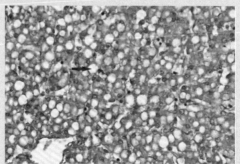

图 1-30　肝脂肪变（×100；×400）
Fig.1-30　Fatty change of liver（×100；×400）

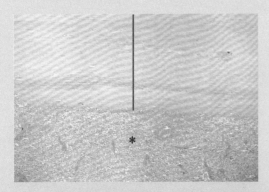

图 1-31　脾包膜玻璃样变（×40；×200）
Fig.1-31　Hyaline degeneration of spleen capsule（×40；×200）

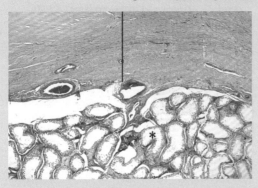

图 1-32　睾丸白膜玻璃样变（×40；×200）
Fig.1-32　Hyaline degeneration of albuginea of testis（×40；×200）

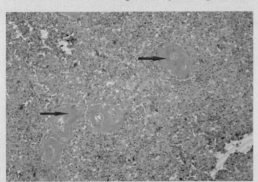

图 1-33　脾小动脉玻璃样变（×200；×400）
Fig.1-33　Hyaline degeneration of central artery in spleen（×200；×400）

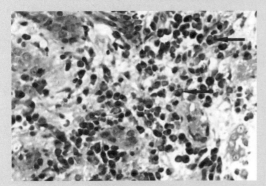
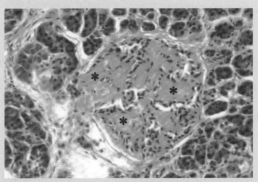

图 1-34　浆细胞玻璃样变（×400）
Fig.1-34　Hyaline degeneration of plasma cells（×400）

图 1-35　胰岛淀粉样变（×200）
Fig.1-35　Amyloid change of pancreatic islets（×200）

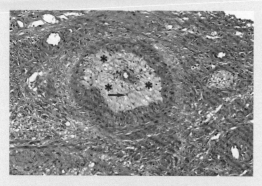

图 1-36　血管壁黏液样变（×200）
Fig.1-36　Mucoid change of vascular wall（×200）

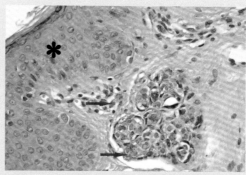

图 1-37　皮内痣（×100）
Fig.1-37　Intradermal nevus（×100）

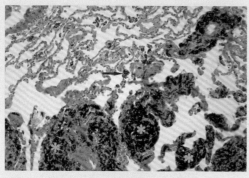

图 1-38　肺炭末沉着（×200）
Fig.1-38　Anthracosis of lung（×200）

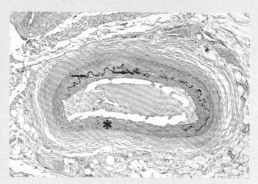

图 1-39　动脉中层钙化（×100）
Fig.1-39　Arterial media calcification（×100）

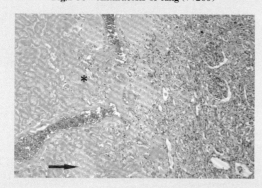

图 1-40　肾凝固性坏死（×100；×200）
Fig.1-40　Coagulative necrosis of kidney（×100；×200）

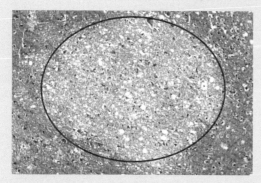
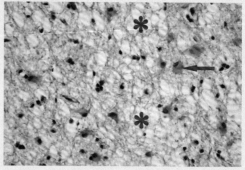

图 1-41　脑液化性坏死（×200；×400）
Fig.1-41　Liquefactive necrosis of brain（×200；×400）

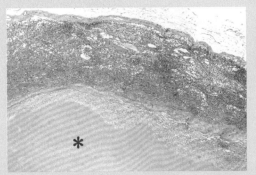
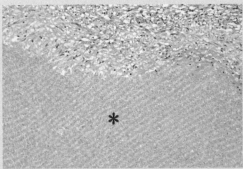

图 1-42 淋巴结干酪样坏死（×40；×200）
Fig.1-42 Caseous necrosis of lymph node（×40；×200）

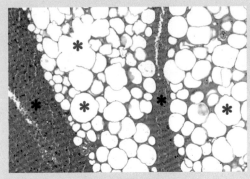
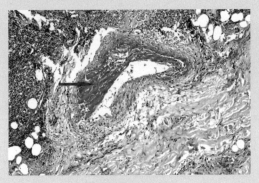

图 1-43 皮下脂肪坏死（×100）
Fig.1-43 Subcutaneous fat necrosis（×100）

图 1-44 血管壁纤维素样坏死（×100）
Fig.1-44 Fibrinoid necrosis of vascular wall（×100）

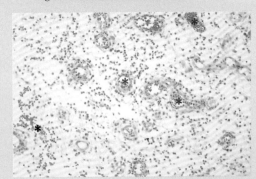

图 1-45 肉芽组织（×200；×400）
Fig.1-45 Granulation tissue（×200；×400）

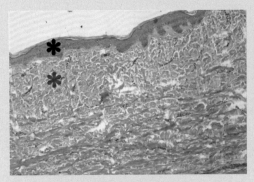
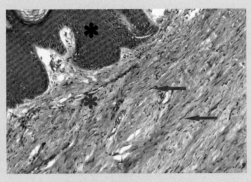

图 1-46 皮肤一期愈合（×100）
Fig.1-46 Healing by first intention of skin（×100）

图 1-47 瘢痕疙瘩（×200）
Fig.1-47 Keloid（×200）

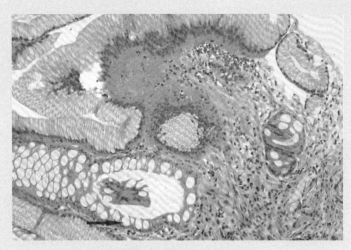

图 1-48　案例 1（×200）

Fig.1-48　Case 1（×200）

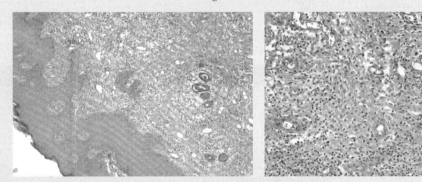

图 1-49　案例 2（×100；×200）

Fig.1-49　Case 2（×100；×200）

卜晓东（Xiaodong Bu）

第二章
局部血液循环障碍

一、目的要求

1. 掌握淤血、血栓形成、栓塞、梗死的概念。
2. 掌握淤血的形态学特征及其对局部组织的影响。
3. 掌握血栓的形态学特征及其结局。
4. 掌握各型梗死的形态学特征及鉴别点。
5. 了解血栓形成、栓塞和梗死的相互关系。

导学

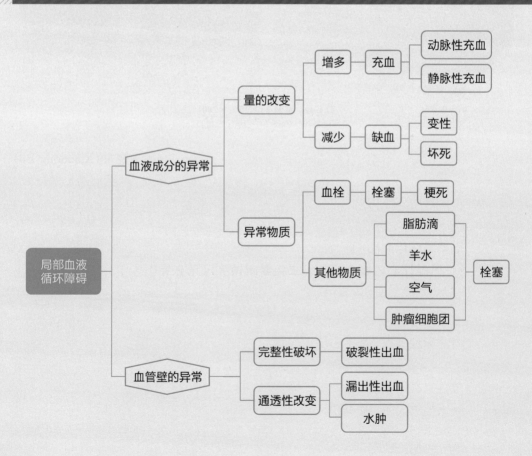

二、大体标本

1. 充血

1.1 阑尾炎性充血（急性阑尾炎）（图 2-1）

阑尾肿大，暗红色，浆膜面血管高度扩张充血，表面因化脓而附有脓性渗出物。

1.2 脑膜炎性充血（图 2-2）

大脑表面及脑底部靠近脑沟处小血管较正常明显增多且扩张充血。

2. 淤血

2.1 慢性肝淤血（槟榔肝）（图 2-3）

肝脏表面光滑，体积增大，切面可见均匀而弥漫分布的暗红色小点，其周围呈灰黄色，部分区域暗红色小点相互融合，形成红黄相间的斑纹状外观。红黄相间斑纹宛如中药槟榔（左上角插图）切面花纹，故称为槟榔肝。

2.2 慢性肺淤血（肺褐色硬变）（图 2-4）

肺膜表面光滑，暗红色，可见黑色斑点。切面肺组织呈红褐色，略带棕色，质地较致密。

2.3 慢性脾淤血（图 2-5）

脾体积明显增大，包膜不规则增厚。切面见脾组织呈灰红色（新鲜时为暗红色，该标本固定较久）。白髓萎缩甚至消失故不易见到，灰白色细丝状脾小梁数目增多。

3. 血栓

3.1 静脉血栓（图 2-6）

静脉腔内见血栓形成。血栓外观干燥粗糙，红白相间（蓝箭）。

3.2 动脉血栓（图 2-7）

腹主动脉下端与右髂动脉内有一血栓，呈黄白及黑褐色，血栓表面干燥粗糙（蓝箭）。

3.3 心脏附壁血栓（图 2-8）

左心房壁上有一个较大的附壁血栓（蓝箭），血栓呈球形，灰白色，易脱落。

3.4 心瓣膜白色血栓（图 2-9）

此为急性风湿性心内膜炎标本。二尖瓣闭锁缘可见有针帽大小的灰白色赘生物（蓝箭），即白色血栓。

4. 梗死

4.1 肾贫血性梗死（图 2-10）

肾切面可见多处灰白色梗死区（黄箭），呈典型的扇面形，尖端指向肾门，基底达包膜，周边有充血出血带。

4.2 脾贫血性梗死（图 2-11）

脾体积增大，切面可见灰白色坏死区，略呈楔形（蓝箭），质地致密而干燥，边界清楚，周围绕有一圈黑褐色的出血带，坏死组织表面见少量纤维素渗出。

4.3　肠出血性梗死（图 2-12）

一段小肠。肠壁增厚、肿胀,暗红色(黄箭)。浆膜面干燥,失去原有光泽。

4.4　肺出血性梗死（图 2-13）

肺下叶近边缘部可见一暗红色楔形梗死病灶(蓝箭),紧贴肺膜,此乃出血梗死灶,试与贫血性梗死比较其形态有何不同。

5.　出血

5.1　脑出血（图 2-14）

大脑的水平切面,经过内囊。一侧内囊有出血,已将内囊破坏(蓝箭),并与侧脑室相通。大脑中线已向对侧移位,注意两侧对比,观察是否对称。

5.2　胸膜淤点（图 2-15）

婴幼儿的肺脏。肺胸膜面有弥漫的或散在的出血点,大如粟粒,小如针头,称为淤点(蓝箭)。

5.3　肾出血（图 2-16）

肾表面和切面可见多数密集的出血灶(蓝箭)。

三、组织切片

1.　淤血

1.1　慢性肝淤血（图 2-17）

肝组织内有多处明显的淤血区(蓝星),呈片状、索状,并有互相连接者,与周围的肝组织相间。淤血区中央可见中央静脉,其附近的肝索因受压变细,或断续,或消失不见,淤血区附近肝细胞可见脂肪变性(蓝箭)。

1.2　慢性肺淤血（图 2-18）

肺泡壁毛细血管数目增多,且极度充血,呈串珠状排列。肺泡腔可见多少不一的圆形或不规则形的巨噬细胞,胞浆内有大量棕褐色的细颗粒物质(含铁血黄素),多见于左心衰竭时,称为心力衰竭细胞(蓝箭)。此外有些肺泡内尚有淡伊红染浆液(水肿液)。

1.3　慢性脾淤血（图 2-19）

脾窦高度扩张充血,脾小梁因结缔组织增生而增宽。有时可在小梁及包膜下见到成团分布、染成淡绿色或棕黄色的结晶物质(此为出血后,铁盐和钙盐之结晶),即含铁小结。脾小体数目减少,体积缩小。慢性脾淤血多由门静脉高压引起。

2.　血栓和栓塞

2.1　混合血栓（图 2-20）

血栓切片见淡伊红染无结构的颗粒状物质,呈明显波浪形的不规则条索,此为崩溃的血小板组成的小梁(蓝星),在其边缘有白细胞附着(黑箭)。位于血小板小梁之间者,为网状结构的纤维素(黑星),有的网眼中充满红细胞。

2.2　血栓机化（图 2-21）

血管腔内可见一混合血栓,其中一侧与血管壁紧密相连(蓝箭),并有肉芽组织长入。

2.3　肺脂肪栓塞（图 2-22）

肺组织广泛水肿，肺小动脉内可见脂滴栓子（蓝箭）。栓子内尚可见骨髓造血细胞，脂滴被二甲苯溶解呈大小不等的空泡状。

3. 梗死

3.1　肾贫血性梗死（图 2-23）

肾组织切片的一侧可见结构不清的伊红染色区，是肾的梗死部分（蓝星），其周围是结构清晰的肾小球及肾小管，二者间有充血出血现象（蓝箭）和炎细胞浸润，即炎症反应带。高倍镜下见梗死区肾小球肾小管的胞核俱消失不见，惟轮廓尚存，故呈一片伊红染色。

3.2　脾贫血性梗死（图 2-24）

脾脏内出现大片伊红染无结构区域即梗死区（蓝星），可见梗死区内组织崩解呈颗粒状，细胞核消失，注意与低倍视野中左侧残留的组织相比较。

3.3　肺出血性梗死（图 2-25）

肺组织可见一深红染的出血性梗死区（蓝星）。梗死区内充满红细胞，肺泡壁固有结构的细胞核消失，肺泡轮廓已难以辨认。梗死区外肺组织肺泡腔大多皆空虚无所见，唯有少数胞浆内含有含铁血黄素的巨噬细胞见于少数肺泡腔。

4. 水肿

肺水肿（图 2-26）

大部分肺泡腔内充满均匀、淡伊红色的水肿液，仅少数肺泡腔内尚含有空气。肺泡壁毛细血管扩张充血。

5. 出血

5.1　肺出血（图 2-27）

几乎所有肺泡腔内均充满红细胞，并可见较多福尔马林色素沉着和少数吞噬含铁血黄素的巨噬细胞。出血区内肺泡壁结构尚存，周边肺组织可见局灶性代偿性肺气肿。

5.2　肾上腺出血（图 2-28）

肾上腺皮质及髓质内均出现大量红细胞，肾上腺皮质结构尚存，部分实质细胞萎缩。

四、临床病理讨论

案例　患者，女性，54 岁，死于心力衰竭，入院诊断为风湿性心脏病伴二尖瓣狭窄与关闭不全。尸检发现扩大的左心房内有一个球形暗红色兼灰白色块状物；肺组织呈红褐色，质地较致密；肝脏体积增大，表面有均匀弥漫分布的暗红色小点，呈红黄相间花斑状；肾脏有一灰白色坏死区略呈扇形，质地致密而干燥，边界清楚，周围有一圈黑褐色的出血带，坏死组织表面见少量纤维素渗出。组织学检查典型图片见图 2-29 所示。

（1）各脏器有何病变？

（2）各脏器病变之间有何相互联系？

（3）简述该患者病变发展的临床病理联系。

五、 思考题

1. 慢性肺、肝、脾淤血有哪些形态特征？其形态发生机制及常见的原因是什么？这些器官淤血可引起什么后果？

2. 血栓的形成条件有哪些？

3. 常见的栓子类型有哪些？

4. 血栓、栓塞、梗死之间有何关联？

5. 名词解释：充血，淤血，心力衰竭细胞，槟榔肝，血栓形成，栓塞，梗死。

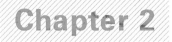

Chapter 2

Hemodynamic Disorders and Abnormalities of Blood Supply

Ⅰ. Aims

1. To grasp the concepts of congestion, thrombosis, embolism, and infarction.

2. To grasp the morphologic characteristics and consequence of congestion.

3. To grasp the morphologic characteristics and outcomes of thrombi.

4. To grasp the morphologic characteristics and identifications of various types of infarcts.

5. To understand the relationship among thrombosis, embolism and infarction.

Guidance to study

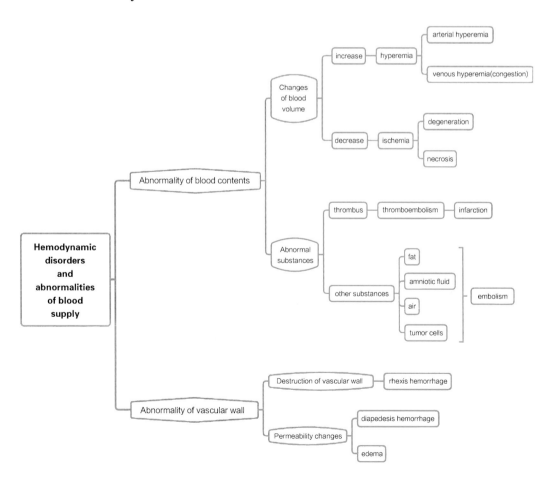

Ⅱ. Gross specimens

1. Hyperemia

1. 1 Inflammatory hyperemia of appendix（Fig.2-1）

The appendix is greatly swollen and dark red. The surface of serosa is covered with fibrinopurulent exudate due to suppurative inflammation and the vessels of serosa are hyperemic.

1. 2 Meningeal hyperemia（Fig.2-2）

The number of small blood vessels is significantly increased near the sulci on the top and bottom of the brain, and the blood vessels are dilated and hyperemic due to inflammation.

2. Congestion

2. 1 Chronic hepatic congestion（Nutmeg liver）（Fig.2-3）

The liver is enlarged with smooth surface. On the cut section, some dark red dots are observed, and the surrounding tissue is yellow, therefore, a red-yellow striped appearance is obvious, which resembles the cut surface of traditional Chinese medicine nutmeg（insert）. This pathological change is known as nutmeg liver.

2. 2 Chronic pulmonary congestion（Fig.2-4）

The lung surface is smooth and dark red with some black spots. The cut section of the lung is brown and firm.

2. 3 Chronic congestion of spleen（Fig.2-5）

The spleen is obviously enlarged and the splenic capsule is irregularly thickened. Its cut section is gray-red after fixation. The white pulp is not easy to be seen due to atrophic change. The number of gray-white filamentous splenic trabeculae increases.

3. Thrombus

3. 1 Thrombus in vein（Fig.2-6）

There is a thrombus in the vein, which is attached firmly to the vessel wall. The thrombus is dry and rough, with alternating pale gray and red areas（blue arrow）.

3. 2 Thrombus in artery（Fig.2-7）

There is a thrombus（blue arrow）between the lower end of abdominal aorta and right iliac artery. The thrombus is yellow-white and dark-brown with dry and rough surface.

3. 3 Mural thrombus in heart（Fig.2-8）

There is a large mural thrombus on the left atrial wall (blue arrow). The thrombus is spherical, gray-white and easy to fall off.

3.4　Pale thrombus of heart valve（Fig.2-9）

This is an acute rheumatic endocarditis specimen. Along the closure line of mitral valve, there are many tiny gray wart-like vegetations (pale thrombi, blue arrows).

4.　Infarct

4.1　Anemic infarct of kidney（Fig.2-10）

The cut section of the kidney shows multiple gray-white infarcts (yellow arrows). The infarcts are typically wedge-shaped, with the apexes pointing towards the renal hilus and the bases reaching the capsule. The margins of infarcts are defined by narrow rims containing hyperemic and hemorrhagic zones.

4.2　Anemic infarct of spleen（Fig.2-11）

The spleen increases in size, and its grayish white necrotic area is slightly wedge-shaped (blue arrow). The necrotic area is dense and dry with clear border. The boundary indicates a dark brown bleeding zone enclosing the necrotic area. A little fibrinous exudate can be seen on the surface of necrotic tissue.

4.3　Hemorrhagic infarct of intestine（Fig.2-12）

This is a segment of the intestine. The intestinal wall is thickened, swollen and dark red (yellow arrows). The serosa surface is dry and loses the original luster.

4.4　Hemorrhagic infarct of lung（Fig.2-13）

A dark red wedge-shaped infarct can be seen in the proximal edge of lower lobe (blue arrow). The infarct is close to the pleura, and belongs to a hemorrhagic infarct. Please compare its morphology with anemic infarct of kidney.

5.　Hemorrhage

5.1　Cerebral hemorrhage（Fig.2-14）

This is a horizontal section of the brain, passing through the internal capsule. A large hemorrhagic lesion has destroyed the right internal capsule (blue arrow) and adjacent lateral ventricle. The septum pellucidum between lateral ventricles has not been destroyed, but shifted to the contralateral side. Please observe the difference between the left and right cerebrum in morphology, and notice whether they are symmetrical.

5.2　Pleural hemorrhage（Fig.2-15）

The lung specimen is from an infant. There are diffuse or scattered hemorragic lesions in the pleura, which is less than 2 mm in diameter. The hemorrhagic foci are called as petechiae (blue arrows).

5.3　Renal hemorrhage（Fig.2-16）

The specimen shows hemorrhagic foci with various sizes (blue arrows) on the surface and cut section of the kidney.

III. Tissue sections

1. Congestion

1.1　Chronic hepatic congestion（Fig.2-17）

There are obvious congested areas (blue asterisks) in the liver tissue, which are flaky, cordlike and connected with each other. The central veins and sinuses are dilated and filled with erythrocytes, and the hepatic cords become thin, intermittent, even disappear because of compression by the congested areas. The adjacent hepatocytes present fatty degeneration (blue arrows).

1.2　Chronic pulmonary congestion（Fig.2-18）

The capillaries in the septa increase in number. The congested and dilated capillaries appear like strings of beads. Alveolar macrophages loaded with brown yellow particles (hemosiderin) are seen in the lumens of the alveoli, and named heart failure cells during chronic heart failure (blue arrows). In addition, some lumens of the alveoli contain eosinophilic fluid (edematous fluid).

1.3　Chronic congestion of spleen（Fig.2-19）

The splenic sinuses are highly dilated and congested, and the spleen trabeculae are widened because of connective tissue hyperplasia. Sometimes, clusters of crystalline materials are dyed with light green or brownish yellow (which is the crystallization of iron and calcium salt after hemorrhage) under the capsule, and referred as to siderotic nodules. The splenic corpuscles are atrophic. Chronic congestion of the spleen is commonly caused by portal hypertension.

2. Thrombus and embolism

2.1　Mixed thrombus（Fig.2-20）

The section of the thrombus displays that unstructured granular material is lightly stained with eosin, showing obvious coral-like irregular trabeculae composed of collapsed platelets (blue asterisks), and white blood cells locate at the trabecular edge (black arrows). There are reticulated fibrins (black asterisk) and erythrocytes among platelet trabeculae.

2.2　Organization of thrombus（Fig.2-21）

One side of the mixed thrombus is closely attached to the vessel wall, and the granulation tissue has grown into and partly organized the thrombus (blue arrows).

2.3　Pulmonary fat embolism（Fig.2-22）

The lung tissue presents extensive edema and a lipid embolus in the branch of pulmonary artery (blue arrow). The embolus is composed of bone marrow hematopoietic cells and a large number of lipid droplets, which are solubilized into different-sized vacuoles by xylene.

3. Infarct

3. 1   Anemic infarct of kidney (Fig.2-23)

There is a slightly eosin-stained area in the slice, which is infarcted area (blue asterisk), and the nearby tissue shows normal glomeruli and renal tubules. The infarcted area is demarcated from normal cortex by a narrow hyperemic zone (blue arrows) containing infiltrating neutrophils, which represents acute inflammatory response. Under high power view, the nuclei of glomeruli and renal tubules in the necrotic area have disappeared, but the outline of them is visible.

3. 2   Anemic infarct of spleen (Fig.2-24)

The large eosin-stained area in the spleen is infarcted area, and it shows that the collapsed necrotic tissue is granular and indistinct (blue asterisks).

3. 3   Hemorrhagic infarct of lung (Fig.2-25)

There is a dark red area with a slightly spherical shape, showing hemorrhagic infarct (blue asterisk). In the infarcted focus, the alveolar cavities are filled with erythrocytes, and the cells of alveolar wall are all necrotic, thus it is difficult to discern the outline of alveoli. While the alveolar lumens outside the necrotic area are mostly vacant, and only a few macrophages containing hemosiderin are found in some alveolar cavities.

4. Edema

Pulmonary edema (Fig.2-26)

Most of the alveolar cavities are filled with homogenous, eosinophilic fluid, and only few alveoli still contain air. The pulmonary capillaries are dilated and congested with erythrocytes.

5. Hemorrhage

5. 1   Pulmonary hemorrhage (Fig.2-27)

Most of the alveolar cavities are filled with erythrocytes with some hemosiderin-laden macrophages and abundant formalin hyperpigmentation. Compensatory emphysema is observed beside the hemorrhagic area. The structures of alveolar septa still remain intact.

5. 2   Adrenal hemorrhage (Fig.2-28)

There are large numbers of erythrocytes in both the adrenal cortex and medulla. The cortical structure still remains intact and some parenchymal cells are atrophic.

Ⅳ. Clinical pathological discussion

Case

A 54-year-old woman died of heart failure. She was admitted to hospital because of rheumatic heart disease with mitral stenosis and insufficiency. Autopsy showed that there was a spherical dark red and grayish white lump in the enlarged left atrium. The lung tissue was brownish red and dense. The liver was enlarged with diffuse dark red dots and presented red and yellow mottled effect. In the kidney, there was a grayish-white necrotic area with slightly fan-shape and clear boundary. The lesion was dense and dry, and surrounded by a dark-brown bleeding zone. Moreover, there was a little fibrin exudate on the necrotic tissue surface. Typical pictures of the histological examination are shown in Fig.2-29.

(1) What pathological diagnoses do you make for these organs?

(2) What's the interrelationship among these organ lesions?

(3) Please briefly describe the relationships among pathological changes of involved organs and possible clinical manifestations.

Ⅴ. Questions

1. What are the morphological characteristics of chronic congestion of lung, liver and spleen? What are the mechanisms and common causes of these lesions? What are the possible consequences of congestion in these organs?

2. Which conditions are included to induce thrombosis?

3. What are common types of emboli?

4. What's the relationship among thrombosis, embolism and infarction?

5. Terms: Hyperemia, Congestion, Heart failure cell, Nutmeg liver, Thrombosis, Embolism, Infarction.

VI. 附图 (Figures)

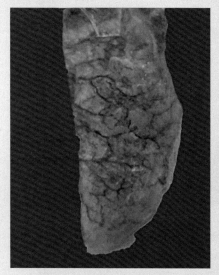

图 2-1　阑尾炎性充血
Fig.2-1　Inflammatory hyperemia
of appendix

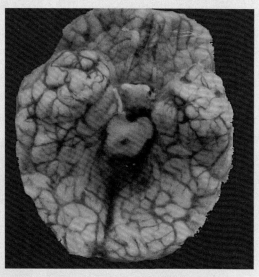

图 2-2　脑膜炎性充血
Fig.2-2　Meningeal hyperemia

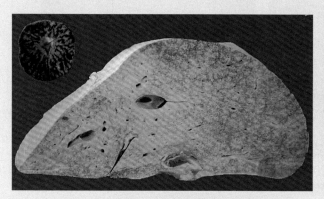

图 2-3　慢性肝淤血
Fig.2-3　Chronic hepatic congestion

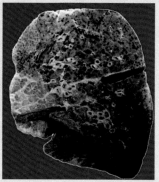

图 2-4　慢性肺淤血
Fig.2-4　Chronic pulmonary
congestion

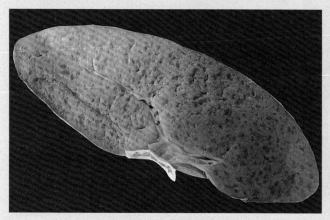

图 2-5　慢性脾淤血
Fig.2-5　Chronic congestion of spleen

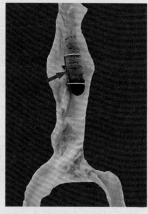

图 2-6　静脉血栓
Fig.2-6　Thrombus in vein

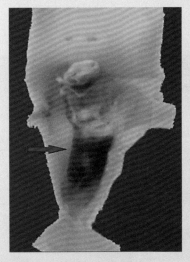

图 2-7　动脉血栓
Fig.2- 7　Thrombus in artery

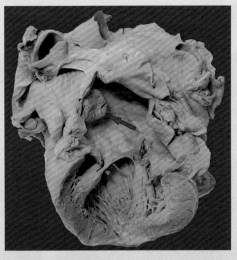

图 2-8　心脏附壁血栓
Fig.2-8　Mural thrombus in heart

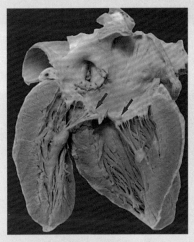

图 2-9　心瓣膜白色血栓
Fig.2-9　Pale thrombus of heart valve

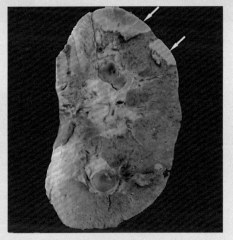

图 2-10　肾贫血性梗死
Fig.2-10　Anemic infarct of kidney

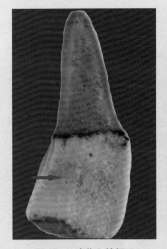

图 2-11　脾贫血性梗死
Fig.2-11　Anemic
infarct of spleen

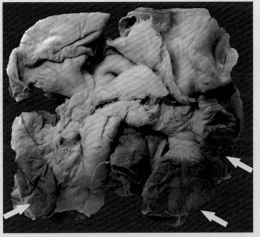

图 2-12　肠出血性梗死
Fig.2-12　Hemorrhagic infarct
of intestine

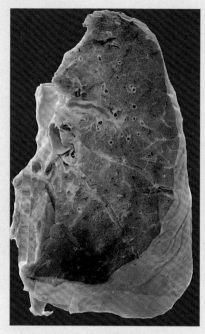

图 2-13 肺出血性梗死
Fig.2-13 Hemorrhagic infarct of lung

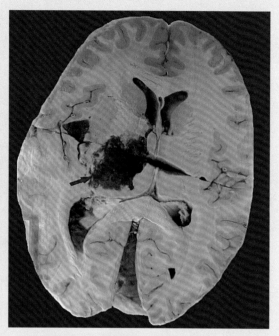

图 2-14 脑出血
Fig.2-14 Cerebral hemorrhage

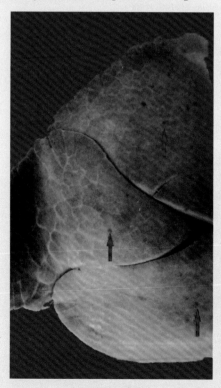

图 2-15 胸膜淤点
Fig.2-15 Pleural hemorrhage

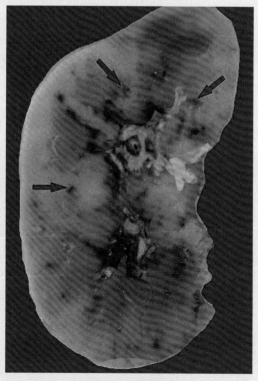

图 2-16 肾出血
Fig.2-16 Renal hemorrhage

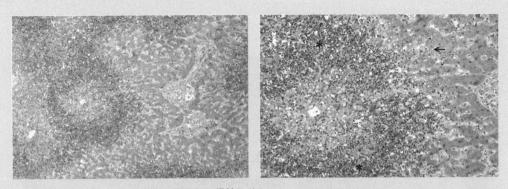

图 2-17 慢性肝淤血（×100；×200）

Fig.2-17 Chronic hepatic congestion（×100；×200）

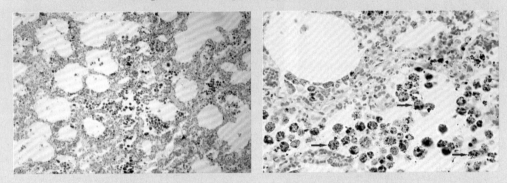

图 2-18 慢性肺淤血（×100；×400）

Fig.2-18 Chronic pulmonary congestion（×100；×400）

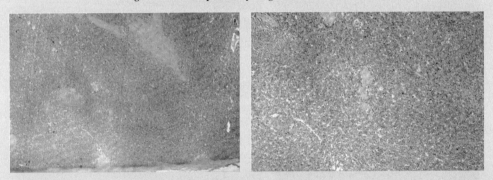

图 2-19 慢性脾淤血（×100；×200）

Fig.2-19 Chronic congestion of spleen（×100；×200）

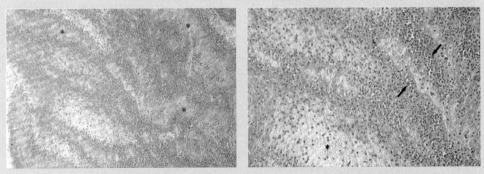

图 2-20 混合血栓（×100；×200）

Fig.2-20 Mixed thrombus（×100；×200）

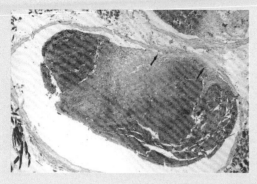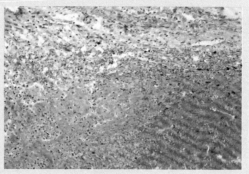

图 2-21　血栓机化（×40；×200）
Fig.2-21　Organization of thrombus（×40；×200）

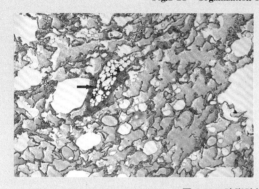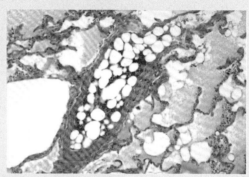

图 2-22　肺脂肪栓塞（×40；×100）
Fig.2-22　Pulmonary fat embolism（×40；×100）

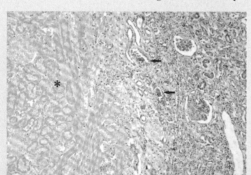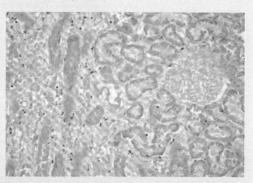

图 2-23　肾贫血性梗死（×100；×200）
Fig.2-23　Anemic infarct of kidney（×100；×200）

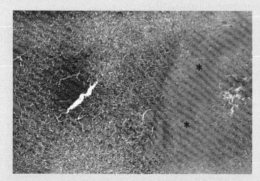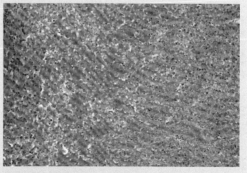

图 2-24　脾贫血性梗死（×40；×200）
Fig.2-24　Anemic infarct of spleen（×40；×200）

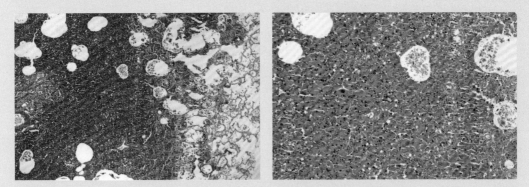

图 2-25　肺出血性梗死（×100；×200）

Fig.2-25　Hemorrhagic infarct of lung（×100；×200）

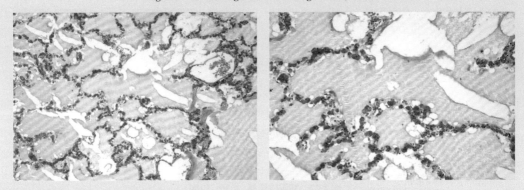

图 2-26　肺水肿（×100；×200）

Fig.2-26　Pulmonary edema（×100；×200）

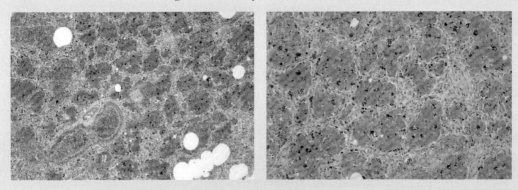

图 2-27　肺出血（×100；×200）

Fig.2-27　Pulmonary hemorrhage（×100；×200）

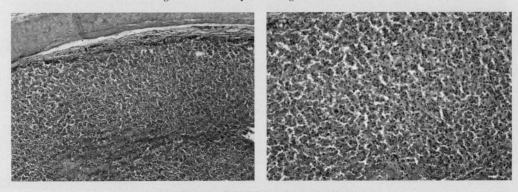

图 2-28　肾上腺出血（×100；×200）

Fig.2-28　Adrenal hemorrhage（×100；×200）

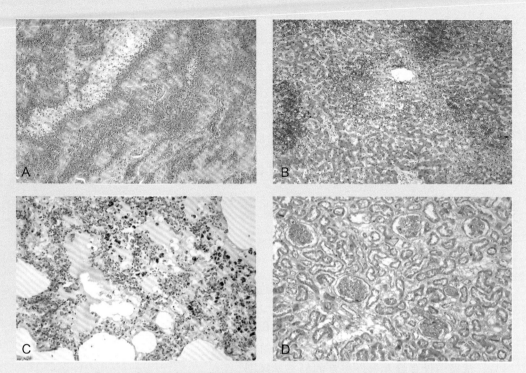

图 2-29 案例（A：左心房球形物 ×100；B：肝 ×100；C：肺 ×200；D：肾 ×100）
Fig.2-29 Case（A：Spherical lump in the left atrium ×100；B：Liver ×100；C：Lung ×200；D：Kidney ×100）

张爱凤（Aifeng Zhang）

第三章

炎　症

一、目的要求

1. 掌握炎症的基本病理变化。
2. 掌握各种炎细胞的形态学特征及其在炎症中出现的意义。
3. 掌握炎症的病理类型及各型的病变特点及其转归。
4. 掌握急性炎症和慢性炎症的形态学区别。

导学

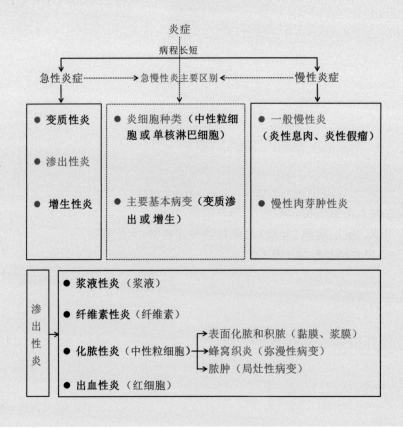

二、 大体标本

1. 变质性炎

急性重型肝炎（图 3-1）

肝体积明显缩小，重量减轻，质地变软，包膜皱缩，边缘锐利；肝表面及切面呈黄色，切面散在分布灰黄色斑块，结构不清，质地疏松。

2. 渗出性炎

2.1 浆液性炎

皮肤浆液性炎（图 3-2）

手烫伤后表皮见一水疱（蓝箭），内为透明的水样浆液。浆液的主要成分为血浆，含少量小分子蛋白质、少许中性粒细胞和纤维素。

2.2 纤维素性炎

2.2.1 纤维素性心包炎（图 3-3）

心包膜粗糙，失去正常光泽，血管模糊不清，被覆灰白、灰黄色膜状纤维素性渗出物（蓝箭）。纤维素性渗出物因心脏搏动的摩擦牵拉而呈绒毛状，故又称"绒毛心"。主要见于感染和风湿病。可结合大体标本推测其可能的转归。

2.2.2 白喉（图 3-4）

喉、气管、支气管连同肺之标本，气管及支气管已从背侧剪开。沿口咽部及扁桃体表面、会厌部、喉部及气管、支气管内均有一层灰白色膜状物。在咽部、扁桃体表面附着甚紧（固膜），在气管及支气管表面假膜卷曲，部分浮于表面，已成剥离状（浮膜，蓝箭）。请思考咽部及气管的假膜病变为何不同，其造成的后果是否也会不同？ 为什么？

2.2.3 纤维素性胸膜炎（图 3-5）

脏层胸膜表面可见纤维素构成的薄苔或灰白、灰红色膜状覆盖物（蓝箭），外观干燥、易撕脱。如渗出的纤维素不能被机体溶解吸收，可能会发展为胸膜纤维性粘连，甚至闭塞性胸膜炎。

2.2.4 闭塞性胸膜炎（图 3-6）

胸膜腔因大量渗出物（绿星）充填而闭塞，其中有大量渗出的纤维素、新生的肉芽组织和纤维组织。脏层胸膜（蓝箭）和渗出物粘连紧密，无法剥离。

2.2.5 肠纤维性粘连（图 3-7）

肠管切开标本，可见肠黏膜肿胀，粗糙无光泽。肠管弯曲，肠管间粘连紧密，无法分离。请思考该病变发生的常见原因及其可能给机体带来的后果。

2.3 化脓性炎

2.3.1 化脓性脑膜炎（图 3-8）

脑表面血管扩张充血，脑膜混浊，蛛网膜下腔内见黄白色脓液积聚，血管周围尤为明显（黄箭），脑沟、脑回结构因大量渗出物积聚而模糊不清，脑回变宽，脑沟变窄。

2.3.2 肾脓肿（图 3-9）

肾脏体积增大，切面可见皮髓质分界尚清，其中散在多个灰黄色小脓肿灶（黄箭），髓质部居多。肾组织因充血、水肿而质地柔软。

2.3.3　肝脓肿（图 3-10）

脓肿主要位于左叶，其周围充血，颜色加深。切面见多个形状不规则、大小不等的脓肿（蓝箭）。脓肿由"脓肿膜"（最内侧为黏稠的脓液，向外依次为增生的肉芽组织及纤维组织）与周围组织分开，大脓肿可能是数个小脓肿融合而成。肝脓肿主要源于化脓菌的血源播散，常为多发。

2.3.4　肺脓肿（图 3-11）

肺组织切面可见多个大小不等的灰黄色脓肿灶（绿星），有的呈现形状不规则的空洞（黄星），其内脓液大部分已流失，内壁不光滑，附着少量残留脓液，外围以"脓肿膜"。

2.3.5　脑脓肿（图 3-12）

标本为脑冠状切面。患侧脑组织肿胀，内有一椭圆形脓肿灶（蓝箭），周围有厚层纤维结缔组织包绕，边界清楚，内壁不光滑，附有少量稠厚脓液。多为细菌血源播散所致。

2.3.6　急性化脓性阑尾炎（图 3-13）

阑尾肿胀，浆膜面覆有纤维素性、脓性渗出物。切面阑尾壁层次结构不清，腔内黏膜有破坏，管腔扩大，内有积脓。注意蓝箭指示部位发生的变化及其原因。

3. 增生性炎

3.1　非特异性慢性炎

3.1.1　慢性阑尾炎（图 3-14）
阑尾体积变小，色灰白，质硬。

3.1.2　慢性胆囊炎（图 3-15）
胆囊体积增大，壁增厚，胆囊腔扩张，黏膜呈粗网状（黄星），有胆汁附着，内见桑葚状结石一枚（绿箭）。

3.1.3　鼻息肉（图 3-16）
鼻腔内取出的结节状组织，灰白色、半透明，表面光滑湿润。常见于慢性鼻炎或过敏性鼻炎。

3.2　肉芽肿性炎

肠血吸虫病（图 3-17）

结肠一段，黏膜面粗糙，可见短小带蒂的息肉（绿箭）或颗粒状隆起，部分区域因萎缩而平坦。

三、组织切片

1. 变质性炎

急性重型肝炎（图 3-18）

肝组织呈现一片"荒凉"景象，肝细胞大片坏死崩解（蓝星）、仅小叶边缘残存少量变性肝细胞。坏死区和汇管区有大量炎细胞浸润，主要为淋巴细胞和巨噬细胞。肝窦明显扩张（蓝箭）、充血甚至出血。

2. 渗出性炎

2.1 纤维素性心包炎（图3-19）

心包膜脏层表面被覆一层伊红染网状结构物质（双向蓝箭），即渗出的纤维素（蓝箭）。纤维素下方的心包膜血管扩张充血，炎细胞浸润（双向绿箭），组织水肿。

2.2 白喉（图3-20）

标本为白喉患者近会厌处咽后壁切片。黏膜上皮消失，被一层淡伊红染的膜样物质取代（假膜，双向绿箭）。主要由丝状纤维素（绿箭）和坏死组织构成，其间有中性粒细胞、坏死脱落的上皮细胞及核碎片。假膜与黏膜下层粘连在一起，黏膜下层血管扩张充血，部分管腔内见大量白细胞。

2.3 化脓性脑膜炎（图3-21）

蛛网膜下腔明显扩大，其内有高度扩张充血的血管（绿箭）和大量炎细胞（绿星）及少许纤维素。炎细胞主要为中性粒细胞和脓细胞（变性坏死的中性粒细胞，蓝箭）。脑实质（蓝星）形态基本正常。

2.4 肾脓肿（图3-22）

蓝星所示的脓肿区肾组织破坏，正常结构消失，代之以密集的中性粒细胞和脓细胞（蓝箭）及核碎片。周围血管扩张充血。绿箭示脓肿周围的肾小球。

2.5 肝脓肿（图3-23）

绿箭所指区域为脓肿区，边界较清楚，肝组织结构消失，代之以大量浸润的炎细胞，主要是中性粒细胞及变性坏死的脓细胞。绿星示周围的肝组织，可见中央静脉及肝小叶结构。

2.6 急性蜂窝织性阑尾炎（图3-24）

阑尾各层结构不清，有大量中性粒细胞和脓细胞弥漫性浸润、血管扩张充血。黏膜上皮细胞大多已变性坏死脱落形成缺损（蓝箭），仅存少许上皮细胞（黑箭）。绿箭示肌层大量浸润的中性粒细胞。

3. 增生性炎

3.1 鼻息肉（图3-25）

组织表面覆以假复层纤毛柱状上皮，上皮下方组织疏松水肿，纤维组织增生，有较多炎细胞浸润，以上皮下和腺体周围较明显。部分腺体因分泌物潴留而呈囊状扩张（蓝箭），腺上皮受压变扁平。

注意识别炎细胞类型。绿箭示嗜酸性粒细胞，细胞圆形，核多为两叶，细胞浆红染、其内见粗大红染嗜酸性颗粒。黑箭示淋巴细胞，细胞圆形，核圆形深蓝染，胞浆很少。红箭示浆细胞，细胞椭圆形，细胞核位于胞浆一侧、境界清楚，核周有空晕，胞浆略嗜碱染色。黄箭示成纤维细胞，细胞较炎细胞体积大，梭形，核卵圆形。

3.2 肠炎性息肉（图3-26）

表面被覆的肠上皮细胞增生，其下方血管扩张充血、毛细血管（红箭）和成纤维细胞

（蓝箭头）增生，急慢性炎细胞浸润，可见中性粒细胞（黑箭）和淋巴滤泡（蓝箭）。

3.3　肺炎性假瘤（图 3-27）

肺组织实变，肺泡结构被破坏，代之以大量新生毛细血管（绿箭）、增生的纤维结缔组织（蓝星）、增生的肺泡上皮细胞（黑箭）和浸润的炎细胞，并可见淋巴滤泡（绿星）。蓝箭示黄色瘤样泡沫细胞。

3.4　慢性胆囊炎（图 3-28）

胆囊黏膜上皮尚保持完整，黏膜上皮可萎缩但多数增生。罗-阿氏窦（蓝箭）常深达肌层甚至穿过肌层（慢性胆囊炎较为特征性的病理改变，注意与肿瘤浸润区别）。囊壁全层有大量炎细胞浸润（蓝星），浸润的细胞以淋巴细胞（黑箭）和浆细胞（黄箭）为主，黏膜层及外膜较为明显。表面金黄色物为胆汁结晶（红箭）。

3.5　慢性扁桃体炎（图 3-29）

扁桃体淋巴滤泡增多、增大，生发中心扩大（蓝星），有慢性炎细胞浸润（蓝箭）。隐窝鳞状上皮内可见组织坏死和炎细胞浸润。

3.6　慢性阑尾炎急性发作（图 3-30）

阑尾分层结构可见，但黏膜下层纤维结缔组织增生；各层均有炎细胞浸润，以黏膜层最明显，包括浆细胞（蓝箭头）、淋巴细胞和中性粒细胞，并可见淋巴滤泡增生（绿星）及大量新生毛细血管（绿箭头）和成纤维细胞（黑箭头）。

3.7　异物性肉芽肿（图 3-31）

标本为横纹肌及周围纤维结缔组织，内见结节状病灶（蓝圈）。结节内可见淡蓝色折光物质，即异物（外科缝线，黑箭头），周围有较多的多核巨细胞（蓝箭和绿箭）。这些异物巨细胞体积大，形状不规则，胞浆丰富、伊红染，核多、分布不规则，部分异物巨细胞（蓝箭）胞浆内见吞噬的异物。

四、临床病理讨论

案例 1　患者，女性，26 岁，孕前体检发现宫颈有一外生性生长的肿物。予以切除并送病理科检查，典型图片见图 3-32。

（1）请给出该宫颈肿物的病理诊断，并说明理由，分析该病变发生的可能原因。

（2）试分析如果未予任何医学干预，该患者宫颈肿物可能的结局。

案例 2　患者，男性，48 岁，进食油腻食物 2 小时后突发右上腹痛，呈阵发性发作并逐渐加重，急诊入院。

体检：腹部平软，强迫弯腰体位，Murphy 征阳性。血常规：白细胞计数 $16 \times 10^9/L$，中性粒细胞比例 80%，余无异常。医生初步诊断为急性胆囊炎，与病人及家属沟通后急诊手术，术中发现胆囊体积增大，充血水肿明显，囊腔内有脓性渗出物，未查见结石。送检病理科后 H.E. 染色，典型图片见图 3-33。

（1）请给出患者胆囊的病理诊断。

（2）为什么患者的 Murphy 征会是阳性？

（3）试分析患者右上腹痛、血常规白细胞和中性粒细胞异常的病理学基础。

五、 思考题

1. 如何从病理形态角度认识炎症？
2. 渗出性炎有哪些类型，各型主要病变特点是什么？
3. 请比较脓肿和蜂窝织炎。
4. 急性和慢性炎症在形态上各有何特征？
5. 炎性肉芽肿和炎性息肉、肉芽组织有何区别？
6. 炎细胞的种类有哪些？ 列出炎症的主要类型及其主要渗出的炎细胞。
7. 名词解释：炎症，渗出物，炎症介质，黏附分子，卡他性炎，假膜性炎，绒毛心，脓肿，溃疡，窦道，瘘管，蜂窝织炎，炎性息肉，炎性假瘤，肉芽肿。

Chapter 3

Inflammation

Ⅰ. Aims

1. To grasp the basic pathological changes of inflammation.

2. To grasp the characteristics and significances of various types of inflammatory cells.

3. To grasp the pathological types of inflammation, corresponding morphology and outcomes.

4. To grasp the difference between acute inflammation and chronic inflammation in morphology.

Guidance to study

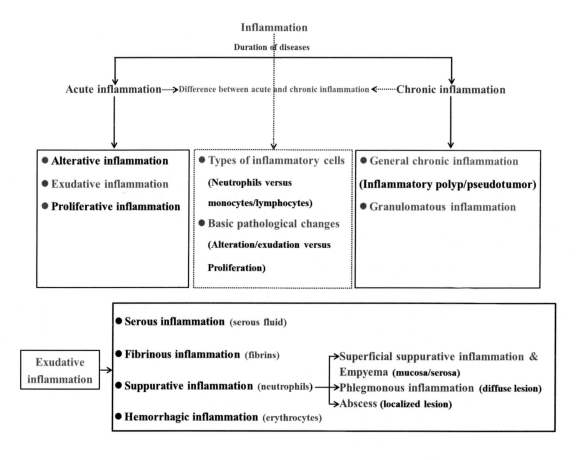

II. Gross specimens

1. Alterative inflammation

Acute fulminant hepatitis (Fig.3-1)

This liver is shrunken, limp, and the capsule is wrinkled. The weight is obviously reduced. The surface and cut surface is gray-yellow or yellow-green. On the cut surface, hepatic tissue becomes desolate with scattered yellow necrotic areas.

2. Exudative inflammation

2.1　Serous inflammation

Serous inflammation of skin (Fig. 3-2)

A big blister with watery fluid (blue arrow) is on the surface of the hand skin burned. The serous fluid is mainly composed of plasma, a small amount of low molecular proteins, fibrin and neutrophils.

2.2　Fibrinous inflammation

2.2.1　Fibrinous pericarditis (Fig. 3-3)

The pericardium is not glistening and smooth but dull with grayish-white, flocky deposits (blue arrows), and the blood vessels are unclear. The deposits were drawn into villi-like due to heart beating. Therefore, it is also called "cor villosum" or "shaggy heart". Fibrinous pericarditis commonly occurs after infection and rheumatic fever.

2.2.2　Diphtheria (Fig. 3-4)

Here is a specimen with the trachea, bronchi, and lung. It shows an extensive pale yellowish-white diphtheritic pseudomembrane (blue arrows) involving the larynx, trachea and bronchi. The pseudomembrane on the surface of trachea and bronchi is insecurely attached and can be readily desquamated and dislodged, however, the pseudomembrane on the surface of larynx and tonsils is attached firmly. Please think about the causes of the difference, and the effects on the host.

2.2.3　Fibrinous pleuritis (Fig. 3-5)

The pleura are covered by gray-white and gray-red fibrin flakes (blue arrows). They can be easily stripped off. Fibrinous pleuritis with abundant exudate may develop into pleural adhesions, even occlusive pleuritis.

2.2.4　Occlusive pleuritis (Fig. 3-6)

The pleural cavity (green stars) is blocked by a large amount of exudate including fibrin, granulation tissue, and fibrous tissue. The visceral (blue arrows) and parietal pleura are adhered too tight to be separated.

2.2.5　Intestinal fibrous adhesion (Fig. 3-7)

The specimen shows extensive peritoneal adhesions with loops of bowel, and the loops are firmly attached each other and difficult to separate.

2.3　Suppurative inflammation

2.3.1　Suppurative meningitis（Fig. 3-8）

The blood vessels on the surface are dilated and congested. Subarachnoid space is filled with yellow-white pus（yellow arrows）, especially around the blood vessels. The shape of gyri and sulci is obscure due to exudate, and the gyri become widened with narrowed sulci.

2.3.2　Renal abscesses（Fig. 3-9）

The kidney is enlarged and soft due to hyperemia and edema. There are multiple small grayish-yellow foci（yellow arrows）on the cut section of the kidney. The demarcation between the cortex and medulla is still clear.

2.3.3　Hepatic abscesses（Fig. 3-10）

The numerous abscesses（blue arrows）are mainly distributed in the left lobe of the liver. Among them, some abscesses present cavities lined with a shaggy greenish-yellow purulent exudate. The abscess membrane can be identified as a yellow-white undulating band including pus, granulation tissue and fibrous tissue from inner to outer. Liver abscesses are commonly caused by hematogenous spread of pyogenic bacteria, and present multiple lesions.

2.3.4　Pulmonary abscesses（Fig. 3-11）

On the cut surface of left lung, the lobes are consolidated with numerous abscesses. Some abscesses are filled with grayish-yellow pus（green stars）, and some abscesses display cavities because pus has been removed through airways（yellow stars）. The walls of abscesses are irregular, somewhat shaggy and still covered with pus.

2.3.5　Brain abscess（Fig. 3-12）

This is a coronal section of the brain. An oval abscess with a cavity（blue arrow）is shown in the brain. The inner wall of the cavity is rough and covered with grayish-yellow purulent exudate, and the abscess is enclosed in a capsule containing granulation tissue, fibrous tissue and reactive glial tissues on histological examination. Brain abscesses usually result from hematogenous spread of bacteria.

2.3.6　Acute suppurative appendicitis（Fig. 3-13）

The vermiform appendix is swollen and covered with fibrinopurulent exudate. On incision, the lumen is dilated with greenish-yellow pus, and the layers of structure are unclear in the appendix wall. It may cause perforation and peritonitis. Note the lesion indicated by blue arrow and identify its pathological changes.

3.　Proliferative inflammation

3.1　Non-specific chronic inflammation

3.1.1　Chronic appendicitis（Fig. 3-14）

The specimen is a firm, grayish-white vermiform appendix.

3. 1. 2   Chronic cholecystitis（Fig. 3-15）

The specimen shows a gallbladder with markedly thickened wall, and a big mulberry-like stone (green arrow) exists inside the dilated gallbladder. Mucous membrane of the gall bladder is rough and appears as reticular structure (yellow star).

3. 1. 3   Nasal polyp（Fig. 3-16）

The polyp is a smooth, shiny semi-translucent and gray-bluish nodule. Nasal polyps most probably result from inflammatory edema and hypertrophy of nasal mucous membrane induced by chronic rhinitis and allergic rhinitis.

3. 2   Granulomatous inflammation

Schistosomiasis of colon（Fig. 3-17）

This is a segment of dissected colon. Multiple pedunculated polyps (green arrows), granular bulges, flattened and atrophied lesions are observed on the surface of mucous membrane.

Ⅲ. Tissue sections

1. Alterative inflammation

Acute fulminant hepatitis（Fig.3-18）

Complete destruction of hepatocytes in contiguous lobules has only left a few dying or died hepatocytes. The necrotic areas (blue stars) are infiltrated by inflammatory cells (mostly for lymphocytes and macrophages). Hepatic sinuses are markedly dilated and congested (blue arrow).

2. Exudative inflammation

2. 1   Fibrinous pericarditis（Fig.3-19）

The exudate (blue bidirectional arrow) is well established on the epicardial aspect of pericardium. Under the exudate, dilated blood vessels and inflammatory cells can be observed in thickened epicardium (green bidirectional arrow). The exudate is made up of dense masses of pink-staining fibrin (blue arrows) and inflammatory cells.

2. 2   Diphtheria（Fig.3-20）

This specimen is from posterior pharyngeal wall adjacent to epiglottic mucosa. The mucous epithelia are replaced by a layer of pseudomembrane (green bidirectional arrow), which consists of a dense network of fibrin (green arrows), leukocytes, and necrotic epithelia. The pseudomembrane has mingled with submucous tissues, which is infiltrated with inflammatory cells.

2. 3　Suppurative meningitis（Fig.3-21）

The subrachnoid space becomes large with mass of infiltrating neutrophils (green star) and a small quantity of fibrin. Green arrows indicate the dilated and congested blood vessels. Some neutrophils present clearly lobulated nuclei, and others are dying or dead (blue arrows) . The cerebral parenchyma (blue star) is not involved.

2. 4　Renal abscesses（Fig.3-22）

There is a relatively localized lesion (blue star) in the renal tissue, which appears as aggregations of neutrophils (blue arrows) and necroses. The surrounding area presents dilated and congested blood vessels, infiltrating inflammatory cells, and residual glomeruli (green arrow).

2. 5　Hepatic abscesses（Fig.3-23）

The abscess indicated by green arrows presents abundant inflammatory cells with clear border, and the original structure disappears. The infiltrating cells are mainly neutrophils and pus cells (degenerative or necrotic neutrophils). The green star indicates the nearby liver tissue with normal central vein and hepatic cords.

2. 6　Acute phlegmonous appendicitis（Fig.3-24）

The inflammatory histological changes exist in all the layers of appendix wall. The mucosal ulceration (blue arrows) becomes more extensive, and few of the mucosal glands (black arrow) remain intact. Large numbers of neutrophils have infiltrated through the submucosa and muscle layer to the serosa. The smooth muscle cells are separated by infiltrating neutrophils (green arrows), thus the intermuscular spaces become widened.

3．Proliferative inflammation

3. 1　Nasal polyp（Fig.3-25）

The nodule is covered with pseudostratified ciliated columnar epithelium and infiltrated by chronic inflammatory cells. Some glands become cystic dilation with flattened epithelial cells due to the retention of secretion (blue arrows). Marked edema and fibroblasts (yellow arrow) are observed in the interstitial tissue.

Please identify the types of inflammatory cells. The black arrow points to a lymphocyte (round cell with little cytoplasm), the green arrow for an eosinophil (round cell with bi-segmented nucleus and eosinophilic granules in the plasma), and the red arrow for a plasma cell (oval cell having an eccentric nucleus with basophilic cytoplasm and perinuclear halo).

3. 2　Intestinal inflammatory polyp（Fig.3-26）

The tissue is covered by proliferative simple columnar epithelia. Under the epithelia, dilated and congested capillaries (red arrows), abundant inflammatory cells (black arrows), lymphoid follicles (blue arrows), and fibroblasts (blue arrowheads) are obviously observed.

3. 3   Pulmonary inflammatory pseudotumor（Fig.3-27）

The lung tissue becomes consolidated, and the damaged alveoli are replaced by large amount of newly formed capillaries (green arrows), proliferative pneumocytes (black arrow) and fibrous connective tissue (blue stars), infiltrating inflammatory cells as well as lymphoid follicles (green stars). The blue arrows point to the xanthoma-like foam cells.

3. 4   Chronic cholecystitis（Fig.3-28）

The tissue shows histological architecture of the gallbladder wall. Mucosal folds are normal or flattening. The gallbladder wall is widened by infiltrating inflammatory cells (blue star), such as lymphocytes (black arrows), plasma cells (yellow arrows), and proliferating connective tissue. The increased pressure in the lumen leads to diverticulum-like outpouchings of the mucous membranes (Rokitansky-Aschoff sinus, a morphological marker for chronic cholecystitis, blue arrow). The red arrows indicate bile crystals.

3. 5   Chronic tonsillitis（Fig.3-29）

The lymphoid tissue in the tonsil reacts to inflammation by lymphoid hyperplasia (blue stars) and inflammatory cells infiltration. The squamous epithelium of crypt is disrupted by infiltrating leukocytes (blue arrow).

3. 6   Chronic appendicitis，acute onset（Fig.3-30）

The appendix shows layer of structure, but submucosal layer is unclear due to proliferative fibrous tissue. All the layers display infiltration of inflammatory cells containing lymphocytes, plasma cells (blue arrowhead), neutrophils, and lymphoid follicles (green stars). Mass of new formed capillaries (green arrowhead) and fibroblasts (black arrowhead) are easily observed.

3. 7   Foreign body granuloma（Fig.3-31）

Some nodules (blue circle) are visible in the skeletal muscle and fibrous connective tissue. Within the nodules, some foreign materials showing light-blue refraction (black arrowheads) are noticed. However, the most notable feature is the presence of many foreign body giant cells (green and blue arrows) which are multinucleated with plentiful cytoplasm. Some giant cells present foreign materials in the cytoplasm (blue arrows).

Ⅳ. Clinical pathological discussion

Case 1

A female aged 26 was found to have an exophytic-growing mass in the cervix when taking her pre-pregnancy physical examination. The mass was removed and investigated by pathologists. After stained by H.E., the typical morphology is shown as Fig.3-32.

(1) Please diagnose the cervix and describe common causes of the mass formation.

(2) Please explain what will possibly occur if no medical intervention was done about the mass.

Case 2

A male aged 48 suddenly complained his up-right abdominal pain after taking a fatty food. The pain was paroxysmal and gradually became worse, thus he was sent to emergency and asked to be hospitalized. Physical examination: his abdomen was flat and soft, but he was keeping a forced bend gesture. His Murphy sign was positive. Blood routine test: leukocytes 16×10^9/L, neutrophils 80%. The doctor primarily diagnosed him as acute cholecystitis. After talking with his family, he underwent immediate surgery. During the operation, his gall bladder was observed to become large with marked congestion and edema. The cavity showed purulent exudate, but not calculus. The removed gallbladder was sent for pathological investigation, and the typical figures are shown as Fig.3-33.

(1) Please give pathological diagnosis of the gall bladder.

(2) What is Murphy sign, and why is the patient positive?

(3) Try to explain the patient's abdominal pain and abnormal results from blood routine test using pathological changes.

V. Questions

1. How to understand inflammation based on pathological changes?

2. How many types is exudative inflammation classified into? List main exudate for each type?

3. Compare the two kinds of suppurative inflammation, abscess and phlegmonous inflammation.

4. What are the morphological characteristics of acute and chronic inflammation?

5. Differentiate inflammatory granulomas from inflammatory polyps and granulation tissues.

6. List the main types of inflammation, and dominant infiltrating inflammatory cells for each type.

7. Terms: Inflammation, Exudate, Inflammatory mediator, Adhesion molecule, Catarrhal inflammation, Pseudomembranous inflammation, Cor villosum, Abscess, Ulcer, Sinus, Fistula, Phlegmonous inflammation, Inflammatory polyp, Inflammatory pseudotumor, Granuloma.

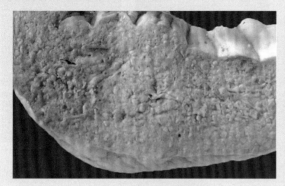

图 3-1　急性重型肝炎
Fig.3-1　Acute fulminant
　　　　hepatitis

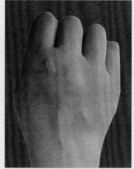

图 3-2　皮肤浆液性炎
Fig.3-2　Serous
　　　　inflammation of skin

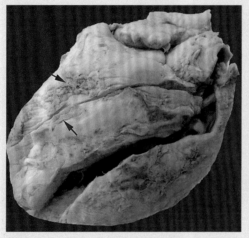

图 3-3　纤维素性心包炎
Fig.3-3　Fibrinous pericarditis

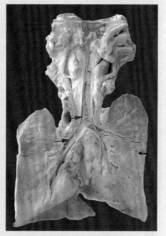

图 3-4　白喉
Fig.3-4　Diphtheria

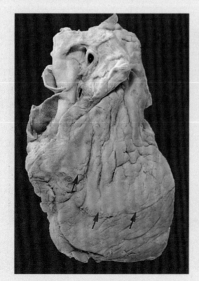

图 3-5　纤维素性胸膜炎
Fig.3-5　Fibrinous pleuritis

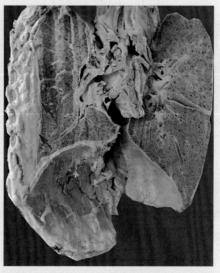

图 3-6　闭塞性胸膜炎
Fig.3-6　Occlusive pleuritis

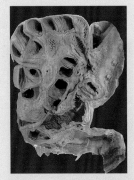

图 3-7 肠纤维性粘连
Fig.3-7 Intestinal fibrous
adhesion

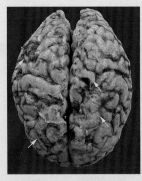

图 3-8 化脓性脑膜炎
Fig.3-8 Suppurative
meningitis

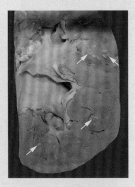

图 3-9 肾脓肿
Fig.3-9 Renal abscesses

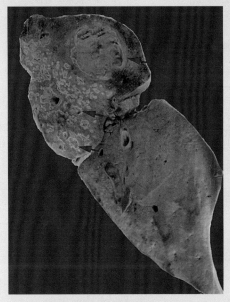

图 3-10 肝脓肿
Fig.3-10 Hepatic abscesses

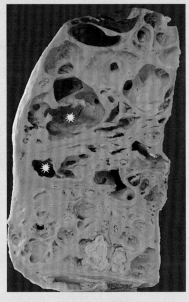

图 3-11 肺脓肿
Fig.3-11 Pulmonary abscesses

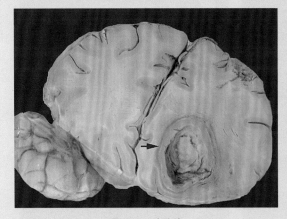

图 3-12 脑脓肿
Fig.3-12 Brain abscess

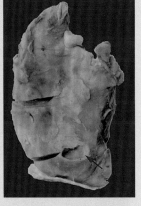

图 3-13 急性化脓性
阑尾炎
Fig.3-13 Acute
suppurative appendicitis

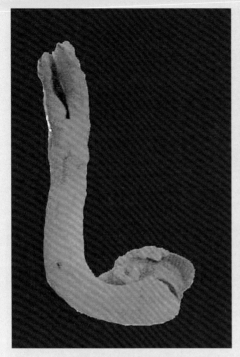

图 3-14 慢性阑尾炎
Fig.3-14 Chronic appendicitis

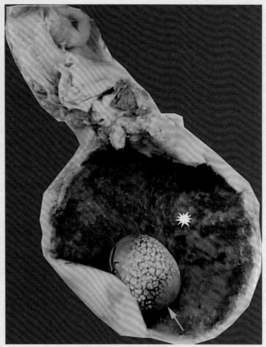

图 3-15 慢性胆囊炎
Fig.3-15 Chronic cholecystitis

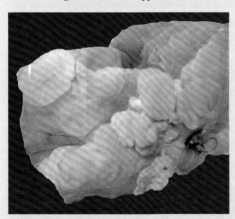

图 3-16 鼻息肉
Fig.3-16 Nasal polyp

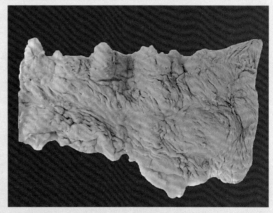

图 3-17 肠血吸虫病
Fig.3-17 Schistosomiasis of colon

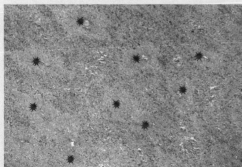

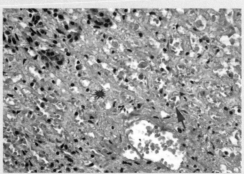

图 3-18 急性重型肝炎（×40；×400）
Fig.3-18 Acute fulminant hepatitis（×40；×400）

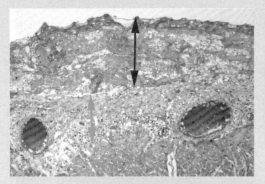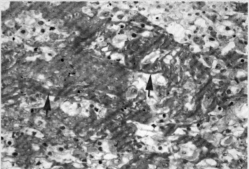

图 3-19　纤维素性心包炎（×100；×400）
Fig.3-19　Fibrinous pericarditis（×100；×400）

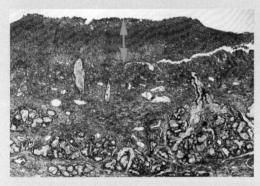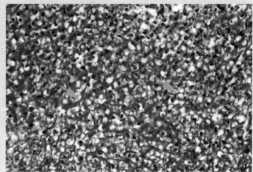

图 3-20　白喉（×100；×400）
Fig.3-20　Diphtheria（×100；×400）

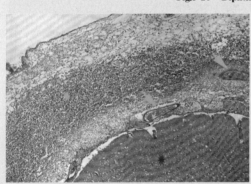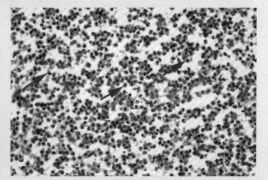

图 3-21　化脓性脑膜炎（×40；×400）
Fig.3-21　Suppurative meningitis（×40；×400）

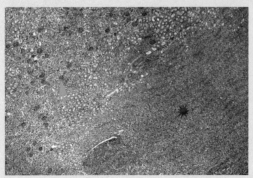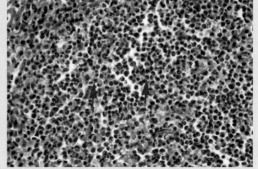

图 3-22　肾脓肿（×100；×400）
Fig.3-22　Renal abscesses（×100；×400）

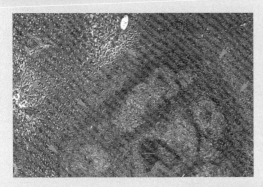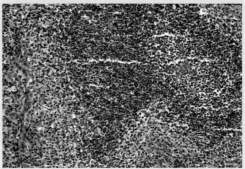

图 3-23　肝脓肿（×40；×200）

Fig.3-23　Hepatic abscesses（×40；×200）

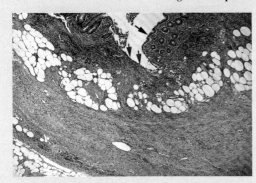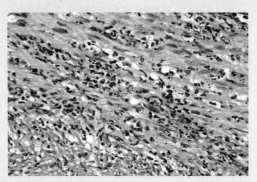

图 3-24　急性蜂窝织性阑尾炎（×40；×400）

Fig.3-24　Acute phlegmonous appendicitis（×40；×400）

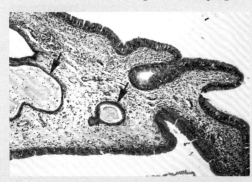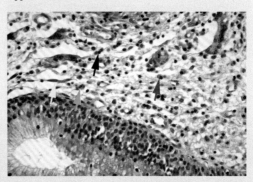

图 3-25　鼻息肉（×100；×400）

Fig.3-25　Nasal polyp（×100；×400）

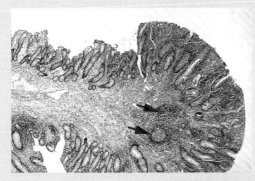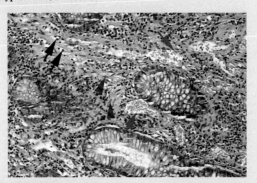

图 3-26　肠炎性息肉（×40；×200）

Fig.3-26　Intestinal inflammatory polyp（×40；×200）

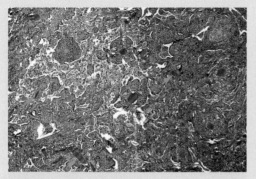
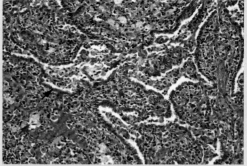

图 3-27 肺炎性假瘤（×40；×200）

Fig.3-27 Pulmonary inflammatory pseudotumor（×40；×200）

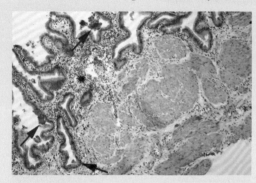
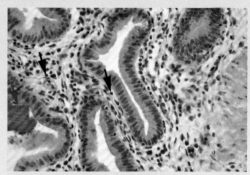

图 3-28 慢性胆囊炎（×100；×400）

Fig.3-28 Chronic cholecystitis（×100；×400）

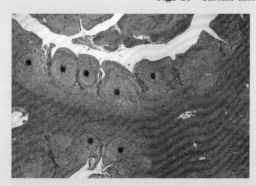
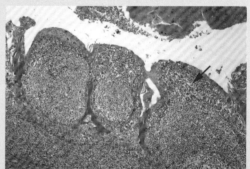

图 3-29 慢性扁桃体炎（×40；×100）

Fig.3-29 Chronic tonsillitis（×40；×100）

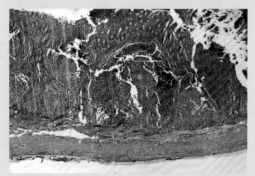
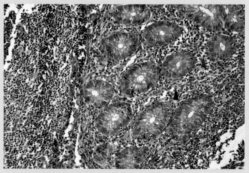

图 3-30 慢性阑尾炎急性发作（×40；×200）

Fig.3-30 Chronic appendicitis，acute onset（×40；×200）

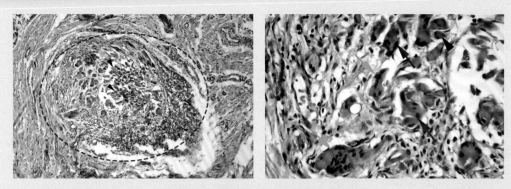

图 3-31　异物性肉芽肿（×100；×400）
Fig,3-31　Foreign body granuloma（×100；×400）

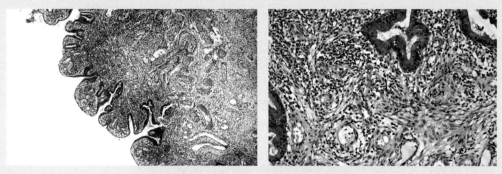

图 3-32　案例 1（×40；×200）
Fig,3-32　Case 1（×40；×200）

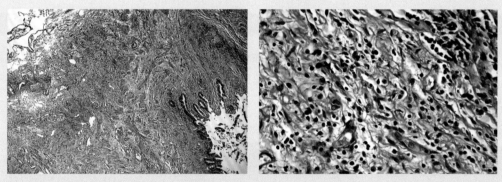

图 3-33　案例 2（×40；×400）
Fig,3-33　Case 2（×40；×400）

李懿萍（Yiping Li）

第四章

肿　　瘤

一、目的要求

1. 掌握常见肿瘤的命名和分类原则。
2. 掌握肿瘤的大体形态特点及生长方式。
3. 掌握肿瘤的异型性。
4. 掌握恶性肿瘤的常见转移途径。
5. 掌握良恶性肿瘤的鉴别要点以及癌与肉瘤的区别。
6. 熟悉常见上皮组织肿瘤和间叶组织肿瘤的基本形态学改变。

导学

　　诊断肿瘤的形态学依据包括大体观察和组织学改变,依据分化程度、有无浸润、转移和坏死分为良性或恶性肿瘤;恶性肿瘤可依据其组织起源初步确定是癌或者肉瘤。

良恶性肿瘤的区别

	良性	恶性
大体形态	息肉状、菜花状、结节状、溃疡性等	息肉状、菜花状、结节状、溃疡性、出血性等
生长方式	外生性、膨胀性	外生性、浸润性
组织结构异型性	有,小	有,明显
细胞形态异型性	不明显(细胞增大、核浆比增高)	明显(细胞和细胞核大小、形态不一;瘤巨细胞和多核瘤巨细胞;核分裂象易见,病理性核分裂象)
肿瘤坏死	不明显	大体、镜下均可见

癌与肉瘤的区别

	癌	肉瘤
组织起源	上皮组织	间叶组织
大体形态	质硬、灰白色	质软、鱼肉状、灰红色
瘤细胞排列方式	巢状、腺样、条索样等	弥漫分布
实质与间质关系	分界清楚	分界不清
网状纤维分布	癌巢周围	瘤细胞之间

二、大体标本

1. 上皮组织肿瘤

1.1 上皮组织良性肿瘤

1.1.1 皮肤乳头状瘤（图 4-1）

完整手术切除的灰红色不规则结节，由许多乳头状突起组成，表面不光滑，未见正常组织与其相连。思考：该结节能被完整切除，说明它是什么样的生长方式？

1.1.2 结肠息肉状腺瘤（图 4-2）

结肠黏膜面可见多个类圆形或不规则、灰白色息肉状结节（蓝星），大小不等，表面光滑或呈菜花状，有蒂（蓝箭）与肠黏膜相连。较大的息肉表面可见出血、坏死。

1.1.3 卵巢乳头状浆液性囊腺瘤（图 4-3）

囊壁样组织一块，外表面基本光滑，散在乳头状突起（蓝箭，左图）。囊内未见分隔，为单房，切开囊壁时浆液样内容物已经流失。囊壁内侧可见大量大小不等的乳头状突起（蓝箭，右图）。

1.1.4 卵巢黏液性囊腺瘤（图 4-4）

椭圆形肿瘤表面光滑，外表面可见多个灰白色半球形隆起（蓝箭）。切面，为多房性，由大小不等的多个囊腔组成。囊内壁光滑，腔内充满灰白灰红色、半透明、胶冻状黏液。

1.1.5 乳腺纤维腺瘤（图 4-5）

卵圆形肿物，包膜不完整，境界清楚，质韧。切面灰白色，边缘清楚，可见细颗粒或由微小裂隙构成地图状外观，部分区域黏液变，切面带有光泽。

1.1.6 腮腺多形性腺瘤（图 4-6）

不规则肿物一块，包膜不完整，表面光滑。切面粗大分叶状，彼此分隔不全，可见半透明胶冻状区域（蓝星）、软骨样区、囊性变区（蓝箭）。

1.2 上皮组织恶性肿瘤

1.2.1 皮肤鳞状细胞癌（图 4-7）

皮肤组织一块，表皮面可见一广基肿物，表面粗糙，呈蕈伞状或菜花状，灰白色，质脆,可见出血、坏死和溃疡。思考:与皮肤乳头状瘤比较,哪些形态说明该肿物是恶性的?肿瘤切除时为什么不能直接贴着皮肤?

1.2.2　阴茎鳞状细胞癌(图 4-8)

手术切除的阴茎和部分阴囊组织,在冠状沟处可见一菜花状、外生性生长的肿物,表面可见出血、坏死。肿瘤基底与组织紧密相连,并向皮肤下组织浸润。

1.2.3　胃癌(息肉型)(图 4-9)

手术切除的胃组织沿胃大弯剪开,胃小弯处可见息肉型肿块,表面粗糙、灰黑色,为肿瘤出血、坏死造成。

1.2.4　直肠癌(息肉型)(图 4-10)

手术切除直肠组织一段,可见一灰红灰白色广基肿物,表面粗糙,呈菜花状,中心因坏死而凹陷。注意该息肉型肿物和息肉状腺瘤的形态区别。

1.2.5　阑尾类癌(图 4-11)

横断切开的管腔样组织一块,管壁各层分界不清(蓝箭),切面致密,未见明显肿块。思考:阑尾类癌是恶性肿瘤吗?

1.2.6　乳腺癌腋窝淋巴结转移(图 4-12)

乳腺手术切除标本,表面皮肤呈橘皮样外观,未见溃疡。切面可见一质硬、不规则、灰白色肿瘤(蓝星),散在少量灰黄色点状坏死区域。肿瘤边缘不规则,有些地方呈尖角状伸入周围组织,有的深达深层浅筋膜。腋窝部位淋巴结可见一灰白色、质硬、卵圆形结节(蓝箭),包膜完整,和周围组织无粘连。

1.2.7　宫颈癌直接蔓延(图 4-13)

全子宫＋双侧附件＋部分阴道＋左肾＋部分乙状结肠、直肠切除标本。从子宫切面可见宫颈肥大,向上累及子宫体至子宫底,正常结构已被完全破坏,被肿瘤所取代(蓝箭)。肿瘤灰白色、质软、切面可见大量小腔隙似蜂窝状,坏死明显。从子宫阴道观察可见宫颈粗糙伴有糜烂。癌组织向两侧浸润阔韧带及附件;向下侵犯阴道壁,向后侵犯直肠、乙状结肠(绿星);向左上方侵犯肾脏(蓝星),导致直肠、左肾和子宫粘连,无法分离。

1.2.8　肺转移性癌(图 4-14)

完整切除肺组织一叶,胸膜面和切面可见散在、不规则分布多个大小不等、圆形、灰白色质实结节,有些结节中心可见坏死。

2. 间叶组织肿瘤

2.1　间叶组织良性肿瘤

2.1.1　软纤维瘤(图 4-15)

有蒂的灰白色、结节状肿物,表面由皱缩的皮肤包绕,质地软。

2.1.2　纤维瘤(图 4-16)

结节状肿块,纤维包膜完整,质地硬,切面致密,灰红色与灰白色纤维条索纵横交错呈编织状,伴有白色反光。

2.1.3　脂肪瘤(图 4-17)

不规则、分叶状的灰黄色肿块,包膜完整,质地软。

2.1.4 子宫平滑肌瘤（图 4-18）

子宫全切标本。子宫体积显著增大，形状不规则，表面可见多个结节状隆起。切面，见子宫肌壁间、浆膜下和内膜下多个大小不等的圆形、类圆形、不规则结节状灰白色质硬肿块，切面呈不规则编织状或漩涡状纹理，与周围正常组织分界明显。因为瘤组织缓慢生长，推挤周围正常组织形成假包膜。

2.1.5 肝海绵状血管瘤（图 4-19）

肝脏组织切面，靠近包膜处可见一暗红色不规则结节，和周围正常组织分界清楚。

2.1.6 皮肤淋巴管瘤（图 4-20）

标本为一半透明、部分纤维组织包膜包裹的不规则肿块。切面见多个囊腔，囊壁薄、半透明、灰白色，囊内容物已经流失。未切开的囊腔内可见清亮液体。

2.2 间叶组织恶性肿瘤

2.2.1 纤维肉瘤（图 4-21）

椭圆形肿块，表面光滑，切面淡粉红色，质软、均匀细腻鱼肉状，无明显包膜。注意和纤维瘤大体形态的区别。

2.2.2 脂肪肉瘤（图 4-22）

椭圆形、灰黄色结节状肿块，边界尚清。切面，部分区域灰黄色（蓝星），是肿瘤分化比较好的区域。部分区域黄白色（绿星），质地均匀细腻、鱼肉样，是肿瘤分化较差区域。

2.2.3 肺平滑肌肉瘤（图 4-23）

巨大、不规则肿瘤，边界尚清楚，部分区域（蓝圈）呈编织状或漩涡状、质地硬，是肿瘤分化较好区域。其他部分（绿圈）呈浅粉红色，质地均匀细腻、鱼肉状，散在多处不规则灰白色坏死灶和囊性变。肿瘤组织内可见残存的肺组织（蓝箭），内有黑色炭末沉着。

3. 其他肿瘤

3.1 足部滑膜肉瘤（图 4-24）

跖骨旁可见一灰白色类圆形肿物，表面皮肤完整，和周围组织部分区域分界不清（蓝箭）。蓝星所示区域有多个囊腔形成。

3.2 神经鞘瘤（图 4-25）

结节状肿物，有完整纤维包膜。切面，灰白色、呈编织状或漩涡状，可见散在小囊腔（绿箭）及出血坏死区（蓝箭）。

3.3 神经纤维瘤（图 4-26）

结节状肿块，无明显包膜，肿瘤表面不光滑，但被完整剥离。切面淡粉红色，夹杂有粗细不等的灰白色条索状分布的组织。

3.4 视网膜母细胞瘤（图 4-27）

标本为眼球的矢状切面。眼球正常结构被破坏，充满灰白色肿瘤组织，有多处不规则灰黑色出血区（蓝箭）。角膜（绿箭）、巩膜（蓝箭头）及其周围软组织均被肿瘤破坏，仅见视网膜的色素层（绿箭头）。

3.5 足蹈趾恶性黑色素瘤（图 4-28）

蹈趾皮肤完整，甲床部位可见黑褐色隆起肿物，境界尚清楚，表面有坏死组织和脓苔附着。切面质地均匀细腻、黑褐色。肿瘤组织在向甲床表面生长的同时,向甲床下方生长,最深处已经接近趾骨皮质(蓝箭)。

3.6 肝转移性恶性黑色素瘤(图 4-29)

部分切除肝组织一块,表面不光滑,结节状隆起(绿箭)。切面可见多个大小不等的黑褐色不规则结节(绿圈),境界清楚,几乎占据整块肝组织。

3.7 皮下转移性恶性黑色素瘤(图 4-30)

皮肤及皮下脂肪组织一块,表皮完整,表皮下可见一圆形灰黑色结节(蓝箭),和周围组织界限清楚,未见包膜。思考:如何判断该肿瘤是转移性的?

3.8 卵巢成熟性囊性畸胎瘤(图 4-31)

囊壁样组织一块,包膜光滑、完整。囊内见一形状不规则结节状突起(头节,蓝星),内壁有牙齿(蓝箭)、毛发等组织附着。

3.9 卵巢未成熟性畸胎瘤(图 4-32)

肿瘤呈不规则结节状,包膜完整、光滑,可见毛发。切面,灰白灰黄色、质地中等,多为实性组织,有多个大小不等的小囊腔,有些囊腔内可见灰黄色皮脂残留。

3.10 下颌骨造釉细胞瘤(图 4-33)

下颌骨的右侧下颌体牙槽侧可见一灰白色卵圆形肿物(蓝圈),包膜完整,质地中等。

三、 组织切片

1. 上皮组织肿瘤

1.1 上皮组织良性肿瘤

1.1.1 皮肤乳头状瘤(图 4-34)

皮肤组织外生性生长形成有蒂的肿瘤(T 肿瘤,N 正常表皮)。肿瘤呈乳头状(蓝圈),被覆鳞状上皮明显增生(蓝星),层数增多、分化良好,基底膜完整。肿瘤细胞异型性不明显,核分裂象不易见,可见过度角化或角化不全。每个乳头都由少量结缔组织间质组成轴心(蓝箭),内含血管、淋巴管,并有慢性炎细胞浸润。

1.1.2 结肠腺瘤(图 4-35)

肿瘤组织主要由密集分支的管状结构组成,形状不规则(蓝星)。腺体上皮细胞为单层柱状上皮,核浆比增大,核浓染,可见核仁,核分裂象不易见。有些腺体上皮分泌亢进,腺腔扩张,其内充满分泌物。瘤体中轴为纤维血管轴心,可见多量慢性炎细胞浸润。

1.1.3 乳腺纤维腺瘤(图 4-36)

结节状肿物(红箭,T)与周围增生的乳腺组织(N)界限清楚。肿瘤主要由增生的纤维间质和腺体组成。腺体由两层细胞围成,腺腔面为单层立方上皮,外侧为肌上皮细胞。间质细胞增生,推挤扩张的腺管,使其呈狭长分支裂隙状,腺上皮受压变扁、萎缩,甚至完全消失(蓝箭)。间质可见广泛的黏液变性,部分间质硬化(蓝星)。周围乳腺组织增生,小叶内腺泡数目增多。

1.1.4 腮腺多形性腺瘤(良性混合瘤)(图 4-37)

实性巢状、腺管状或条索状排列的细胞团(蓝星),散布于黏液软骨样间质(绿星)

中。腺管状排列的瘤细胞多由两层细胞构成,内层为扁平、立方或低柱状上皮细胞,胞浆嗜伊红染色,外层为胞浆淡染的肌上皮细胞,肌上皮细胞与黏液软骨样的间质成分相互移行。

1.2　上皮组织恶性肿瘤

1.2.1　皮肤鳞状细胞癌（图4-38）

皮肤表面被覆完整的鳞状上皮（蓝箭）,在其下方可见癌细胞呈巢状、片状或条索状排列（癌巢,红箭）,浸润至真皮和皮下组织,和周围的纤维结缔组织（蓝星）分界清楚。部分癌巢中心可见癌珠形成（癌巢中央呈同心圆性层状排列、嗜酸性的角化物,也称作角化珠,蓝箭头）。癌细胞呈多边形,大小不一,胞浆丰富,嗜酸性染色。细胞边界清楚,有些细胞间可见细胞间桥（蓝五角星之间）。胞核大,大小和形状不一,核仁大而清楚,染色质粗,核分裂象易见。间质可见慢性炎细胞浸润。

1.2.2　结肠腺癌（图4-39）

癌细胞柱状或高柱状（蓝五角星）,复层密集排列呈腺管状、筛孔状,核浆比增大,形状不一,核仁明显。核分裂象易见（蓝箭）。可见瘤巨细胞（红箭）。间质血管丰富（红五角星）。正常肠黏膜和癌交界处,可见移行现象。

1.2.3　宫颈高级别鳞状上皮内病变（HSIL）（图4-40）

低倍镜,可见肿瘤组织从正常组织移行特点（蓝实线左侧为肿瘤T,右侧为正常宫颈上皮N）。非肿瘤区组织被覆正常极向分布的鳞状上皮细胞,肿瘤区组织鳞状上皮细胞层数增多,排列紊乱,细胞极性消失。病变累及上皮全层,基底膜完整。高倍镜,癌细胞大小不一,核浆比增大,胞浆嗜碱性染色。核大小、形状不规则,染色深,核仁明显,核分裂象易见且在上皮全层均可见到（蓝箭）。

1.2.4　淋巴结转移性鳞状细胞癌（图4-41）

淋巴结结构大部分被破坏,由癌组织取代（蓝圈）。癌细胞呈巢团状排列,部分癌巢内可见角化珠（蓝箭）,癌细胞间可见细胞间桥（红箭）。高倍镜下癌细胞异型性明显,可见病理性核分裂象。

1.2.5　淋巴结转移性腺癌（图4-42）

淋巴结仅见少量淋巴组织（蓝圈）,大部分结构被癌组织取代。癌细胞形成大小不等、形态不一的腺样结构（蓝星）。癌细胞大小不一,胞浆染色较淡,可见较多分泌空泡（蓝箭）,核大深染、大小不等,并见病理性核分裂象。

2.　间叶组织肿瘤

2.1　间叶组织良性肿瘤

2.1.1　皮下脂肪瘤（图4-43）

肿瘤由弥漫分布的成熟脂肪细胞组成,细胞体积大,胞浆内有一个大脂滴,核小、深染、不规则（蓝箭）。

2.1.2　子宫平滑肌瘤（图4-44）

肿瘤组织呈结节状（T肿瘤）,有明显的假包膜包绕,与周围组织（N正常）界限清楚。瘤细胞呈束状、编织状排列（绿星纵切,蓝星横切）,失去正常子宫肌层的结构层次。瘤细胞大小一致,胞浆丰富、红染,核杆状,两端钝圆呈雪茄烟形,核分裂象不易见。瘤细胞之间有不等量的纤维组织。

2.1.3　肝海绵状血管瘤（图 4-45）

肝组织内可见由大片互相吻合、大小不一、形状不规则的薄壁血管构成的肿瘤组织，血管内充满血液，管壁为单层内皮细胞，血管间有少量的纤维组织分隔。肿瘤组织和周围肝组织（蓝圈）界限清楚，无明显包膜。

2.2　间叶组织恶性肿瘤

2.2.1　腹膜后脂肪肉瘤（图 4-46）

肿瘤呈浸润性生长，周围正常组织被破坏，可见残存的正常骨骼肌组织（红箭）。肿瘤细胞弥漫分布，分化不一致（图 4-46A）。部分区域呈现脂肪分化方向（蓝圈），可见不同分化阶段和异型性的脂肪母细胞（蓝箭，图 4-46D）。脂肪母细胞最具特征的是细胞核被两个或两个以上边缘清晰、较大的空泡挤压、凹陷，边缘呈锯齿状。部分区域呈现纤维（绿星）和神经分化（绿圈），细胞排列呈编织状或漩涡状，弥漫分布，细胞梭形，胞浆嗜伊红染色，细胞核异型性明显。肿瘤中可见瘤巨细胞（绿箭），核分裂象可见。部分区域有间质黏液变性（蓝星）和丛状血管。

2.2.2　平滑肌肉瘤（图 4-47）

肿瘤境界不清，无包膜，呈弥漫、浸润性生长。肿瘤组织分化程度不一致。分化差的区域（绿星），瘤细胞弥漫分布，编织状结构不明显，瘤细胞有明显异型性，少数可见肌原纤维，核异型性明显（红箭），核分裂象易见，甚至一个高倍视野可见 2~5 个核分裂，并可见病理性核分裂（蓝箭），单核或多核瘤巨细胞（绿圈）易见。分化较好的区域（蓝星）主要由梭形细胞束构成，细胞束纵横交错排列，细胞密度大；瘤细胞胞浆丰富，含有肌原纤维。核较大、棒状、不规则形，有一定程度异型性，核分裂象易见。瘤组织可见凝固性坏死（蓝圈）、黏液变性等改变。间质不明显，血管扩张、壁薄，少量慢性炎细胞浸润。

2.2.3　多形性未分化肉瘤（图 4-48）

肿瘤细胞弥漫分布，部分区域呈条索状或席纹状排列（图 4-48A），部分区域弥漫分布（图 4-48B）。肿瘤细胞主要由明显异型的梭形细胞和多形性细胞混合组成，瘤巨细胞易见（绿箭）。细胞核形态不规则、深染、核分裂象易见（红箭、蓝箭），包括病理性核分裂（蓝箭）。肿瘤间质伴有程度不等的胶原化和局灶性黏液变性，有不等量炎细胞浸润。

3. 其他肿瘤

3.1　皮肤恶性黑色素瘤（图 4-49）

肿瘤破坏表皮（红箭），向下浸润皮下组织。肿瘤细胞呈巢状、腺泡状分布，甚至聚集成较大的结节状（蓝星）。肿瘤细胞体积较大、可见瘤巨细胞，多边形或卵圆形、界限清楚，胞浆丰富、淡伊红染。有些细胞胞浆内含有多少不等的细颗粒状黑褐色色素，大量色素可覆盖细胞核着色（蓝箭）。核大、异型性明显，可见核仁。间质内可见慢性炎细胞浸润。

3.2　卵巢成熟性囊性畸胎瘤（图 4-50）

囊壁内衬复层扁平上皮（蓝圈），囊壁及瘤组织内可见成熟的皮脂腺、毛发、脂肪组织、神经组织（蓝星）、假复层纤毛柱状上皮、单层柱状上皮、骨组织、软骨组织等。肿瘤由三个胚层的各种类型的组织混杂构成。思考：在该切片中观察到的成熟组织分别属于哪个胚层？

四、 临床病理讨论

案例 1 患者,女性,65 岁,主诉:绝经 15 年后阴道流血 1 个月。

现病史:1 个月前无明显诱因出现少量阴道流血,暗红色、无凝血块、无异味、无发热等,遂入院求诊。

查体:一般情况可。妇科检查宫颈内口有一 1.0 cm×0.9 cm 新生物,表面呈菜花状,触之易出血,无举痛及摇摆痛。双侧附件区未及明显异常。

临床诊断:宫颈占位。

患者手术切除全子宫＋双侧附件,组织送病理检查,子宫颈组织学典型视野见图 4-51。

(1) 请给出该患者的病理诊断,并说明理由。

(2) 尝试用病理学变化解释患者的阴道流血症状。

案例 2 患者,男性,55 岁,主诉:进食后胸骨后疼痛 15 天。

现病史:15 天前患者进食较硬食物后出现胸骨后疼痛感,饮水后症状消失,未予注意。在此期间多次出现进食较硬食物后胸骨后疼痛感,无呕血、便血、明显消瘦、食欲减退等。为明确诊断,入院就诊。

查体:一般情况可,无贫血貌。心肺无明显异常。

胃镜:距门齿 30 cm 处可见食管黏膜有一 1.5 cm×1.2 cm 黏膜糜烂区,触之易出血。取活检。

该患者后经手术切除病变食管,并送病理检查,组织学典型视野见图 4-52。

(1) 请给出该患者的病理诊断,并说明理由。

(2) 尝试用病理学变化解释患者出现的临床表现和胃镜检查发现。

五、 思考题

1. 什么是肿瘤? 肿瘤性增生和非肿瘤性增生的区别是什么?

2. 肿瘤的异型性主要体现在哪些方面?

3. 简述肿瘤的命名和分类原则。

4. 肿瘤常见的生长方式有哪些?

5. 恶性肿瘤转移方式有哪些?

6. 肿瘤对机体的影响有哪些?

7. 如何区别良恶性肿瘤、癌和肉瘤。

8. 什么是癌前病变? 举例说明。

9. 名词解释:肿瘤,肿瘤实质,肿瘤间质,肿瘤的分化,异型性,浸润,肿瘤的演进,肿瘤的异质性,直接蔓延,转移,种植性转移,恶病质,副肿瘤综合征,癌珠,癌前疾病(或病变),原位癌,癌基因,病毒癌基因,原癌基因,肿瘤抑制基因。

Chapter 4

Neoplasia

Ⅰ. Aims

1. To grasp the principle of the nomenclature and classification of neoplasms.

2. To grasp the gross features and growth patterns of neoplasms.

3. To grasp the atypia of neoplasms in morphology.

4. To grasp the metastatic pathways of malignant neoplasms.

5. To grasp the differences between benign and malignant tumors, carcinoma and sarcoma.

6. To understand the pathologic features of common epithelial and mesenchymal neoplasms.

Guidance to study

To diagnose neoplasms, morphological evidences based on macroscopical and microscopical findings should be required. Further define that neoplasms are benign or malignant, which needs the detailed morphology associated with differentiation, invasion, metastasis, and necrosis. Malignant tumors are preliminarily judged as carcinoma or sarcoma according to their originating tissue.

Differences between benign and malignant tumors

	Benign tumors	Maligant tumors
Gross	Polypous, cauliflower-like, nodular, ulcerating, etc.	Polypous, cauliflower-like, nodular, ulcerating, hemorrhage etc.
Growth	Exophytic, expansile	Invasive, exophytic
Architectural atypia	Yes, not obvious	Yes, obvious
Celluar atypia	Not obvious (size increased, nuclear-to-cytoplasmic ratio increased)	Obvious (pleomorphism of cells and nuclei in size and shape, tumor giant cells and multinucleated giant cells, mitotic figures increased, pathological mitoses)
Necrosis	Not obvious	Obvious

Differences between carcinoma and sarcoma

	Carcinoma	Sarcoma
Originating tissue	Epithelial tissue	Mesenchymal tissue
Gross characteristics	Grey-white, firm	Grey-red, fleshy, soft
Arrangement	Nests, glands, cord-like	Diffuse
Demarcation between parenchyma and stroma	Clear	Unclear
Reticular fiber	Around cancerous nests	Among tumor cells

II. Gross specimens

1. Epithelial tumors

1. 1   Benign epithelial tumors

1. 1. 1   Papilloma of skin (Fig. 4-1)

The irregular, intact, grey-red nodule is composed of many fingerlike or papillary protuberances. The surface is cauliflower-like.

1. 1. 2   Polypoid adenoma of colon (Fig. 4-2)

There are many round or irregular, grey-white, and polypoid nodules (blue stars) with different sizes on the mucosa of colon. The nodules are pedunculated (blue arrows) or sessile, with the surface having a texture resembling velvet and raspberry. On the surface of the larger nodules, hemorrhage and necrosis can be observed.

1. 1. 3   Serous papillary cystadenoma of ovary (Fig. 4-3)

The tumor appears as a cystic wall and has basically smooth outer surface except the area with exophytic excrescences (blue arrow). On cut section, the serous fluid in the cystic cavity has flowed away. The inner surface is covered by papillary patterns (blue arrows), that have various diameters.

1. 1. 4   Mucinous cystadenoma of ovary (Fig. 4-4)

The grey-white oval tumor is smooth with some protrusions (blue arrows) on the outer surface. The outer surface is attached by partial oviduct and multiple hemispherical projections. On the cut surface, the tumor presents multiple cysts with variable sizes, and the cysts are filled by grey-white, sticky, and gelatinous mucus.

1. 1. 5   Fibroadenoma of breast (Fig. 4-5)

The tumor is a firmly elastic grey-white nodule. On the cut surface, some areas show fine particles and slit-like spaces, with shining myxomatous and edematous stroma.

1. 1. 6   Pleomorphic adenoma of parotid gland (Fig. 4-6)

It appears as an irregular, well-demarcated mass without intact capsule. The cut surface shows multiple grey-white incompletely separated lobules. Some areas are translucent and myxoid (blue stars), some are cartilage-like stroma, and others are cystic (blue arrows).

1. 2　Malignant epithelial tumors

1. 2. 1　Squamous cell carcinoma of skin (Fig. 4-7)

The broad-based tumor presents a grey-white heaped-up mass with coarse surface on the skin, and it is brittle with ulcer, necrosis and hemorrhage. How do we distinguish it from papilloma of skin? Why are the surrounding normal tissues excised?

1. 2. 2　Squamous cell carcinoma of penis (Fig. 4-8)

The glans penis has been destroyed and occupied by an irregular, cauliflower-like mass with hemorrhage and necrosis. The broad-based tumor has closely adhered to the surrounding tissue and infiltrated into the deeper tissue of the skin.

1. 2. 3　Gastric carcinoma (Polyp type) (Fig. 4-9)

The polypoid tumor locates in the gastric lesser curvature of the subtotal gastrectomy specimen. The grey-black tumor is cauliflower-like with hemorrhage and necrosis.

1. 2. 4　Carcinoma of rectum (Polyp type) (Fig. 4-10)

The tissue is from the rectum. The grey-red and grey-white cauliflower-like tumor is broad-based with central ulcer. Notice the differences between the polypoid adenoma and carcinoma of colon in morphology.

1. 2. 5　Carcinoid of appendix (Fig. 4-11)

One piece of luminal tissue was cut in transverse direction. The layers of the appendix are difficult to be distinguished (blue arrow). The cut surface is solid without obvious nodular formation. Is carcinoid of appendix malignant tumor?

1. 2. 6　Breast cancer with metastatic lymph nodes (Fig. 4-12)

The specimen from modified radical mastectomy shows orange peel-like skin due to skin retraction. Beneath the depressed nipple, there is an irregular, grey-white, firm, and solid nodule (blue star) on the cut surface. The tumor infiltrates into adjacent normal tissue, even superficial fascia. Another well-circumscribed oval nodule in the axillary lymph nodes (blue arrow) presents the same morphological features as the nodule in the breast.

1. 2. 7　Carcinoma of cervix with direct spread (Fig. 4-13)

The specimen of total uterus and bilateral adnexectomy is accompanied with left kidney, rectum and partial sigmoid. Observing from the uterus, the enlarged cervix has spread directly to the corpus and fundus of the uterus (blue arrows). Many slit-like spaces are on the cut surface. Observing from the vagina, the cervix becomes enlarged, cauliflower-like with necrosis. The tumor has infiltrated into two sides of broad ligaments and adnexa uteri, vagina, rectum, partial sigmoid (green stars), left kidney (blue stars), so the adhesion of involved organs is too tight to be separated.

1. 2. 8   Metastatic carcinoma of lung (Fig. 4-14)

Many round, grey-white nodules scatter on the cut surface of the lung with median texture and different sizes. The nodules are sharply circumscribed with the surrounding tissue. Some nodules show necroses.

2. Mesenchymal tumors

2. 1   Benign mesenchymal tumors

2. 1. 1   Soft fibroma (Fig. 4-15)

The soft, grey-white nodule is sharply demarcated by crimpled intact skin.

2. 1. 2   Fibroma (Fig. 4-16)

The nodule is well-circumscribed, firm and solid. The cut surface is grey-red admixed with grey-white and presents whorled fibrous bundles. The fibrous trabeculae are prominent in the white glistening area.

2. 1. 3   Lipoma (Fig. 4-17)

The sharply defined mass is irregular, lobulated, and soft with intact capsule.

2. 1. 4   Leiomyomas of uterus (Fig. 4-18)

The specimen of uterus becomes enlarged and irregular. Some grey-white, firm, and round nodules discretely locate within the myometrium, beneath the endometrium or under the serosa. The characteristic whorled pattern of smooth muscle bundles on the cut surface usually makes these lesions to be identified easily. The nodules expansively grow and compress the adjacent tissue to form pseudocapsule.

2. 1. 5   Cavenous hemangioma of liver (Fig. 4-19)

The cavernous hemangioma appears as a dark-red, irregular and soft nodule near the capsule.

2. 1. 6   Lymphangioma of skin (Fig. 4-20)

Subcutaneous tissue is distended by a multiple cystic mass containing watery fluid. The irregular mass is soft, translucent, spongy, and well-circumscribed with incomplete capsule.

2. 2   Malignant mesenchymal tumors

2. 2. 1   Fibrosarcoma (Fig. 4-21)

The tumor is a nonencapsulated ovoid mass. The cut surface is soft, light-pink, and homogeneous. Notice the difference between fibroma and fibrosarcoma in morphology.

2. 2. 2   Liposarcoma (Fig. 4-22)

The tumor is a well-circumscribed ovoid mass without true capsule. On the cut surface, some areas are yellow (blue star), and the others are ill-defined greyish-white masses (green stars).

2. 2. 3   Leiomyosarcoma of lung (Fig. 4-23)

The soft, ill-defined tumor is a bulky irregular-mass which has destroyed the normal organ. On the cut surface, some areas(blue circle)are well-differentiated with whorled pattern similar to leiomyoma, and other areas (green circle) are poor-differentiated which are fleshy and pinky with necroses and cysts. Some black dusts deposit in the residual lung tissue (blue arrows).

3. Other tumors

3.1　Synovial sarcoma of foot（Fig.4-24）

A grey-white round-like mass is observed and covered by intact skin near the metatarsal bone. It is poorly defined from the adjacent tissue(blue arrows). The blue stars show multiple cysts.

3.2　Schwannoma（Fig.4-25）

The nodule is an encapsulated mass with clear boundary. The grey-white tumor shows whorled or weaving cut surface with hemorrhage and necrosis(blue arrows). There are some cysts(green arrows) within the nodule.

3.3　Neurofibroma（Fig.4-26）

The irregular mass is well-delineated but unencapsulated nodular lesion with rough surface. The cut surface is pink with grey-white fibrous bundles.

3.4　Retinoblastoma（Fig.4-27）

The specimen is the eyeball sagittally opened. The eyeball has been filled with grey-white tumor tissue, which has destroyed the normal architecture. There are multiple, scattered, irregular, and grey-black hemorrhage areas(blue arrows). The cornea(green arrow)and sclera (blue arrowheads) are infiltrated by the retinoblastoma, and only pigmented layer of retina (green arrowheads)can be observed.

3.5　Malignant melanoma of foot hallex（Fig.4-28）

The skin of the hallex is intact. There is a black-brown cauliflower-like mass in the nail bed with necrosis and purulent exudate. On the cut surface, the tumor is black-brown and homogenous. The tumor grows into the surface of the nail bed and deeper tissue, involving the cortex of the bone(blue arrow).

3.6　Metastatic malignant melanoma of liver（Fig.4-29）

The outer surface of the liver becomes swollen (green arrows) with many well-defined nodules(green circles). On the cut surface, the black-brown nodules scatter throughout the liver with round or oval in shape(green circles).

3.7　Metastatic malignant melanoma of subcutaneous tissue（Fig.4-30）

It is a piece of skin and subcutaneous tissue. A round and grey-black nodule is well-circumscribed within the subcutaneous tissue (blue arrow), and the skin is intact. Consider why the tumor is metastatic.

3. 8　Mature cystic teratoma of ovary（Fig.4-31）

It is an opened unilocular cyst, and the outer surface is smooth and intact. Within the cyst, a solid smooth nodule is noticed, which is referred to as the Rokitansky's protuberance (blue stars). On the inner wall, hair, sebaceous materials, and teeth(blue arrow) are observed.

3. 9　Immature teratoma of ovary（Fig.4-32）

The tumor is irregular with intact and smooth capsule and hair. On cut section, most area is solid with multiple small cysts, and gray-yellow sebaceous materials are observed within the cysts.

3. 10　Ameloblastoma of mandible（Fig.4-33）

An oval and grey-white nodule (blue circle) is well-circumscribed with medium texture in the right mandibular alveolar side of mandible.

Ⅲ. Tissue sections

1.　Epithelial tumors

1. 1　Benign epithelial tumors

1. 1. 1　Papilloma of skin（Fig. 4-34）

The tumor is cauliflower-like protrusions on the skin surface (T-tumor, N-normal skin). The tumor is composed of multiple slender, fingerlike projections (blue circle) with the fibrovascular cores containing chronic inflammatory cells, blood vessels, and lymph vessels (blue arrow). The projections are lined with thickened stratified squamous epithelia with hyperkeratosis and parakeratosis, and they are well differentiated(blue stars).

1. 1. 2　Adenoma of colon（Fig. 4-35）

The tumor is composed by hyperplastic glands with excessive branches(blue stars). The glands are lined by simple columnar epithelial cells with increased nuclear-to-cytoplasmic ratio. The nuclei show dark-stained hyperchromatin, and mitotic figures are seldom. Some enlarged glands are filled with mucus by hypersecretion. The interior of the tumor consists of fibrovascular tissue with chronic inflammatory cells.

1. 1. 3　Fibroadenoma of breast（Fig. 4-36）

A nodule (red arrows) without capsule is separated with surrounding breast tissue (T-tumor tissue, N-normal tissue). The parenchyma of the tumor includes fibrous tissue and glands. The glands are composed of two layers of cells. Simple luminal epithelium is the inner layer, and polygonal, light stained myoepithelial cells are outer layer adjacent to the stroma. The hyperplastic stroma compresses glandular ducts into elongated, branching and slit-like structure. The epithelia become flatten and atrophic, even disappear(blue arrows). The stroma shows extensive myxoid changes with partial sclerosis(blue stars).

1.1.4　Pleomorphic adenoma of parotid gland（Fig. 4-37）

The tumor cells are arranged as nests, glands, cord-like structures（blue stars）, and scattered in the myxoid extracellular matrix（green stars）. The glands are composed of two layers of cells. The inner are cuboidal or low-columnar cells with eosinophilic cytoplasm, and the outer are myoepithelial cells with irregular, light cytoplasm. The transition morphology is noticed from myoepithelial cells to myxoid stroma or chondroid stroma.

1.2　Malignant epithelial tumors

1.2.1　Squamous cell carcinoma of skin（Fig. 4-38）

The surface squamous epithelia are intact with hyperplasia（blue arrows）. The tumor cells showing intercellular bridges, arrange in nests, sheets or cord-like pattern（cancerous nest, red arrows）, which extends into the dermis, even infiltrates the subcutaneous tissue. The tumor nests are surrounded by stroma with chronic inflammatory cells（blue stars）. Intracellular keratinization and keratin pearl are observed. Keratin pearl（blue arrowheads）indicates concentric layered of eosinophilic keratinization in the center of the cancerous nests, and it is also called as cancerous pearl. The polygonal tumor cell has abundant eosinophilic cytoplasm and a large, vesicular nucleus with obvious nucleolus. Mitoses are visible.

1.2.2　Adenocarcinoma of colon（Fig. 4-39）

The columnar or tall-columnar tumor cells arrange in tubular or cribriform with stratification（blue stars）. The tumor cells show irregular, vesicular nuclei with obvious nucleoli and increased mitotic figures（blue arrow）. Tumor giant cells（red arrows）are frequently seen. Lymphocytes and plasma cells infiltrate into the desmoplastic stroma of the tumor（red stars）. The tissue presents transitional area in the tumor cells conjunction with the adjacent non-tumor tissue.

1.2.3　High-grade squamous intraepithelial lesion（HSIL）of cervix（Fig. 4-40）

The normal cervical tissue is covered by squamous epithelium, and HSIL shows multiple layers of epithelia without polarity（T-tumor,N-normal cervical epithelium）. The neoplastic lesion has destroyed the whole epithelia but the basement membrane is intact. The HSIL cells show increased nuclear-to-cytoplasmic ratio and basophilic cytoplasm. The nuclei are large, pleomorphic, and hyperchromasia with obvious nucleoli. Mitotic figures（blue arrow）may be seen within the epithelia.

1.2.4　Metastatic squamous cell carcinoma in lymph node（Fig. 4-41）

The architecture of the lymph node has been destroyed and replaced by tumor nests（blue circle）with necroses. The tumor nests show solid pattern with some keratin pearls（blue arrows）and intercellular bridges（red arrow）. The polygonal tumor cells have abundant eosinophilic cytoplasm and large, vesicular nuclei with obvious atypia. Mitotic figures are easily observed.

1.2.5　Metastatic adenocarcinoma in lymph node（Fig. 4-42）

Most of the lymph node has been destroyed and occupied by tubular（blue stars）or solid tumor nests. Only a small amount of lymph tissue is residual (blue circle). The tumor cells are large with light stained cytoplasm containing secretory vacuoles (blue arrows). The irregular nuclei are vesicular with obvious nucleoli and increased mitotic figures including pathological mitoses.

2. Mesenchymal tumors

2. 1   Benign mesenchymal tumors

2. 1. 1   Subcutaneous lipoma (Fig. 4-43)

The tumor is composed of diffusely distributed adipocytes. The adipocytes are mature showing big lipid droplets and little, dark-stained, irregular nuclei (blue arrows).

2. 1. 2   Leiomyoma of uterus (Fig. 4-44)

At low magnification, there is a well-circumscribed, round nodule (T-tumor) separated with the normal tissue (N-normal tissue) by the pseudocapsule. The tumor cells arrange in bundles or whorled pattern (longitudinal section-green stars, transverse section-blue stars). The tumor cells are uniform with eosinophilic cytoplasm. Mitoses are rare. There is hyaline degeneration in some areas. The tumor compresses the surrounding myometrium by exophytic growth, and results in atrophy of normal smooth muscle cells, which contributes to pseudocapsule formation.

2. 1. 3   Cavenous hemangioma of liver (Fig. 4-45)

The tumor consists of large amount of thin-walled vascular channels in different size, and the channels are lined by endothelial cells, and filled with blood. The tumor has no capsule, but it is demarcated from the surrounding liver tissue (blue circles).

2. 2   Malignant mesenchymal tumors

2. 2. 1   Retroperitoneal liposarcoma (Fig. 4-46)

The tumor has destroyed skeletal muscle and only a small piece of tissue has remained (red arrows). The tumor cells diffusely distributed with various differentiation (Fig.4-46A). Some areas present atypic lipoblasts appearing as adipocytes at various differentiating stages (blue circles in Fig.4-46A and blue arrows in Fig.4-46D). Characteristic of lipoblasts is atypic nuclei compressed by large cytoplasmic vacuoles in the center or aside of the cells. The nuclear edges of some tumor cells are hackly. Some areas differentiate into fibrous tissue (green stars) and nerve tissue (green circles). The spindle cells diffusely distribute and arrange in whorled or weaving patterns. The spindle cells have eosinophilic cytoplasm with obvious atypic nuclei and mitotic figures. Tumor giant cells (green arrows) can be observed. Mucoid degeneration (blue stars) and arborizing capillaries are in the stroma.

2. 2. 2   Leiomyosarcoma (Fig. 4-47)

The tumor tissue shows infiltrating growth pattern and a variant degree of differentiation. The poorly differentiated areas (green star) consist of round or polygonal cells with eosinophilic cytoplasm. The nuclear pleomorphism is obvious with increased nuclear-to-cytoplasmic ratio and mitotic figures, even pathological mitoses (blue arrows). Few cells contain myofibril fibers. Mononucleated or multinucleated tumor giant cells (green circle) are easily visible. The well differentiated areas arrange in interweaving fascicles, and consist of eosinophilic fusocellular cells with blunt, pleomorphic, and hyperchromatic nuclei, but the cytological atypia is not obvious. Tumor tissue presents coagulative necrosis (blue circle) and myxoid degeneration. The dilated thin-wall vessels and chronic inflammatory cells are observed in the stroma.

2. 2. 3　Undifferentiated pleomorphic sarcoma (Fig. 4-48)

The large, anaplastic spindle to polygonal tumor cells arrange in diffuse sheets, fascicular or storiform pattern (Fig.4-48A, B). The tumor cells have a high nuclear-to-cytoplasmic ratio with irregular, sometimes bizarre and hyperchromatic giant nuclei. Mononucleated and multinucleated tumor giant cells are easily observed (green arrows). Mitotic figures (red and blue arrows), including pathological mitoses (blue arrows), are abundant. Collagen deposition and myxoid degeneration exist in the stroma infiltrated by inflammatory cells.

3. Other tumors

3. 1　Cutaneous malignant melanoma (Fig.4-49)

The tumor has destroyed the skin (red arrows) and invaded into subcutaneous tissue. The tumor cells arrange in nests and acini (blue star). The polygonal or oval tumor cells are large with abundant light-eosinophilc cytoplasm. The granular black-brown melanin locates in the cytoplasm, even covers the nucleus (blue arrows). The large vacuolated nuclei are round, oval or irregular with obvious round nucleoli. The atypia of nuclei is prominent. There are infiltrating chronic inflammatory cells in the stroma.

3. 2　Mature cystic teratoma of ovary (Fig.4-50)

The cyst wall consists of stratified squamous epithelia (blue circle) with sebaceous glands, hair, fatty tissue, nervous tissue (blue star), pseudostratified columnar epithelium, simple columnar epithelium, bone tissue, and cartilage, etc. The various mature tissues are derived from three germ cell layers. Please clarify the corresponding relationship between three germ layers and corresponding mature tissues in the section.

Ⅳ. Clinical pathological discussion

Case 1

A 65 years old female has suffered vaginal bleeding for 1 month. But she has been postmenopause for 15 years. The bleeding amount is slight, and the blood is red, without clot and peculiar smell. She has no fever. On gynecological examination, there is a 1 cm diameter cauliflower-like mass on the ectocervix, which becomes bleeding when touched. The patient has not felt any pain. The bilateral ovaries are not involved. She was clinically diagnosed as cervical nodule. After operation, the uterus and bilateral accessories were sent for pathological examination. Microscopic findings are shown in Fig.4-51.

(1) To make a pathologic diagnosis of the mass and clarify the reasons.

(2) Please explain vaginal bleeding based on the pathologic changes.

Case 2

A 55 years old male complained that he got the pain behind the sternum after swallowing hard and dry food 15 days ago. The symptom disappeared after drinking water. The patient didn't see his doctor at that time. But the symptom occurred repeatedly without haematemesis, hematochezia, obvious weight loss, and decreased appetide.

Physical examination showed that he had no anemic face, and his lung and heart were normal in auscultation. There was a 1.5 cm×1.2 cm area of erythematous and erosive mucosa 30 cm below the teeth examined by upper gastrointestinal endoscopy. The lesion became bleeding when touched. The lesion was removed by endoscopic submucosal dissection(ESD). Microscopic pictures of the lesion are shown in Fig.4-52.

(1) To diagnose the lesion and list the diagnostic key points.

(2) Please explain the abnormal clinical manifestation and endoscopic findings according to the pathologic changes.

Ⅴ. Questions

1. What is neoplasm? Please differentiate neoplastic proliferation from non-neoplastic proliferation.

2. What are the features of neoplastic atypia?

3. What are the principles of tumors nomenclature and classification?

4. Please list growth patterns of tumors.

5. Which pathways are common for malignant tumors dissemination to distal organs?

6. What facets of the tumors can affect hosts?

7. What are the differences between benign and malignant tumor, carcinoma and sarcoma?

8. What are precancerous diseases? Please list some examples.

9. Terms: Neoplasm, Parenchyma of tumor, Stroma of tumor, Differentiation, Neoplastic atypia, Invasion, Progression of tumor, Heterogeneity, Direct spreading, Metastasis, Transcoelomic metastasis, Cachexia, Paraneoplastic syndrome, Keratin pearl, Precancerous disease(precancerous lesion), Carcinoma in situ, Oncogene, Viral oncogene, Proto-oncogene, Tumor suppressor gene.

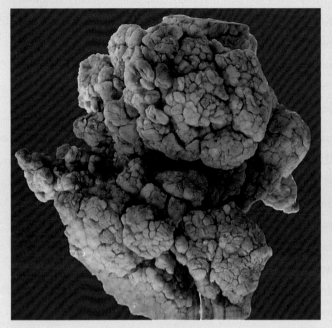

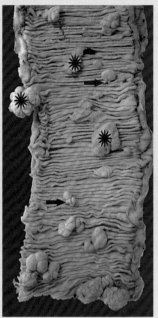

图 4-1　皮肤乳头状瘤
Fig.4-1　Papilloma of skin

图 4-2　结肠息肉状腺瘤
Fig.4-2　Polypoid adenoma
　　　　of colon

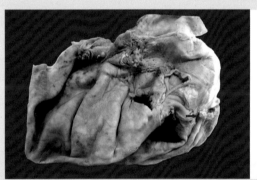

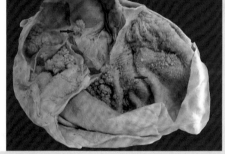

图 4-3　卵巢乳头状浆液性囊腺瘤
Fig.4-3　Serous papillary cystadenoma of ovary

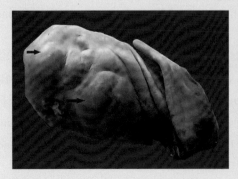

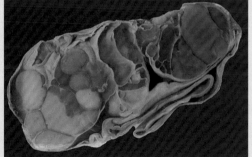

图 4-4　卵巢黏液性囊腺瘤
Fig.4-4　Mucinous cystadenoma of ovary

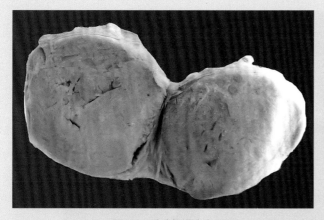

图 4-5　乳腺纤维腺瘤
Fig.4-5　Fibroadenoma of breast

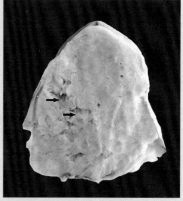

图 4-6　腮腺多形性腺瘤
Fig.4-6　Pleomorphic adenoma
of parotid gland

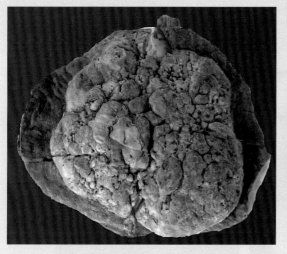

图 4-7　皮肤鳞状细胞癌
Fig.4-7　Squamous cell carcinoma of skin

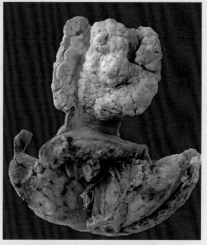

图 4-8　阴茎鳞状细胞癌
Fig.4-8　Squamous cell carcinoma of penis

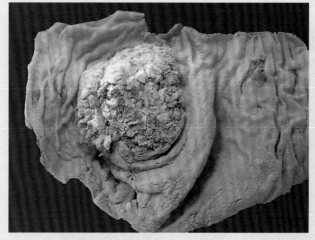

图 4-9　胃癌（息肉型）
Fig.4-9　Gastric carcinoma（Polyp type）

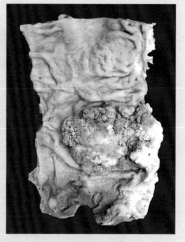

图 4-10　直肠癌（息肉型）
Fig.4-10　Carcinoma of rectum
（Polyp type）

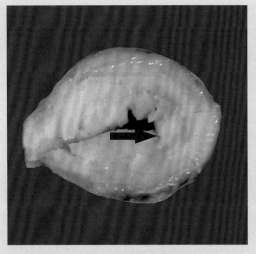
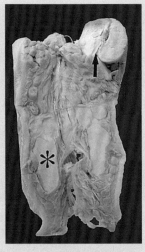

图 4-11　阑尾类癌
Fig.4-11　Carcinoid of appendix

图 4-12　乳腺癌
腋窝淋巴结转移
Fig.4-12　Breast cancer
with metastatic lymph nodes

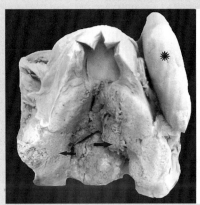
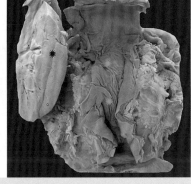

图 4-13　宫颈癌直接蔓延
Fig.4-13　Carcinoma of cervix with direct spread

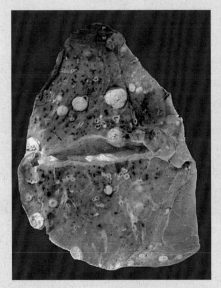
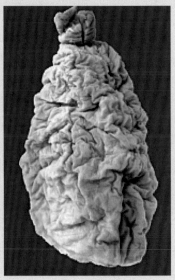

图 4-14　肺转移性癌
Fig.4-14　Metastatic carcinoma of lung

图 4-15　软纤维瘤
Fig.4-15　Soft fibroma

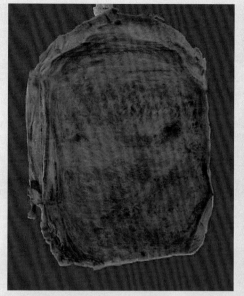

图 4-16 纤维瘤
Fig.4-16 Fibroma

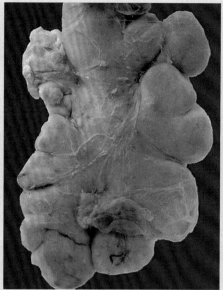

图 4-17 脂肪瘤
Fig.4-17 Lipoma

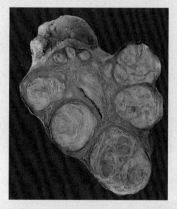

图 4-18 子宫平滑肌瘤
Fig.4-18 Leiomyomas of uterus

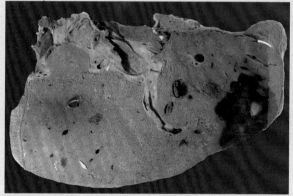

图 4-19 肝海绵状血管瘤
Fig.4-19 Cavenous hemangioma of liver

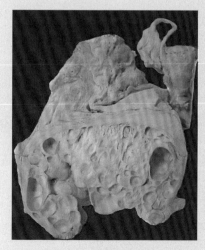

图 4-20 皮肤淋巴管瘤
Fig.4-20 Lymphangioma of skin

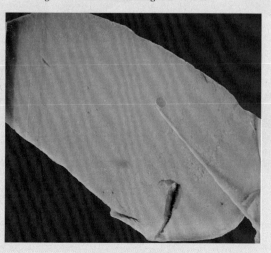

图 4-21 纤维肉瘤
Fig.4-21 Fibrosarcoma

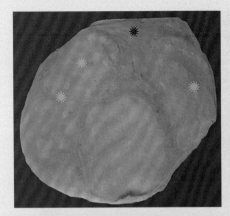

图 4-22 脂肪肉瘤
Fig.4-22 Liposarcoma

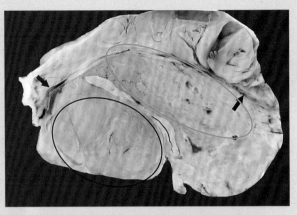

图 4-23 肺平滑肌肉瘤
Fig.4-23 Leiomyosarcoma of lung

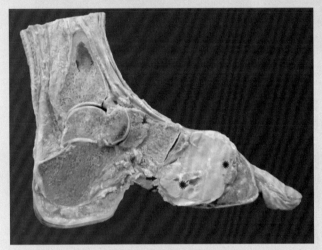

图 4-24 足部滑膜肉瘤
Fig.4-24 Synovial sarcoma of foot

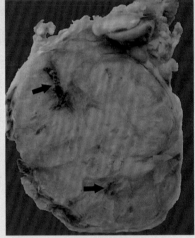

图 4-25 神经鞘瘤
Fig.4-25 Schwannoma

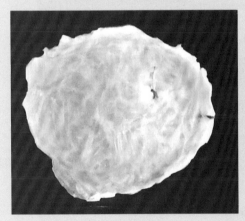

图 4-26 神经纤维瘤
Fig.4-26 Neurofibroma

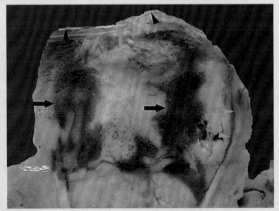

图 4-27 视网膜母细胞瘤
Fig.4-27 Retinoblastoma

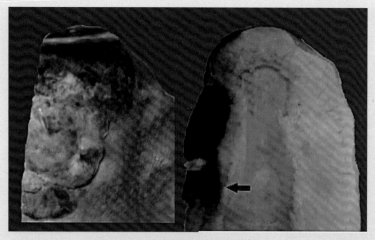

图 4-28　足踇趾恶性黑色素瘤
Fig.4-28　Malignant melanoma of foot hallex

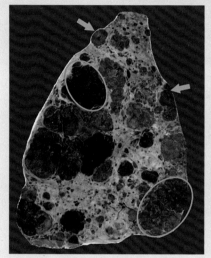

图 4-29　肝转移性恶性黑色素瘤
Fig.4-29　Metastatic malignant
melanoma of liver

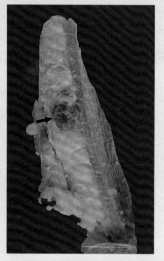

图 4-30　皮下转移性恶性黑色素瘤
Fig.4-30　Metastatic malignant
melanoma of subcutaneous tissue

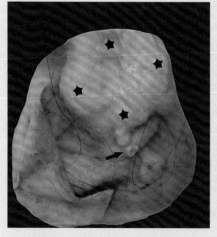

图 4-31　卵巢成熟性囊性畸胎瘤
Fig.4-31　Mature cystic teratoma of ovary

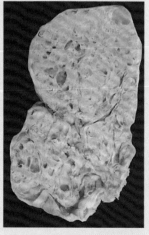

图 4-32　卵巢未成熟性畸胎瘤
Fig.4-32　Immature
teratoma of ovary

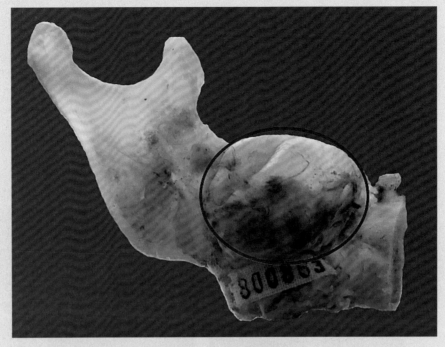

图 4-33　下颌骨造釉细胞瘤
Fig.4-33　Ameloblastoma of mandible

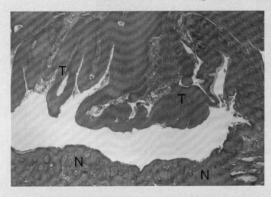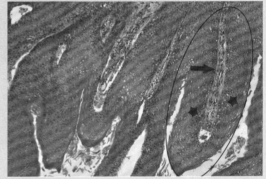

图 4-34　皮肤乳头状瘤（×40；×100）
Fig.4-34　Papilloma of skin（×40；×100）

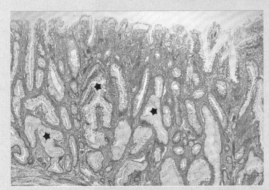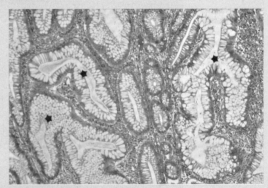

图 4-35　结肠腺瘤（×40；×100）
Fig.4-35　Adenoma of colon（×40；×100）

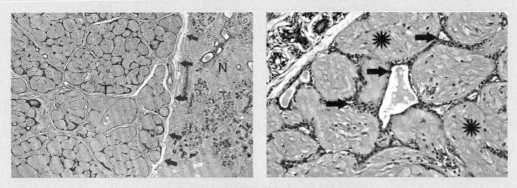

图 4-36　乳腺纤维腺瘤（×40；×200）

Fig.4-36　Fibroadenoma of breast（×40；×200）

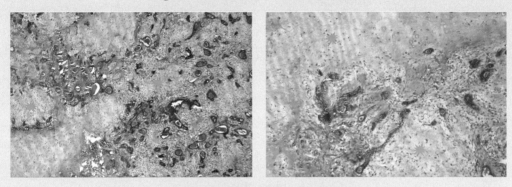

图 4-37　腮腺多形性腺瘤（×40；×100）

Fig.4-37　Pleomorphic adenoma of parotid gland（×40；×100）

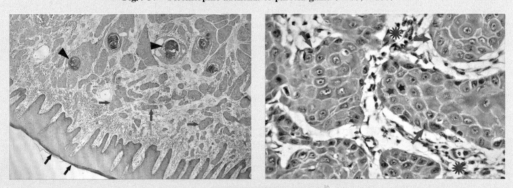

图 4-38　皮肤鳞状细胞癌（×40；×400）

Fig.4-38　Squamous cell carcinoma of skin（×40；×400）

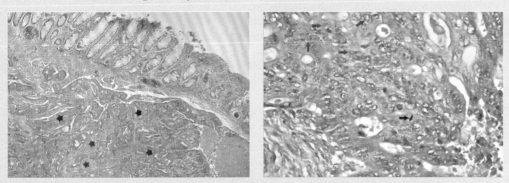

图 4-39　结肠腺癌（×40；×400）

Fig.4-39　Adenocarcinoma of colon（×40；×400）

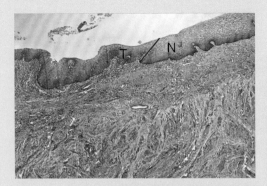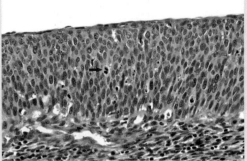

图 4-40　宫颈高级别鳞状上皮内病变（×40；×400）
Fig.4-40　High-grade squamous intraepithelial lesion of cervix（×40；×400）

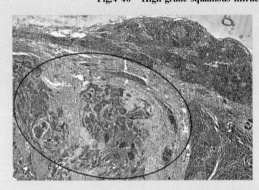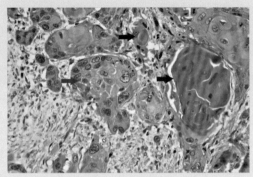

图 4-41　淋巴结转移性鳞状细胞癌（×40；×400）
Fig.4-41　Metastatic squamous cell carcinoma in lymph node（×40；×400）

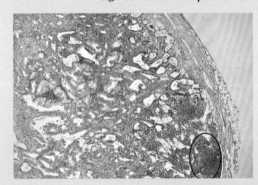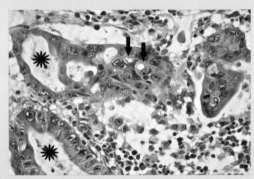

图 4-42　淋巴结转移性腺癌（×40；×400）
Fig.4-42　Metastatic adenocarcinoma in lymph node（×40；×400）

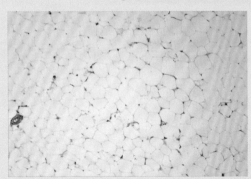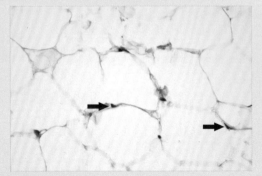

图 4-43　皮下脂肪瘤（×100；×400）
Fig.4-43　Subcutaneous lipoma（×100；×400）

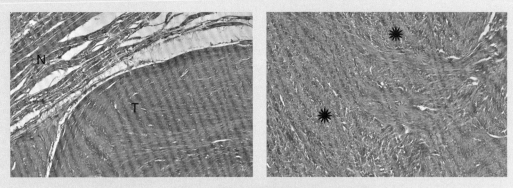

图 4-44　子宫平滑肌瘤（×40；×100）
Fig.4-44　Leiomyoma of uterus（×40；×100）

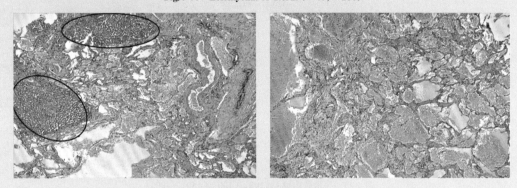

图 4-45　肝海绵状血管瘤（×40；×40）
Fig.4-45　Cavenous hemangioma of liver（×40；×40）

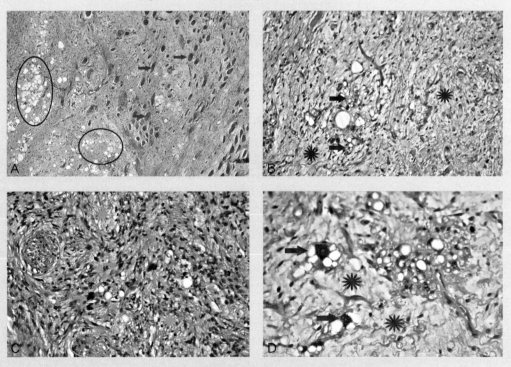

图 4-46　腹膜后脂肪肉瘤（×40；×200；×200；×400）
Fig.4-46　Retroperitoneal liposarcoma（×40；×200；×200；×400）

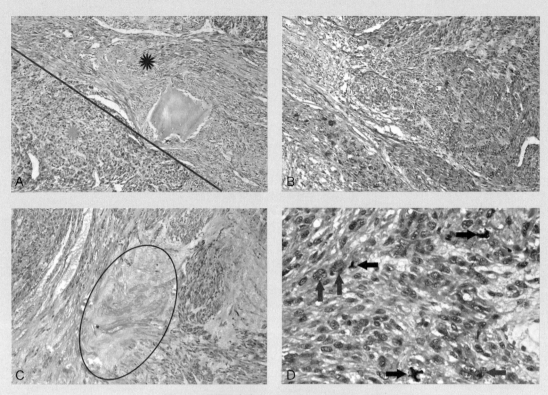

图 4-47　平滑肌肉瘤（×100；×100；×100；×400）
Fig.4-47　Leiomyosarcoma（×100；×100；×100；×400）

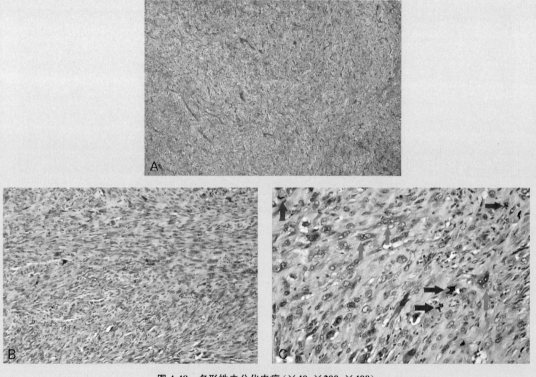

图 4-48　多形性未分化肉瘤（×40；×200；×400）
Fig.4-48　Undifferentiated pleomorphic sarcoma（×40；×200；×400）

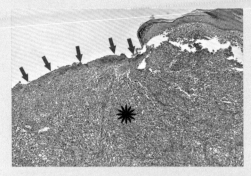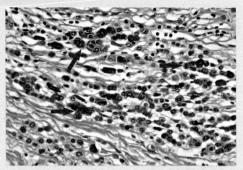

图 4-49　皮肤恶性黑色素瘤（×40；×400）
Fig.4-49　Cutaneous malignant melanoma（×40；×400）

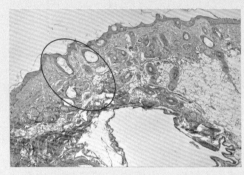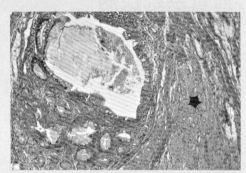

图 4-50　卵巢成熟性囊性畸胎瘤（×40；×100）
Fig.4-50　Mature cystic teratoma of ovary（×40；×100）

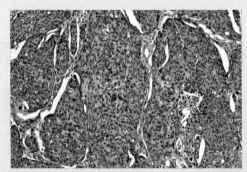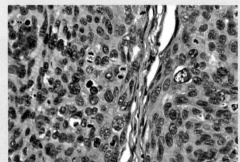

图 4-51　案例 1（×40；×400）
Fig.4-51　Case 1（×40；×400）

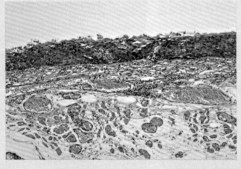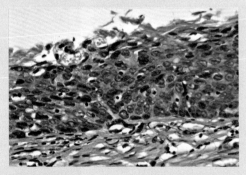

图 4-52　案例 2（×100；×400）
Fig.4-52　Case 2（×100；×400）

盛蓁（Zhen Sheng）

第五章

心血管系统疾病

一、目的要求

1. 掌握动脉粥样硬化的病变特点,理解其发生发展及其在不同脏器所引起的各种后果。

2. 掌握高血压病的形态特征、其累及主要脏器的病理改变和后果。

3. 掌握风湿病的基本病变特点、发生发展及其后果。

4. 熟悉风湿性心脏病的形态特点及其对机体的危害性。

5. 了解感染性心内膜炎赘生物的形态特点、风湿性心内膜炎与感染性心内膜炎赘生物的形态区别。

6. 了解心肌病、心肌炎的基本形态特点。

导学

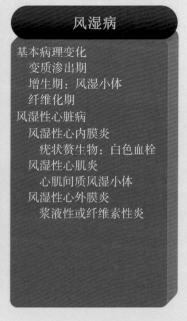

动脉粥样硬化	高血压病	风湿病
基本病理变化	良性高血压病	基本病理变化
脂纹	功能紊乱期	变质渗出期
纤维斑块	动脉病变期	增生期:风湿小体
粥样斑块	细小动脉硬化	纤维化期
继发性病变	内脏病变期	风湿性心脏病
斑块内出血	心:左心室肥大	风湿性心内膜炎
斑块破裂	肾:原发性颗粒性固缩肾	疣状赘生物:白色血栓
血栓形成	脑:脑水肿脑软化脑出血	风湿性心肌炎
钙化	视网膜:中央动脉硬化	心肌间质风湿小体
动脉瘤	恶性高血压病	风湿性心外膜炎
血管腔狭窄	坏死性细动脉炎	浆液性或纤维素性炎
冠状动脉粥样硬化性心脏病	增生性小动脉硬化	
心绞痛		
心肌梗死		
心肌纤维化		
冠状动脉性猝死		

二、大体标本

1. 动脉粥样硬化

1.1　主动脉粥样硬化（图 5-1）

标本为沿纵轴剪开的两段主动脉，左侧标本可见主动脉内膜粗糙不平，有散在浅黄色斑纹及黄白色蜡滴状隆起的斑块（蓝箭）；右侧标本上可见斑块破溃形成的溃疡灶（蓝圈）。

1.2　冠状动脉粥样硬化（图 5-2）

切取心脏含有左冠状动脉横断面的部分组织，可见心外膜下冠状动脉内壁一侧增厚，黄白色病灶向管腔内呈半月状凸出（蓝箭），导致管腔狭窄（黑星）。

1.3　脑动脉粥样硬化（图 5-3）

脑底椎动脉及基底动脉粗细不匀，管壁厚薄不均，厚处可见大小不等的淡黄色粥样硬化斑块（蓝箭）。思考：透过管壁外膜肉眼为何能看到该血管内膜下的病灶？

1.4　主动脉瘤（图 5-4）

于主动脉弓降部开始处，部分动脉壁呈球形向外膨出，内腔与动脉腔相通，此为动脉瘤，其内有附壁血栓（蓝箭）存在。注意观察该段主动脉内膜是否光滑。

2. 高血压病

2.1　高血压性心脏病（图 5-5）

两例心脏体积均明显增大，左侧为代偿期改变，左心室壁明显增厚，乳头肌和肉柱增粗变圆，左心室腔无明显扩张。注意与右侧另一例高血压性心脏病失代偿期改变相比较。

2.2　原发性颗粒性固缩肾（图 5-6）

肾体积缩小，包膜已剥离，表面呈细颗粒状，切面皮质变薄，皮髓质分界不清，叶间小动脉壁较厚，变硬（蓝箭）。

2.3　脑出血（图 5-7）

大脑的水平切面，可见侧脑室内巨大的血凝块，高血压病患者内囊、基底节区的出血灶已经破入侧脑室（蓝箭）。

3. 风湿病及风湿性心瓣膜病

3.1　急性风湿性心内膜炎（二尖瓣疣状赘生物）（图 5-8）

二尖瓣闭锁缘上有灰白或灰黄色细小的赘生物（蓝圈），瓣膜灰白色，半透明，无明显增厚，腱索仍纤细，无明显缩短或融合，心内膜尚光滑。

3.2　慢性风湿性心瓣膜病（二尖瓣病变）（图 5-9）

左心室腔无明显扩大，二尖瓣增厚（蓝圈），粗糙不平，失去光泽，质硬，瓣膜周径缩小，腱索明显变粗缩短，乳头肌肥厚。左心房明显扩大，心内膜增厚较粗糙。

3.3　慢性风湿性心瓣膜病（重度二尖瓣狭窄）（图 5-10）

自剖开的心房面观察二尖瓣，见二尖瓣显著增厚，瓣叶互相粘连，瓣膜口呈鱼口状或漏斗状狭窄（蓝箭）。

3.4　慢性风湿性心瓣膜病（主动脉瓣病变）（图 5-11）

左心室壁增厚，心腔扩大，主动脉瓣增厚卷曲（蓝箭）、变硬、无光泽。

4. 感染性心内膜炎

4.1　急性感染性心内膜炎（二尖瓣病变）（图 5-12）

二尖瓣前叶心房面有粗大赘生物附着（蓝圈），质粗糙而松脆易碎，病变瓣膜尚无明显的增厚粘连。注意与急性风湿性心内膜炎的疣状赘生物相比较。

4.2　亚急性感染性心内膜炎（主动脉瓣病变）（图 5-13）

主动脉瓣边缘可见粗大的灰黄色赘生物（蓝箭），部分已脱落，瓣膜受损，结构不完整。

5. 心脏肿瘤

左心房黏液瘤（图 5-14）

左心房内壁上可见一个质软，灰白色，分叶状的黏液瘤附着（蓝圈），部分出血区域呈现暗红色。黏液瘤是心脏最常见的原发肿瘤，一般可通过外科手术切除。

三、组织切片

1. 动脉粥样硬化

1.1　主动脉粥样硬化（图 5-15）

主动脉内膜呈纤维性增厚，部分区域玻璃样变。纤维帽的深部有大量无定形物质（蓝星），为细胞外脂质和坏死物，其中可见多数针形、菱形的胆固醇结晶的裂隙（黑箭）。粥样病灶周围可见多数泡沫细胞（蓝箭）及斑块内出血。绿星和黑星分别示主动脉中膜和外膜。

1.2　冠状动脉粥样硬化（图 5-16）

冠状动脉分支横断面可见一侧管壁半月形增厚病灶（蓝星），已阻塞约二分之一的管腔，注意与正常管壁（绿星）结构相对比。粥样病灶中可见大量的无定形物质，蓝箭示制片过程中溶解的胆固醇结晶裂隙，绿箭示颗粒状的钙盐沉积。

1.3　陈旧性心肌梗死（图 5-17）

梗死的心肌组织已经被肉芽组织机化，伊红染的残存心肌细胞周围有数量不等的纤维结缔组织（蓝星）穿插包绕。结缔组织内主要见大量成纤维细胞和胶原纤维，以及少量的血管和炎细胞，残存的心肌细胞（蓝箭）呈现波浪状，排列较紊乱。

2. 高血压病

肾小动脉硬化（图 5-18）

肾间质中可见小动脉管壁增厚、管腔狭窄（蓝箭），增厚的动脉管壁呈现均质红染的玻璃样变性。部分肾小管上皮细胞肿胀，蓝星示肾小球内毛细血管袢。

3. 风湿病

风湿性心肌炎（图 5-19）

在心肌（蓝星）间质小血管（黑星）附近可见略呈梭形的风湿小体（蓝圈），即

Aschoff 小体。注意观察风湿细胞（蓝箭）的特征,细胞体积大,胞浆丰富均质,核大,圆形或卵圆形,核膜清晰,细丝状染色质,可为单核、双核或多核。绿箭示纤维素样坏死灶。思考:风湿细胞的来源是何种细胞?

4. 感染性心内膜炎

亚急性感染性心内膜炎（图 5-20）

病变瓣膜为二尖瓣,可见瓣叶明显增厚（黑星）,胶原化,瓣膜边缘附着一形态不完整的巨大赘生物（蓝圈）,部分已脱落,赘生物内可见大量蓝染密集的细菌集落（蓝星）。该病例是在慢性风湿性心瓣膜病基础之上并发了细菌感染所致。

5. 心肌病

扩张性心肌病（图 5-21）

心肌细胞排列紊乱,不均匀性肥大（蓝箭）,横纹尚可见,细胞核大而深染,核形态不规则,部分心肌细胞胞浆内可见空泡变性。

6. 心肌炎

细菌性心肌炎（图 5-22）

心肌间质中可见数量不等的炎细胞浸润（蓝星）,以中性粒细胞（蓝箭）为主,部分心肌细胞胞浆染色不均,呈现变性改变。细菌性心肌炎多由金黄色葡萄球菌、链球菌等感染所致。

四、临床病理讨论

案例　患者,女,54 岁,在家中与人交谈时突然倒地死亡。病理尸检中显示,左心室侧壁可见约 15 mm 长的破裂口,心包腔内大量积血,左心室侧壁组织镜下所见如图 5-23 所示。

（1）该患者左心室侧壁组织的病理诊断是什么?

（2）该病变可能会引起哪些常见的并发症? 该患者的死亡原因是什么?

五、思考题

1. 动脉粥样硬化的基本病理变化有哪些? 其好发于哪些部位的血管?

2. 良性高血压病晚期可能引起哪些严重后果?

3. 风湿病特征性的基本病变是什么? 为何风湿性心脏病会引起较严重的后果?

4. 风湿性心内膜炎及亚急性感染性心内膜炎各有何形态特点? 两者间有何关系?

5. 试论述二尖瓣狭窄可能引起的血流动力学及心脏变化。

6. 名词解释:脂纹,粥瘤,动脉瘤,心肌梗死,室壁瘤,向心性肥大,原发性颗粒性固缩肾,风湿小体,风湿细胞。

Chapter 5

Diseases of Cardiovascular System

Ⅰ. Aims

1. To grasp the pathological characteristics of atherosclerosis and understand its various consequences in different organs.

2. To grasp the pathological characteristics of hypertension, the pathological changes and consequences of the main organs involved.

3. To grasp the basic pathological changes, development and consequences of rheumatism.

4. To familiarize with the pathological characteristics of rheumatic heart disease and its damage to the body.

5. To understand the morphological characteristics of vegetations in infective endocarditis and distinguish it from rheumatic endocarditis.

6. To understand the morphological characteristics of cardiomyopathy and myocarditis.

Guidance to study

Atherosclerosis	Hypertension	Rheumatism
Basic morphology	Benign hypertension	Basic morphology
Fatty streak	Dysfunctional phase	Alteration,exudation
Fibrous plaque	Arterial lesion phase	Proliferation:Aschoff body
Atheromatous plaque	Hyaline aeteriolosclerosis	Fibrosis
Complications	Visceral lesion phase	Rheumatic heart disease
Hemorrhage	Left ventricular hypertrophy	Endocarditis
Rupture	Arteriolar nephrosclerosis	Platelet-fibrin thrombi
Thrombosis	Cerebral edema	Myocarditis
Calcification	Encephalomalacia	Aschoff bodies
Aneurysm formation	Cerebral hemorrhage	Pericarditis
Narrowed lumen	Retinal arteriolosclerosis	Serous or fibrinous exudate
Coronary artery disease	Malignant hypertension	
Angina pectoris	Necrotizing arteriolitis	
Myocardial infarction	Hyperplastic arteriolosclerosis	
Myocardial fibrosis		
Sudden coronary death		

Ⅱ. Gross specimens

1. Atherosclerosis

1. 1　Aortic atherosclerosis（Fig.5-1）

The specimens are two sections of aortae cut along the longitudinal axis. The aortic intima on the left is rough and uneven, with scattered yellow fatty streaks and yellow white wax dripping-like raised plaques(blue arrow). Ulceration foci(blue circle)formed by plaque rupture can be seen on the right specimen.

1. 2　Coronary atherosclerosis（Fig.5-2）

This is a part of the cardiac wall containing the cross section of the left coronary artery. It can be observed that one side of the coronary arterial wall under epicardium is thickened, and the crescentic yellow white plaque protrudes into the lumen (blue arrow), resulting in lumen narrowing(black asterisk).

1. 3　Cerebral atherosclerosis（Fig.5-3）

Different sizes of fatty streaks and plaques (blue arrows) of the vertebral and basilar arteries are visible at the bottom of the brain, resulting in thickened walls and narrowed lumens. Why can the lesions under the intima of the vessel be observed through the adventitia?

1. 4　Aortic aneurysm（Fig.5-4）

A large bulge can be seen at the descending area of aortic arch, and the outward cavity is connected with the lumen of aorta. This is an aneurysm with mural thrombus (blue arrow). Pay attention to observe whether the aortic intima is smooth.

2. Hypertension

2. 1　Hypertensive heart disease（Fig.5-5）

In both specimens, the cardiac volumes increase. The left ventricular wall and the papillary muscle are thickened, but there is no significant dilatation of the cavity during the compensatory period(left). Pay attention to the obvious dilatation of left ventricular cavity in the other hypertensive heart disease accompanying decompensated cardial function(right).

2. 2　Primary granular atrophy of kidney（Fig.5-6）

The capsule of kidney has been stripped. It decreases in size with fine granular surface. On the section, the cortex is thin, and the boundary between cortex and medulla is unclear. The walls of arterioles become thickened(blue arrow).

2. 3　Cerebral hemorrhage（Fig.5-7）

On the horizontal section of the brain, a huge blood clot is in the lateral ventricle. The bleeding focus in the internal capsule and basal ganglia of a patient with hypertension has broken into the lateral ventricle (blue arrow).

3. Rheumatism and rheumatic valvular diseases

3.1 Acute rheumatic endocarditis (verrucous vegetations of mitral valves) (Fig.5-8)

There are gray or yellow white vegetations (blue circles) on the closure line of mitral valves. The leaflets are still translucent, without obvious thickening. The chordae tendineae are thin without shortening or fusion, and the endocardium is still smooth.

3.2 Chronic rheumatic valvular disease (mitral valves) (Fig.5-9)

The mitral valves are thickened (blue circle), rough, and the perimeter of the valves is reduced. The chordae tendineae are significantly shortened and fused together. The left atrium is enlarged and the endocardium is also thickened.

3.3 Chronic rheumatic valvular disease (severe mitral stenosis) (Fig.5-10)

Observing the mitral valves from the opened left atrium, the mitral valves are dramatically thickened, the leaflets adhere to each other, showing a fish-mouth or funnel shaped stricture (blue arrow).

3.4 Chronic rheumatic valvular disease (aortic valves) (Fig.5-11)

The left ventricular wall is thickened, and the cardiac cavity is dilated. The aortic cusps are thickened (blue arrow), curled, and opaque.

4. Infective endocarditis

4.1 Acute infective endocarditis (mitral valves) (Fig.5-12)

There is a large vegetation (blue circle) attached to the anterior mitral valve leaflet. The vegetation is rough and fragile. There is no obvious thickening and adhesion of the diseased valves. Note the difference from verrucous vegetations in acute rheumatic endocarditis.

4.2 Subacute infective endocarditis (aortic valves) (Fig.5-13)

Irregular, grayish yellow vegetations (blue arrow) are seen on the edge of the aortic cusps, and some of which have detached from the valves. The normal structure of valves has been destroyed.

5. Cardiac tumor

Left atrial myxoma (Fig.5-14)

There is a soft, pale, lobulated myxoma (blue circle) attached to the wall of left atrium. Dark red bleeding areas are observed. It is the most common primary tumor of heart and can usually be treated by surgical resection.

III. Tissue sections

1. Atherosclerosis

1.1   Aortic atherosclerosis (Fig.5-15)

The intima of aorta shows fibrous thickening and hyaline degeneration in some areas. There are amorphous substances (blue asterisk) deep beneath the fibrous cap, composed of extracellular lipids and cellular debris, in which most needle or diamond shaped cholesterol crystal cracks (black arrow) can be seen. Most foam cells (blue arrow) and bleeding in the plaque are around the lesion. The green asterisk and black asterisk show the tunica media and adventitia of the aorta, respectively.

1.2   Coronary atherosclerosis (Fig.5-16)

In the cross section of the coronary artery branch, a crescentic thickened plaque (blue asterisks) can be observed at one side of the wall, which has blocked about half of the lumen. Note that it is different from the adjacent normal wall (green asterisk) in morphology. A great amount of amorphous substance can be seen in the atherosclerotic plaque. The blue arrow shows the crack of cholesterol crystal, and the green arrow indicates granular calcification.

1.3   Old myocardial infarction (Fig.5-17)

The infarcted myocardium has been organized by granulation tissue. The residual cardiomyocytes (blue arrow) stained with eosin are wavy and arranged in disorder. They are surrounded by fibrous connective tissues (blue asterisks) composed of a large number of fibroblasts and fibers, some blood vessels and inflammatory cells.

2. Hypertension

Renal arteriolosclerosis (Fig.5-18)

The arteriolar walls in renal interstitium are thickened and the lumens are narrow (blue arrows). The walls present homogeneous eosin-stained hyaline degeneration. Renal tubular epithelial cells are swollen, and the blue asterisks show the capillary loop in the glomerulus.

3. Rheumatism

Rheumatic myocarditis (Fig.5-19)

A spindle shaped rheumatic body (blue circle), namely Aschoff body, can be seen near the interstitial small vessel (black asterisk) of myocardium (blue asterisks). Pay attention to the characteristics of rheumatic cells (Aschoff cells, blue arrows). The Aschoff cell has rich and homogeneous cytoplasm, large round or oval nucleus, clear nuclear membrane and filamentous chromatin. They can be mononuclear, binuclear or multinuclear. The green arrow shows fibrinoid necrosis. Which cell does the rheumatic cell come from?

4. Infective endocarditis

Subacute infective endocarditis（Fig.5-20）

It is the mitral valve with obvious thickening (black asterisks) and collagenization of the leaflet. A large vegetation (blue circle) is attached to the edge of the leaflet, and some of which have detached. Clusters of blue stained bacterial colonies (blue asterisks) can be seen in the vegetation. This case was caused by subacute infective endocarditis on the basis of chronic rheumatic valvular heart disease.

5. Cardiomyopathy

Dilated cardiomyopathy（Fig.5-21）

The unevenly hypertrophic cardiomyocytes (blue arrows) arrange disorderly, and the transverse striations are still visible. The basophilic-stained nuclei of cardiomyocytes are large and irregular. Vacuolar degeneration can be observed in the cytoplasm of some cardiomyocytes.

6. Myocarditis

Bacterial myocarditis（Fig.5-22）

Mass of inflammatory cells (blue asterisks) are examined in the myocardial interstitium, and the dominant infiltrating leukocytes are neutrophils (blue arrows). The cytoplasm of some cardiomyocytes is stained unevenly and presents degeneration. Bacterial myocarditis is commonly caused by staphylococcus aureus and streptococcus infections.

IV. Clinical pathological discussion

Case

A 54 years old female suddenly fell to the ground and died while talking with others at home. The pathological autopsy showed that there was a 15 mm rupture (blue circle) in the left ventricular lateral wall, and a large amount of blood accumulated in the pericardial cavity. The morphology of the left ventricular lateral wall is shown in the Fig.5-23.

(1) What is the pathological diagnosis of the patient's left ventricular lateral wall?

(2) What are the common complications of this disease? What is the leading cause of death of this patient?

V. Questions

1. What are the basic morphological changes of atherosclerosis? Which parts of the blood

vessels are prone to be involved?

2. Please describe the pathologic characteristics and clinical features of hypertensive heart disease.

3. What are the characteristic lesions of rheumatism? Why does rheumatic heart disease cause more serious consequences?

4. Please distinguish the vegetations of rheumatic endocarditis from infective endocarditis.

5. Please describe the hemodynamic and cardiac changes caused by mitral stenosis.

6. Terms: Fatty streak, Atheroma, Aneurysm, Myocardial infarction, Ventricular aneurysm, Concentric hypertrophy, Primary granular atrophy of kidney, Aschoff body, Aschoff cell.

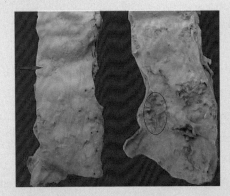

图 5-1 主动脉粥样硬化
Fig.5-1 Aortic atherosclerosis

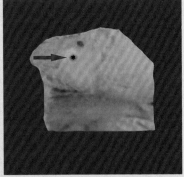

图 5-2 冠状动脉粥样硬化
Fig.5-2 Coronary atherosclerosis

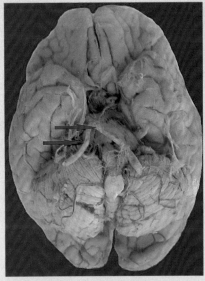

图 5-3 脑动脉粥样硬化
Fig.5-3 Cerebral atherosclerosis

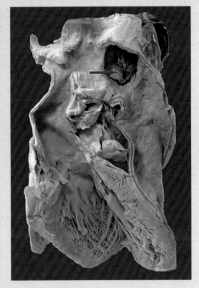

图 5-4 主动脉瘤
Fig.5-4 Aortic aneurysm

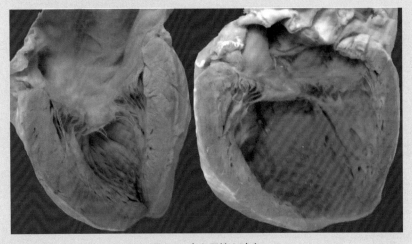

图 5-5 高血压性心脏病
Fig.5-5 Hypertensive heart disease

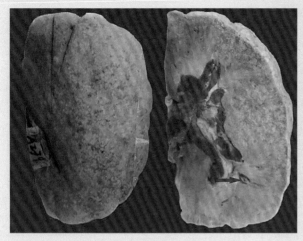

图 5-6　原发性颗粒性固缩肾
Fig.5-6　Primary granular atrophy of kidney

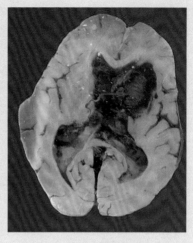

图 5-7　脑出血
Fig.5-7　Cerebral hemorrhage

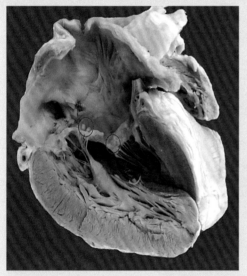

图 5-8　急性风湿性心内膜炎（二尖瓣疣状赘生物）
Fig.5-8　Acute rheumatic endocarditis（verrucous
vegetations of mitral valves）

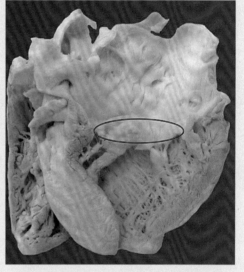

图 5-9　慢性风湿性心瓣膜病（二尖瓣病变）
Fig.5-9　Chronic rheumatic valvular disease
（mitral valves）

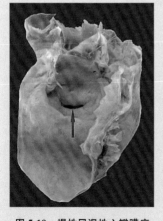

图 5-10　慢性风湿性心瓣膜病
（重度二尖瓣狭窄）
Fig.5-10　Chronic rheumatic
valvular disease（severe mitral stenosis）

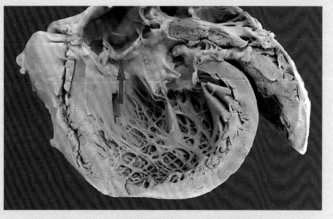

图 5-11　慢性风湿性心瓣膜病（主动脉瓣病变）
Fig.5-11　Chronic rheumatic valvular disease
（aortic valves）

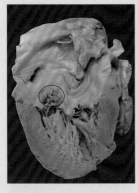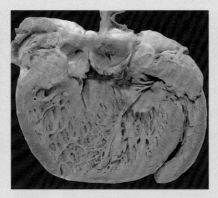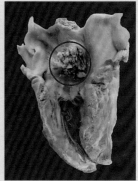

图 5-12　急性感染性心内
膜炎（二尖瓣病变）
Fig.5-12　Acute infective
endocarditis（mitral valves）

图 5-13　亚急性感染性心内膜炎
（主动脉瓣病变）
Fig.5-13　Subacute infective endocarditis
（aortic valves）

图 5-14　左心房黏液瘤
Fig.5-14　Left atrial
myxoma

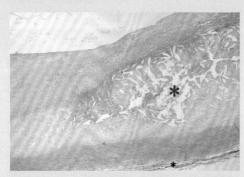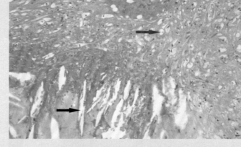

图 5-15　主动脉粥样硬化（×40；×200）
Fig.5-15　Aortic atherosclerosis（×40；×200）

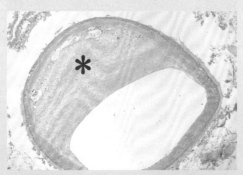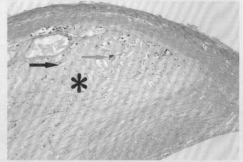

图 5-16　冠状动脉粥样硬化（×40；×100）
Fig.5-16　Coronary atherosclerosis（×40；×100）

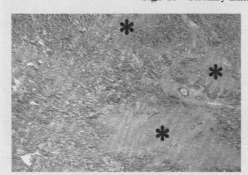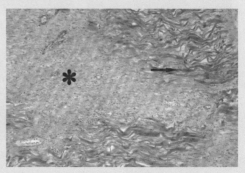

图 5-17　陈旧性心肌梗死（×40；×100）
Fig.5-17　Old myocardial infarction（×40；×100）

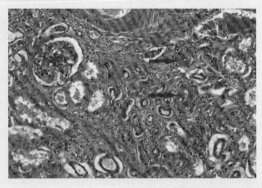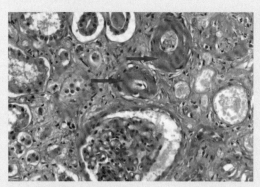

图 5-18　肾小动脉硬化（×200；×400）
Fig.5-18　Renal arteriolosclerosis（×200；×400）

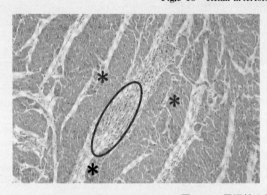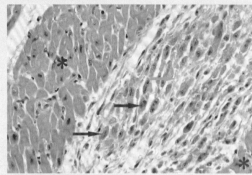

图 5-19　风湿性心肌炎（×100；×400）
Fig.5-19　Rheumatic myocarditis（×100；×400）

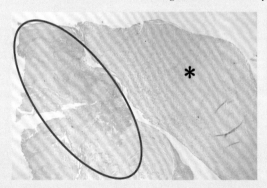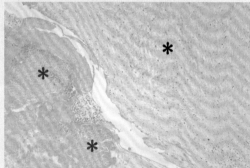

图 5-20　亚急性感染性心内膜炎（×40；×100）
Fig.5-20　Subacute infective endocarditis（×40；×100）

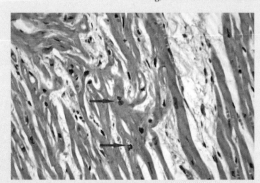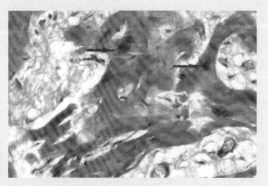

图 5-21　扩张性心肌病（×200；×400）
Fig.5-21　Dilated cardiomyopathy（×200；×400）

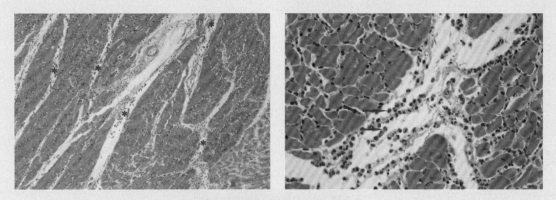

图 5-22　细菌性心肌炎（×100；×400）
Fig.5-22　Bacterial myocarditis（×100；×400）

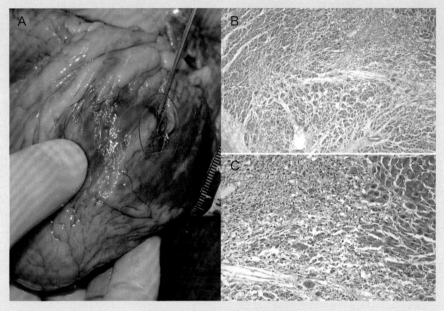

图 5-23　案例（B：×100；C：×200）
Fig.5-23　Case（B：×100；C：×200）

卜晓东（Xiaodong Bu）

第六章

呼吸系统疾病

一、目的要求

1. 掌握大叶性肺炎、小叶性肺炎的形态特点及二者的区别。
2. 掌握慢性支气管炎、肺气肿、支气管扩张的形态特点及常见的病因和后果。
3. 掌握硅肺的形态特点及其产生原因。
4. 掌握原发性肺癌的形态特点及临床病理联系。

导学

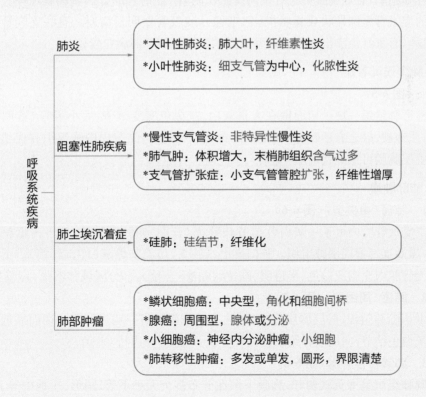

呼吸系统疾病
- 肺炎
  - *大叶性肺炎：肺大叶，纤维素性炎
  - *小叶性肺炎：细支气管为中心，化脓性炎
- 阻塞性肺疾病
  - *慢性支气管炎：非特异性慢性炎
  - *肺气肿：体积增大，末梢肺组织含气过多
  - *支气管扩张症：小支气管管腔扩张，纤维性增厚
- 肺尘埃沉着症
  - *硅肺：硅结节，纤维化
- 肺部肿瘤
  - *鳞状细胞癌：中央型，角化和细胞间桥
  - *腺癌：周围型，腺体或分泌
  - *小细胞癌：神经内分泌肿瘤，小细胞
  - *肺转移性肿瘤：多发或单发，圆形，界限清楚

二、 大体标本

1. 肺炎

1.1　大叶性肺炎（图6-1）

肺脏体积增大，上叶胸膜表面可见灰白灰红色纤维素性渗出物（蓝箭）。切面，灰白色，有灰黑色颗粒散在分布，质地致密如肝脏，略呈颗粒状。支气管未见明显病变。思考：该病变处于大叶性肺炎的哪一期？胸部X线检查会是什么表现？

1.2　小叶性肺炎（图6-2）

左肺散在分布大小不等、梅花状或不规则、灰白灰黄色实变区，部分病变中心可见细小支气管横断面（蓝箭），下叶的病灶相互融合成片。病灶周围肺组织可见气肿。

2. 阻塞性肺疾病

2.1　肺气肿（图6-3）

肺体积明显增大，灰白色，边缘变钝，肋骨压迹明显（红箭）。上叶靠近肺门的胸膜下可见一含气大囊泡，此为肺大疱，囊壁完整，壁薄半透明（红圈）。肺组织切面蜂窝状，可见大量过度含气囊腔。

2.2　支气管扩张（图6-4）

一叶肺组织，脏层胸膜可见纤维结缔组织附着（红箭），部分区域胸膜增厚。切面靠近胸膜的支气管呈圆柱状或囊状扩张（蓝箭），支气管壁明显增厚。有些支气管内壁粗糙、无光泽，有灰红色渗出物覆盖内壁或充填管腔。肺下部病变较重。

3. 肺尘埃沉着症

硅肺（图6-5）

不整形肺组织一块。切面散在大量灰白、灰黑色实变结节，大小不等（蓝圈），形状不规则，质地硬、触之有沙砾感（因继发纤维化和钙化）。结节周围肺组织有代偿性气肿形成。脏层胸膜可见灶状增厚（蓝箭）。

4. 肺部肿瘤

4.1　肺癌（中央型）（图6-6）

右主支气管腔内可见一灰白色结节状肿块（蓝圈）向腔内生长，几乎占据整个支气管腔，并累及支气管周围肺组织。肺门淋巴结肿大，切面灰黑灰白色（红箭）。下部肺组织的支气管腔内充满灰白色、半透明、圆柱状黏液（蓝箭），部分区域肺不张（绿箭）。

4.2　肺癌（周围型）（图6-7）

手术切除肺组织，脏层胸膜完整，肿块靠近胸膜处一明显凹陷。切面靠近胸膜处可见一灰白色结节，向周围肺组织浸润性生长，边缘呈花边状（蓝箭）。

4.3　肺转移性肿瘤（图6-8）

左侧肺组织呈书页状切开，胸膜下散在分布多个大小不等、圆形、质地中等、灰白色结节，边界清楚，部分结节中心可见坏死（蓝箭）。

三、组织切片

1. 肺炎

1.1　大叶性肺炎（图 6-9）

病变弥漫性分布,肺泡腔扩大,充满渗出物,渗出物为大量中性粒细胞和纤维素,以及少量单核细胞和红细胞。肺泡腔内纤维素连接成网,并通过肺泡间孔与相邻肺泡腔内的纤维素相连（蓝箭）。肺泡壁变薄,毛细血管受压变窄。

1.2　小叶性肺炎（图 6-10）

病变呈多灶性、散在分布,以细支气管为中心（蓝星）,累及周围肺组织。细支气管壁上皮细胞变性、坏死、脱落（蓝圈）,细支气管管腔、管壁及周围肺泡内充满渗出物,以中性粒细胞为主,还有少量纤维素、淋巴细胞等;病灶周围肺组织代偿性气肿。思考:其和大叶性肺炎形态上有哪些不同。

1.3　羊水吸入性肺炎（图 6-11）

病变呈多灶性、散在分布（蓝圈）。病灶处肺泡腔内可见少量浆液、中性粒细胞渗出,部分肺泡腔内可见片状或层状、伊红染物质,为角化物（蓝箭）;部分肺泡腔内可见毳毛、皮脂等。肺泡间隔增宽,毛细血管扩张、充血、炎细胞渗出。

2. 阻塞性肺疾病

2.1　气管慢性炎（图 6-12）

气管壁被覆的假复层纤毛柱状上皮细胞坏死、脱落,杯状细胞数量显著减少,上皮下可见淋巴细胞浸润（蓝箭）,基底膜节段性显著增厚及玻璃样变（红箭）。黏膜下层水肿,间质纤维结缔组织增生及玻璃样变（蓝星）,血管扩张、充血,可见散在淋巴细胞、浆细胞和单核细胞浸润。

2.2　肺气肿（图 6-13）

肺泡扩张（蓝星）,肺泡间隔变窄并断裂（蓝箭）,导致邻近肺泡相互融合形成较大的囊腔,肺泡间隔内毛细血管受压狭窄或闭塞。

2.3　支气管扩张症（图 6-14）

切片取材自图 6-4 中扩张的支气管壁。支气管的假复层纤毛柱状上皮细胞坏死、脱落（蓝箭）,纤毛粘连、倒伏（红箭）,上皮内可见炎细胞浸润。支气管腔内可见坏死脱落的上皮细胞、红细胞和炎性渗出物（黄星）。上皮下可见大量淋巴细胞、浆细胞和中性粒细胞浸润（蓝星）,血管扩张、充血（绿星）、出血。

3. 肺尘埃沉着症

硅肺（图 6-15）

肺组织内可见散在大小不等的结节状病灶（蓝圈）,中央可见小血管（蓝箭）。有的结节主要由吞噬硅尘颗粒的巨噬细胞组成（细胞性硅结节,红箭）;有的结节中央可见成纤维细胞和沉积的胶原纤维（纤维性硅结节,图 6-15C）;也有的结节中央由同心圆或漩涡状排列的胶原纤维组成,可发生玻璃样变、病理性钙化（红星）。相邻结节融合后肉眼可见。肺间质纤维结缔组织弥漫性增生,肺泡间隔变宽。

4　肺癌

4.1　肺鳞状细胞癌（图 6-16）

肿瘤组织内癌细胞巢团状排列,可见明显坏死（蓝星）,并向周围组织浸润性生长（蓝箭）。癌细胞多边形,大小不一,可见瘤巨细胞。细胞边界清楚,胞浆丰富,嗜酸性,可见细胞间桥和细胞内角化（红箭）。核浆比增大,细胞核大小和形状不一,核仁略嗜酸、大而明显,染色质粗,核分裂象易见。间质纤维组织增生,慢性炎细胞浸润。

4.2　肺腺癌（图 6-17）

癌细胞呈腺泡状或条索状排列（红箭）,部分可见微乳头形成,浸润周围肺组织（蓝箭）。癌细胞呈柱状、高柱状或不规则形,大小不一,胞浆中等量、嗜酸性染色,部分细胞可见分泌空泡（绿箭）。核浆比增大,细胞核大小和形状不一,染色质粗（图 6-17C）,核分裂象易见。间质可见多量炎细胞浸润。

4.3　肺小细胞癌（图 6-18）

肿瘤细胞呈巢状、片状、小梁状生长（红圈）,伴单个或者小灶状癌细胞坏死。癌细胞小,圆形或卵圆形,胞浆稀少,类似淋巴细胞。细胞核深染,染色质呈细颗粒状,核仁不明显,核分裂象易见。间质增生的纤维结缔组织伴有玻璃样变（绿圈）。

四、临床病理讨论

案例　患者,男性,60 岁。5 天前患者出现发热、咳嗽、咳痰,白色泡沫样痰,量中等,体温 38.3℃。血常规检查:白细胞计数 12.5×10^9/L,中性粒细胞比例 84%,C 反应蛋白 58 mg/L。给予抗生素治疗后,上述症状未见好转。3 天前痰液转变为黄绿色、黏稠、量大,体温在 39℃ 左右波动。30 分钟前出现呼吸骤停,抢救无效后死亡。患者肺部的形态学检查所见如图 6-19。

（1）请给出该患者的病理诊断,并说明理由。

（2）尝试用病理学变化解释患者出现的临床表现。

五、思考题

1. 如何区别大叶性肺炎和小叶性肺炎?

2. 慢性支气管炎、肺气肿和支气管扩张症各自有何形态特征?

3. 简述肺癌的大体和组织学分类及其病变特点。

4. 名词解释:肺肉质变,大叶性肺炎,小叶性肺炎,病毒包涵体,透明膜,严重急性呼吸综合征,慢性阻塞性肺疾病,肺气肿,支气管扩张症,硅肺,硅结节,慢性肺源性心脏病。

Chapter 6

Diseases of Respiratory System

Ⅰ. Aims

1. To grasp the difference between lobar pneumonia and lobular pneumonia, especially in morphology.

2. To grasp the morphological features, and common causes of chronic bronchitis, emphysema and bronchiectasis.

3. To grasp the basic pathological changes and pathogenesis of silicosis.

4. To grasp the morphological characteristics and clinicopathological relationship of lung cancers.

Guidance to study

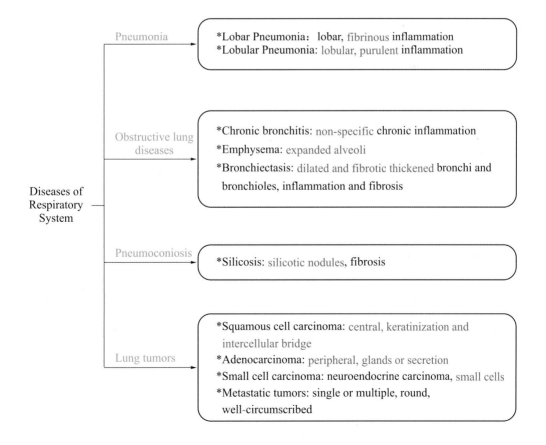

Pneumonia
*Lobar Pneumonia: lobar, fibrinous inflammation
*Lobular Pneumonia: lobular, purulent inflammation

Obstructive lung diseases
*Chronic bronchitis: non-specific chronic inflammation
*Emphysema: expanded alveoli
*Bronchiectasis: dilated and fibrotic thickened bronchi and bronchioles, inflammation and fibrosis

Diseases of Respiratory System

Pneumoconiosis
*Silicosis: silicotic nodules, fibrosis

Lung tumors
*Squamous cell carcinoma: central, keratinization and intercellular bridge
*Adenocarcinoma: peripheral, glands or secretion
*Small cell carcinoma: neuroendocrine carcinoma, small cells
*Metastatic tumors: single or multiple, round, well-circumscribed

Ⅱ. Gross specimens

1. Pneumonia

1.1　Lobar pneumonia（Fig.6-1）

Two lobes of the lung are enlarged. Pleural surface of upper lobe is covered with grey-white and grey-red fibrinous exudation（blue arrow）. The upper lobe is completely consolidated and presents liver-like texture. The lower lobe is not uniformly consolidated. The bronchi are not involved. Try to identify the pathological stage of the upper lobe with lobar pneumonia. What is the sign you can see by chest X-ray?

1.2　Lobular pneumonia（Fig.6-2）

There are some scatteredly swollen gray-white and gray-yellow areas beneath the pleura. They are irregular and consolidated on the cut surface, which are centered on the bronchioles（blue arrows）. The patchy lesions become confluent in the lower lobe, and the adjacent tissues show compensatory emphysema.

2. Obstructive lung diseases

2.1　Emphysema（Fig.6-3）

The left lung is large, grey-white, with obviously sternal impression（red arrows）. There is a large bulla in the upper lobe（red circle）. Many emphysematous spaces are observed with different diameters, especially in the area next to pleura.

2.2　Bronchiectasis（Fig.6-4）

The bronchi and bronchioles are cylindrical or cystic dilated with thickened walls（blue arrows）, especially near the pleura. Grey-red exudate is noticed in the lumens of the fibrotic bronchi and bronchioles. The pleura become partially thickened accompanying proliferated fibrotic tissue（red arrows）.

3. Pneumoconiosis

Silicosis（Fig.6-5）

It is a piece of lung tissue. On cut section, there are many grey-white or grey-black, round nodules（blue circle）. The nodules are hard and brittle due to secondary fibrosis and calcification. The compensatory emphysema and local thickened pleura（blue arrow）are visible.

4. Lung tumors

4.1　Lung cancer（central type）（Fig.6-6）

A grey-white nodule（blue circle）has invaded and occluded the bronchus. On the cut surface, the enlarged hilar lymph nodes are grey-white and grey-black(red arrows). The lower bronchi are filled with grey-white, translucent mucus(blue arrows). The green arrow indicates atelectasis.

4. 2　Lung cancer(peripheral type)(Fig.6-7)

The specimen from pneumonectomy shows a well-circumscribed nodule under the intact pleura. This cancerous nodule is irregular, grey-white and has infiltrated into the adjacent tissue(blue arrow), and the involved pleura presents depression.

4. 3　Metastatic tumor of lung(Fig.6-8)

There are many round and gray-white nodules(blue arrows)beneath the bulged pleura of left lung. The nodules are well circumscribed with normal tissue and some nodules present necrotic change.

Ⅲ. Tissue sections

1. Pneumonia

1. 1　Lobar pneumonia(Fig.6-9)

All the alveoli on the tissue slice are almost involved and appear as enlarged alveolar spaces filled with exudates, largely neutrophils, fibrin and erythrocytes. The fibrin forms meshwork through the alveolar pores(blue arrows). The septa of the alveoli have become thin because of compressed capillaries.

1. 2　Lobular pneumonia(Fig.6-10)

Lobular pneumonia is also called bronchopneumonia. The lesions are multiple, scattered and bronchioles-centered(blue stars), involving adjacent tissue. The epithelia of the injured bronchioles are alterative and detached(blue circle). The bronchioles and adjacent alveoli are filled with abundant neutrophils, a little fibrin and lymphocytes. Pulmonary compensatory emphysema is visible around the foci. Please consider the differences between lobar pneumonia and lobular pneumonia.

1. 3　Amniotic fluid aspiration pneumonia(Fig.6-11)

The foci are scattered and multiple(blue circle). Some alveolar spaces are filled with a little serous fluid, neutrophils and patchy or lamellar eosinophilic keratose(blue arrows). Hair and sebum can be seen in some alveolar spaces, bronchial and bronchilolar cavities. The septa of alveoli are dilated with congested capillaries and infiltrating inflammatory cells.

2. Obstructive lung diseases

2. 1　Chronic inflammation of bronchus(Fig.6-12)

The bronchial epithelia arc necrotic and detached with atrophic goblet cells, and infiltrated by lymphocytes and plasma cells (blue arrows). The basement membrane is segmentally thickened with hyaline degeneration (red arrows). The submucosa is edematous. The stroma shows fibrous tissue proliferation and hyaline degeneration (blue stars) with infiltrating chronic inflammatory cells, such as lymphocytes, plasma cells and monocytes.

2. 2　Emphysema (Fig.6-13)

The alveoli are dilated due to hyperinflation (blue stars), and the septa become thin with narrowed, even occlusive capillaries due to compression (blue arrows). Some neighbouring alveoli are confluent to form larger cysts.

2. 3　Bronchiectasis (Fig.6-14)

The tissue section has been made from the dilated bronchial wall described in Fig.6-4. The pseudostratified ciliated columnar epithelia display necrosis and desquamation (blue arrow) with adhesive and lodging cilia (red arrow). There are many lymphocytes, plasma cells and neutrophils in the bronchial walls (blue stars). The exudation and necrosis can be observed in the lumens (yellow star). The blood vessels are dilated, congested (green star), or hemorrhagic.

3. Pneumoconiosis

Silicosis (Fig.6-15)

Numerous irregular nodules (blue circles) and diffuse fibrous connective tissue proliferation are shown in the lung tissue, and some nodules center around blood vessels (blue arrows). Some nodules consist of macrophages with silica particles only (cellular silicotic nodule, red arrows), some nodules are composed of fibroblasts and collagen (fibrous silicotic nodule, Fig.6-15C), and other nodules present whorled or concentric collagen fibers with hyaline degeneration and calcification (red star). Some adjacent nodules merge into larger nodules.

4. Lung tumors

4. 1　Squamous cell carcinoma of lung (Fig.6-16)

The tumor cells are arranged in nests with obvious necroses (blue stars), and have infiltrated into the adjacent non-tumor tissue (blue arrows). The polygonal tumor cells have abundant eosinophilic cytoplasm and large, vesicular nuclei with clear nucleoli, and mitotic figures as well as pathological mitoses can be observed. The intracellular keratinization and intercellular bridges, indicators of squamous cells, are present (red arrow). There are chronic inflammatory cells infiltration and fibrotic proliferation in the stroma.

4. 2　Adenocarcinoma of lung (Fig.6-17)

The columnar or polygonal tumor cells arrange in tubular or cord-like structures (red arrows) with partial micropapillaries. The tumor cells show abundant eosinophilic cytoplasm containing vesicular secretion (green arrows). They present increased ratio of nucleus to cytoplasm, and irregular nucleoli with coarse chromatin (Fig. 6-17C). Mononucleated or multinucleated tumor giant cells are frequently seen. The mitoses are easily visible. The cancer cells have invaded the adjacent lung tissue (blue arrows).

4. 3   Small cell carcinoma of lung (Fig.6-18)

The tumor cells arrange in nests, sheets and trabecular (red circle) with fibroblast proliferation and hyaline degeneration in the stroma (green circles). The round, oval, and spindle-shaped tumor cells are relatively small cells with scant cytoplasm as lymphocytes, finely granular nuclear chromatin and inconspicuous nucleoli. Mitotic figures are easily observed.

Ⅳ. Clinical pathological discussion

Case

A 60-year-old male suffered fever (body temperature 38. 3℃), and coughed with white-foam sputum 5 days ago. The routine blood test shows that white blood cell count is 12.5×10^9/L, the percentage of neutrophils for 84%, and CRP for 58 mg/L. Antibiotics had been administrated, but the symptoms became worse 3 days ago. The sputum was yellow-green and too thick to expectorate. The rescue was ineffective and the patient died. The autopsy was performed and the morphological changes of lung are shown in Figure 6-19.

(1) What is the pathological diagnosis of the lung, and why?

(2) Please explain the symptoms and signs according to the pathological changes.

V. Questions

1. Describe the differences between lobar pneumonia and lobular pneumonia in morphology.

2. Describe the morphological features of chronic bronchitis, emphysema and bronchiectasis.

3. Please list macroscopical and microscopical classifications of lung cancers and corresponding morphological characteristics.

4. Terms: Pulmonary carnification, Lobar pneumonia, Lobular pneumonia, Virus inclusion body, Hyaline membrane, Severe acute respiratory syndrome, Chronic obstructive pulmonary diseases, Emphysema, Bronchiectasis, Silicosis, Silicotic nodule, Chronic cor pulmonale.

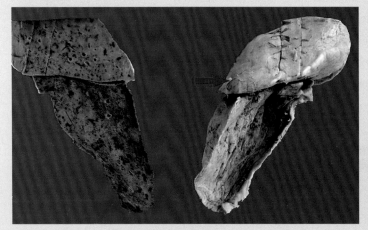
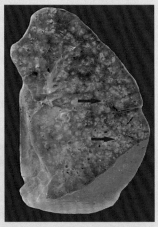

图 6-1　大叶性肺炎
Fig.6-1　Lobar pneumonia

图 6-2　小叶性肺炎
Fig.6-2　Lobular pneumonia

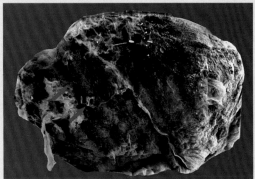
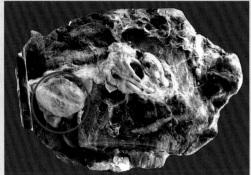

图 6-3　肺气肿
Fig.6-3　Emphysema

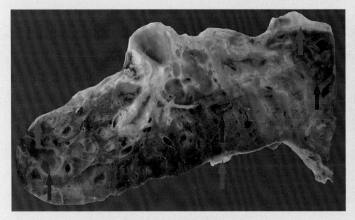
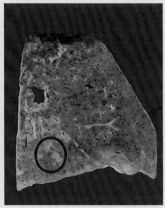

图 6-4　支气管扩张症
Fig.6-4　Bronchiectasis

图 6-5　硅肺
Fig.6-5　Silicosis

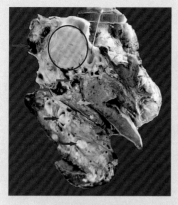 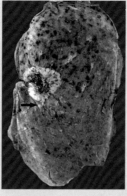 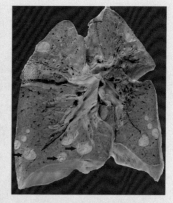

图 6-6　肺癌（中央型）　　　图 6-7　肺癌（周围型）　　　图 6-8　肺转移性肿瘤
Fig.6-6　Lung cancer　　　　Fig.6-7　Lung cancer　　　　Fig.6-8　Metastatic tumor
　　　（central type）　　　　　　　（peripheral type）　　　　　　　of lung

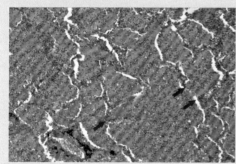 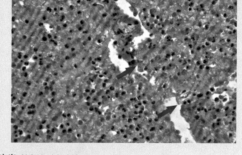

图 6-9　大叶性肺炎（×40；×400）
Fig.6-9　Lobar pneumonia（×40；×400）

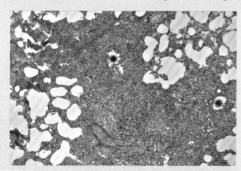 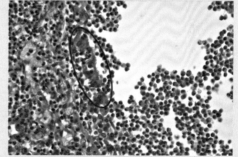

图 6-10　小叶性肺炎（×40；×400）
Fig.6-10　Lobular pneumonia（×40；×400）

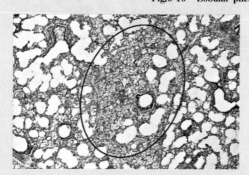 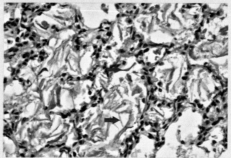

图 6-11　羊水吸入性肺炎（×40；×400）
Fig.6-11　Amniotic fluid aspiration pneumonia（×40；×400）

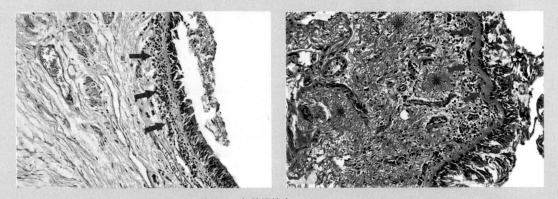

图 6-12　气管慢性炎（×200；×200）
Fig.6-12　Chronic inflammation of bronchus（×200；×200）

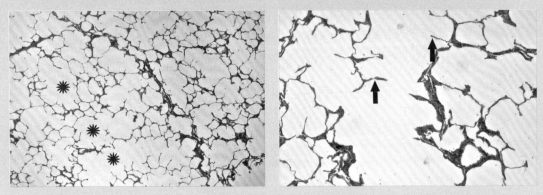

图 6-13　肺气肿（×40；×100）
Fig.6-13　Emphysema（×40；×100）

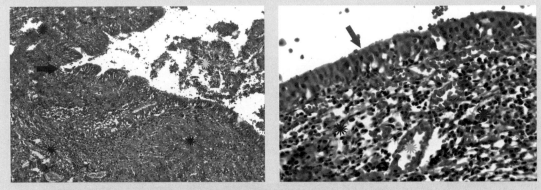

图 6-14　支气管扩张症（×100；×400）
Fig.6-14　Bronchiectasis（×100；×400）

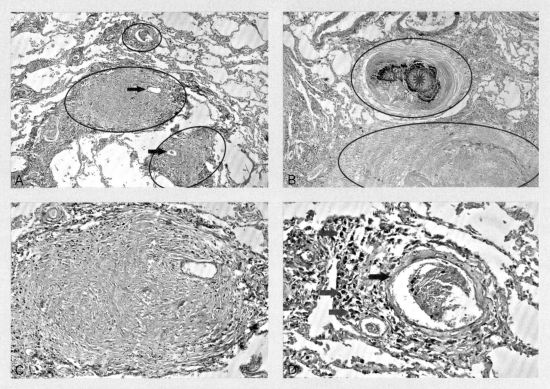

图 6-15　硅肺（A：×40；B：×40；C：×100；D：×200）
Fig.6-15　Silicosis（A：×40；B：×40；C：×100；D：×200）

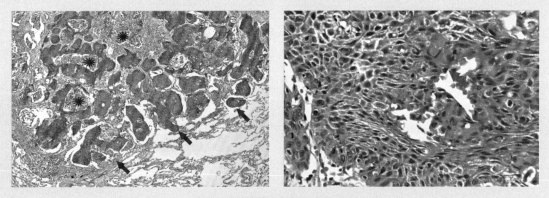

图 6-16　肺鳞状细胞癌（×40；×400）
Fig.6-16　Squamous cell carcinoma of lung（×40；×400）

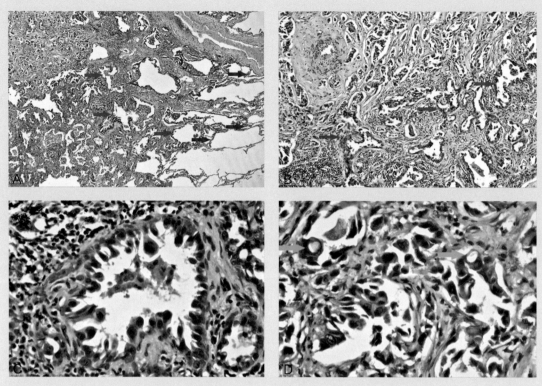

图 6-17　肺腺癌（A：×40；B：×100；C：×400；D：×400）
Fig.6-17　Adenocarcinoma of lung（A：×40；B：×100；C：×400；D：×400）

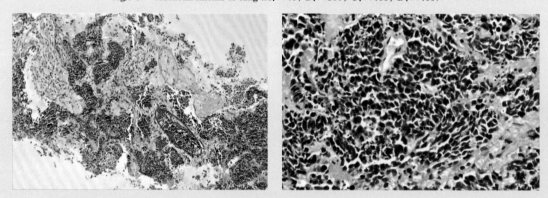

图 6-18　肺小细胞癌（×100；×400）
Fig.6-18　Small cell carcinoma of lung（×100；×400）

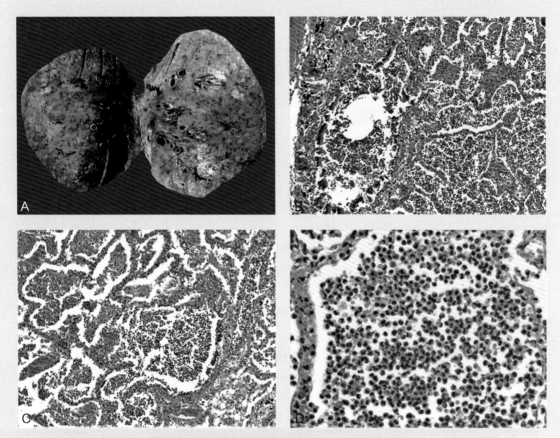

图 6-19　案例（A：大体；B：×100；C：×100；D：×400）
Fig.6-19　Case（A：Gross；B：×100；C：×100；D：×400）

盛蓁（Zhen Sheng）

第七章

消化系统疾病

一、目的要求

1. 掌握慢性消化性溃疡的病理特点。
2. 掌握各型病毒性肝炎的病变特点及临床病理联系。
3. 掌握各种肝硬化的病理特点及其后果，小结节性与大结节性肝硬化的异同点。
4. 掌握消化系统常见肿瘤的形态特征和临床病理联系。
5. 熟悉溃疡性结肠炎和克罗恩病的组织学特点。
6. 了解急慢性胃炎的组织学特点。

导学

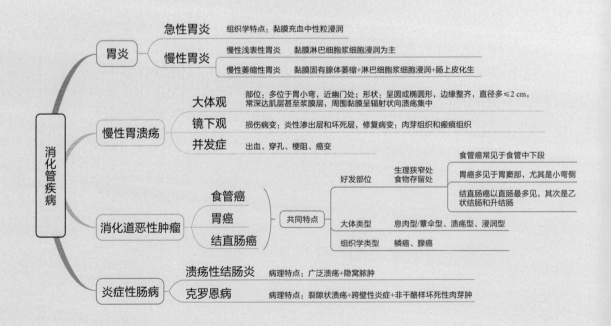

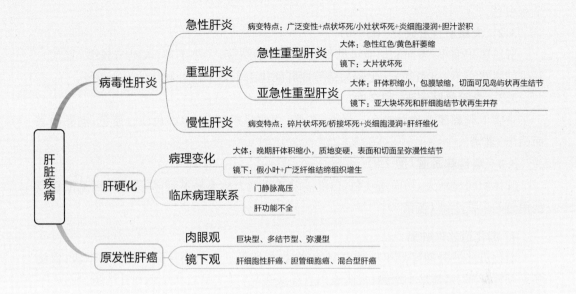

二、大体标本

1. 胃溃疡

1.1　急性胃溃疡（图 7-1）

次全切除胃标本沿胃大弯剪开，黏膜面散在大小不等、形态不规则的浅溃疡及糜烂（蓝箭），溃疡底多呈黑褐色，浆膜面未见明显异常。

1.2　慢性胃溃疡（图 7-2）

次全切除胃标本沿胃大弯剪开，溃疡位于胃小弯，近幽门处（蓝箭）；圆或椭圆形，直径小于 2 cm，深达肌层甚至浆膜层；边缘整齐如刀割状，贲门侧呈潜掘状，幽门侧呈斜坡状；周围黏膜呈辐射状向溃疡集中。

2. 病毒性肝炎

2.1　急性重型肝炎（图 7-3）

肝体积缩小，重量减轻，质软，包膜皱缩，边缘较锐。肝表面及切面呈黄绿色。切面见肝组织疏松，并有散在分布的灰黄色境界不清斑块（肝细胞坏死区）。因肝脏呈黄色，故旧称急性黄色肝萎缩。肝脏充血出血明显者，也称为急性红色肝萎缩。

2.2　亚急性重型肝炎（图 7-4）

肝脏体积缩小，表面略呈结节状，黄褐色，包膜皱缩，边缘锐利，质软。切面散布大小不等的土黄色斑块或结节。

3. 肝硬化

3.1　小结节性肝硬化（图 7-5）

肝脏体积缩小、变形、边缘变锐、重量减轻、质地变硬；表面及切面呈细颗粒状或小结节状，结节大小较一致（蓝箭），直径一般≤3 mm；结节间纤维间隔宽度≤2 mm（黄箭）。

结节可呈黄褐色（肝细胞脂肪变性）或黄绿色（含较多的胆色素），结节间纤维间隔纤细呈灰白色。

3.2　大结节性肝硬化（图7-6）

肝脏体积缩小，表面和切面可见弥漫性分布的结节，大小不等，大结节较多（蓝箭），纤维间隔宽窄不一（黄箭）。比较大结节性肝硬化与小结节性肝硬化的形态差异。

3.3　食管静脉曲张（图7-7）

食管下段黏膜下静脉吻合支淤血、扩张，弯曲呈蚯蚓状，暗红色或青紫色，向黏膜表面凸出（蓝箭）。

3.4　慢性脾淤血（图7-8）

脾体积明显增大，切面暗红色，白髓萎缩甚至消失故不易见到，局部区域可见散在呈深褐色的含铁小结（蓝箭）。

4.　消化道恶性肿瘤

消化道恶性肿瘤好发于生理狭窄处、食物存留处。食管癌常见于食管中下段；胃癌多见于胃窦部，尤其是小弯侧；大肠癌以直肠最多见，其次是乙状结肠和升结肠。

4.1　早期胃癌（图7-9）

次全切除胃标本示癌肿位于胃窦小弯侧，癌变处黏膜层缺损，称为"癌性糜烂"（蓝箭），边缘略不规则。思考：何谓早期胃癌，它的形态学含义是什么？

根据肿瘤生长方式、间质的多少以及坏死脱落等情况，进展期肿瘤大体形态可归为以下几种类型：

4.2　息肉型或蕈伞型（图7-10～图7-12）

食管、胃和结肠腔内可见肿瘤以外生性生长为主，形成息肉状、蕈伞状或巨块状肿块突入腔内（蓝箭），表面可坏死脱落；肿瘤组织浸润管壁较浅，常累及管壁周径的一部分。

4.3　溃疡型（图7-13～图7-15）

食管、胃部和结肠腔内均可见癌组织向管壁深层生长，累及管壁周径一部分，表面坏死脱落形成溃疡（蓝箭）。溃疡底部凹凸不平，溃疡边缘在食管常参差不齐，微向腔内突出；在胃或大肠则边缘呈结节状凸起或呈环堤状（如火山喷口状）。

4.4　弥漫浸润型或缩窄型（图7-16～图7-18）

癌组织弥漫浸润于消化管全周径的各层，无或伴有明显的间质结缔组织增生，管壁增厚僵硬导致食管、胃、肠管局部环形狭窄（蓝箭）。癌组织弥漫浸润于胃壁称革囊胃。

5.　肝脏肿瘤

5.1　原发性肝癌（巨块型）（图7-19）

整个肝脏体积明显增大，肝右叶可见一个明显的肿块（蓝圈），体积巨大，切面中心有出血坏死，瘤体周围出现了多个卫星状癌结节。

5.2　原发性肝癌（多结节型）（图7-20）

肝质地变硬，切面散在分布多个大小不等不规则癌结节（蓝箭）。

5.3　原发性肝癌（弥漫型）（图7-21）

癌组织弥散分布于全肝内，整个肝脏切面粗糙，无明显结节，但有散在的出血坏死。

三、 组织切片

1. 非肿瘤性疾病

1.1 胃炎

1.1.1 急性胃炎（图7-22）

胃镜活检黏膜组织。部分胃浅表黏膜上皮细胞变性坏死,灶性出血,固有层内血管扩张充血,大量炎细胞浸润,其间可见较多的中性粒细胞浸润（黄箭）。

1.1.2 慢性浅表性胃炎（图7-23）

胃镜活检黏膜组织。胃黏膜固有层内少量炎细胞浸润,以淋巴细胞和浆细胞为主。

1.1.3 慢性萎缩性胃炎（图7-24）

胃镜活检黏膜组织。胃黏膜固有腺体萎缩,局部腺上皮有肠上皮化生（蓝箭）,固有层水肿,有炎细胞浸润,可见淋巴滤泡形成。

1.2 慢性胃溃疡（图7-25）

切片中央见一凹陷即溃疡所在处,镜下见溃疡处胃黏膜、黏膜下层及部分肌层缺损形成溃疡,溃疡底部由浅向深大致可分为四层：① 炎性渗出物；② 坏死组织；③ 新鲜肉芽组织（绿箭）；④ 陈旧瘢痕组织,其中血管内膜常有增殖性动脉内膜炎（蓝星）,神经纤维常变性断裂、小球状增生（蓝箭）。溃疡边缘可见黏膜腺体增生,固有层有慢性炎细胞浸润；黏膜肌与肌层粘连。

1.3 病毒性肝炎

1.3.1 急性重型肝炎（图7-26）

肝组织广泛性大片状坏死（蓝星）,小叶内肝细胞消失,可见少量淋巴细胞浸润（蓝箭）。

1.3.2 慢性肝炎（图7-27）

肝组织内见明显的桥接坏死（蓝箭）,坏死区内主要以淋巴细胞浸润为主,伴有巨噬细胞和浆细胞。汇管区纤维结缔组织增生（黄箭）。一些肝细胞胞浆内充满嗜酸性细颗粒物质,不透明似毛玻璃样改变,称之为毛玻璃样肝细胞（黑箭）,主要见于HBsAg阳性时。

1.4 肝硬化

1.4.1 小结节性肝硬化（图7-28）

肝内有广泛的纤维结缔组织增生、破坏了肝小叶的正常结构,代之以大小不等的再生肝细胞结节——假小叶（蓝星）。假小叶内中央静脉常偏位、缺如或有两个以上的中央静脉；肝细胞板由多层肝细胞组成（正常肝板为单层）,排列紊乱；再生肝细胞体积较大、胞浆丰富略呈嗜碱性,核大深染,可有双核；有的区域肝细胞呈现不同程度萎缩、变性、坏死、淤胆,有的区域肝细胞基本正常。假小叶周围为增生的纤维结缔组织包绕,纤维间隔宽窄比较一致（绿星）,其中含有新生的细小胆管和假胆管,并有一定量的淋巴细胞、单核细胞浸润。

1.4.2 大结节性肝硬化（图7-29）

大结节性肝硬化病变与小结节性肝硬化类似,肝内有广泛的纤维结缔组织增生（绿星）和假小叶形成（蓝星），但假小叶内肝细胞变性坏死更为明显，纤维间隔宽窄不一，纤维间隔内炎细胞浸润和胆管增生更为显著。

1.5　炎症性肠病

1.5.1　溃疡性结肠炎（图7-30）

结肠黏膜有广泛溃疡形成（蓝箭），黏膜及黏膜下层可见中性粒细胞、淋巴细胞、浆细胞及嗜酸性粒细胞浸润，肠隐窝有微小脓肿形成（黄箭）。

1.5.2　克罗恩病（图7-31）

肠壁各层有明显炎症性病变。黏膜层可见溃疡，深达肌层，固有层水肿、淋巴管扩张、淋巴组织增生（黄星），局部肉芽肿形成。

2　消化系统恶性肿瘤

2.1　早期胃癌（图7-32）

癌组织局限在黏膜层内，未突破黏膜肌层。癌细胞形成不规则腺样结构，有的腺体扩张，腔内充满大量红染无结构的坏死物质（蓝星）。

2.2　食管鳞状细胞癌（图7-33）

癌组织形成不规则的癌巢（黑箭），浸润食管管壁全层，侵及外膜。一侧可见被覆鳞状上皮的食管黏膜组织（蓝箭）。

2.3　胃腺癌（图7-34）

胃壁组织，癌细胞呈不规则腺管状排列。部分腺腔内有脱落的肿瘤细胞（黑星）。癌组织已突破黏膜肌层，浸润黏膜下层及肌层。一侧可见正常胃黏膜（蓝箭）。

2.4　结肠腺癌（图7-35）

结肠壁内癌组织呈浸润性生长达浆膜层。癌细胞呈腺管状排列，部分腺腔内有癌细胞分泌的黏液样物。

2.5　肝细胞性肝癌（图7-36）

癌组织由不同分化的肿瘤细胞组成。分化好的区域癌细胞呈索状排列（蓝星），核大、异型性明显，周边为血窦。分化差的区域癌细胞呈团块状，胞浆弱嗜碱性，偶见胆汁颗粒。癌组织挤压周围肝组织，与肝组织分界相对清楚。

2.6　肝转移性腺癌（图7-37）

切片取自肝组织，正常的肝脏结构大部分被破坏，由癌组织占据。癌细胞来源于腺上皮，形成大小不等、形态不一、排列不规则的腺样结构（蓝星）。黑星示少量未被完全破坏的肝组织。

四、临床病理讨论

案例　1　患者，女性，35岁。上腹部隐痛3年余，去年起腹痛加剧，经常呕吐。两个月来，面部及手足水肿，尤以左上肢为显著，尿量减少，食欲极差。半小时前，排黑色大便，呕吐大量鲜血，突然昏倒而急诊入院。体检：消瘦，面色苍白，四肢厥冷，血压60/40 mmHg，心音快而弱。两侧颈部，左锁骨上及腋下淋巴结显著肿大。血红蛋白90 g/L，血浆总蛋白42 g/L，白蛋白14 g/L。抢救无效死亡。

尸检摘要:左上肢极度水肿,两下肢及背部亦见水肿。胸腹腔内分别有 1 000 ml 及 500 ml 淡黄色澄清液体。胃小弯幽门区有一 4 cm×5 cm×5 cm 肿块,质硬,表面溃疡、出血。镜检为腺癌(图 7-38A,B)。胃周围淋巴结、颈部及腋下淋巴结均见腺癌组织(图 7-38C,D)。肝肿大,淡黄色,质较软,肝细胞内充满圆形空泡,核被挤在一侧(图 7-38E,F)。肾小管上皮细胞内充满粉红色颗粒。

(1)患者入院时的临床表现是何原因引起?

(2)本例水肿与积水的原因是什么?

(3)肝脏与肾脏可能有何病变? 分析其原因。

(4)试按疾病发展过程写出病理诊断。

案例 2 患者,男性,26 岁。因发热、上腹饱胀及乏力 6 天入院。患者于 6 天前感觉发冷发热,并有上腹部饱胀及乏力。第二天症状加剧,尿黄。第三天全身皮肤发黄,乏力明显,伴恶心呕吐。

体检:肝肋下未及,肝上界第 6 肋间。实验室检查:血清总胆红素 330 μmol/L(正常< 34 μmol/L),谷丙转氨酶 1 050 U/L(正常< 100 U/L),HBsAg(+),凝血酶原时间 148 秒(正常 13 秒)。

住院经过:入院后黄疸进行性加深。次日下午出现神经精神症状。第三天神志昏迷,肝脏进行性缩小,消化道持续不断出血,量多。第五天体温骤升至 40℃,持续抽搐,肝肾功能衰竭而死亡。

尸检摘要:巩膜和全身皮肤高度黄染。肝脏体积明显缩小,右叶居肋弓以内,左叶在剑突以上,重 730 g(正常 1 500 g 左右)。包膜皱缩,表面暗红并黄染,质地柔软可以卷曲,尤以左叶为甚。切面黄绿色,小叶结构不清。镜检:肝细胞大片坏死,仅残留汇管区周围少量肝细胞,有广泛出血(图 7-39)。肾组织见肾小管上皮细胞变性坏死,尤以远端小管明显,管腔堵塞、充满管型。肺组织有广泛出血。心外膜亦见出血。

(1)患者所患肝炎为哪种类型?

(2)患者是身强力壮的青年,抵抗力较好,为什么肝炎却如此严重?

(3)患者为什么全身出血? 为什么发生肾衰竭?

五、 思考题

1. 比较良性胃溃疡和恶性胃溃疡的肉眼形态差异。

2. 试分析慢性胃溃疡不易愈合的原因及常见并发症。

3. 重型病毒性肝炎的病理变化有何特点? 试讨论其临床表现的病理基础。

4. 肝硬化的基本病变及其对机体的影响如何?

5. 简述肝硬化主要累及的侧支循环及并发症。

6. 试述肝炎、肝硬化与肝癌之间的关系。

7. 试述消化管恶性肿瘤的共同形态学特征。

8. 名词解释:嗜酸性小体,点状坏死,碎片状坏死,桥接坏死,肝硬化,假小叶,毛玻璃样肝细胞,早期胃癌,革囊胃。

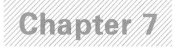

Diseases of Digestive System

Ⅰ. Aims

1. To grasp the pathological features of peptic ulcer.

2. To grasp the characteristics and clinicopathologic relationship of various types of viral hepatitis.

3. To grasp the pathological features and their consequences in various types of liver cirrhosis, and the difference between micronodular cirrhosis and macronodular cirrhosis.

4. To grasp the morphologic features of the common malignant tumors of digestive system.

5. To familiarize with the histological characteristics of ulcerative colitis and Crohn's disease.

6. To understand the histological features of acute and chronic gastritis.

Guidance to study

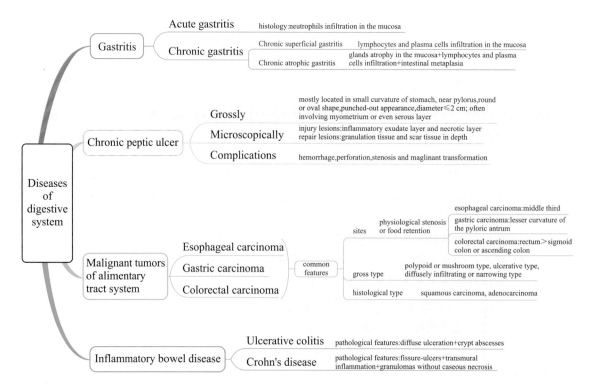

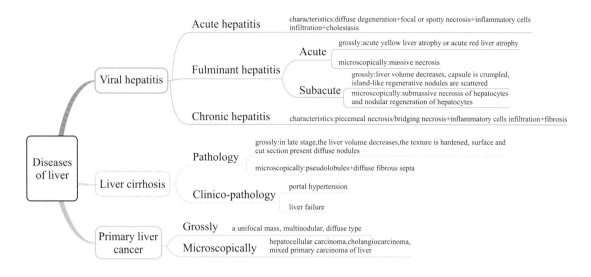

II. Gross specimens

1. Gastric ulcer

1.1　Acute gastric ulcer（Fig.7-1）

This is a subtotal gastrectomy specimen cut along greater curvature. Superficial ulcers and erosions with various sizes（blue arrows）scatter on the mucosa, and the bases of the ulcers are mostly pitchy.

1.2　Chronic gastric ulcer（Fig.7-2）

This is a subtotal gastrectomy specimen cut along greater curvature. Chronic peptic ulcer （blue arrow）locates in the lesser curvature and closes to pyloric antrum. The diameter of the oval ulcer is less than 2 cm, and the edge is neat with a shape like to be cut by a knife. The cardia side is burrowing, and the pylorus side is sloping. The mucosal folds around the ulcer radiate outwards from the center of the ulcer.

2. Viral hepatitis

2.1　Acute fulminant hepatitis（Fig.7-3）

The liver is shrunken and limp with decreased weight. The capsule is wrinkled. Both the surface and cut section are yellowish-green. On cut section, hepatic tissue becomes loosen with scattered yellow necrotic area, which is also named acute yellow/red hepatic atrophy because of the changes of congestion/necrosis in the liver.

2.2　Subacute fulminant hepatitis（Fig.7-4）

The liver is shrunken and yellowish-brown, while the surface displays slightly nodularity with a wrinkled capsule. On cut section, isabelline plaque or regenerative nodules with unequable sizes scatter in the liver.

3. Liver cirrhosis

3. 1　Micronodular cirrhosis（Fig.7-5）

The liver is shrunk and deformed with sharp edge and reduced weight. The surface and cut surface show small nodules（blue arrow）, which is uniform in size with the diameter of less than 3 mm. The width of grayish white fibrous septa between nodules is thinner than 2 mm（yellow arrow）. The nodules are yellowish brown（fatty degeneration of liver cells）or yellowish green（containing more bile pigments）.

3. 2　Macronodular cirrhosis（Fig.7-6）

The liver is reduced in size. Both the surface and cut surface present diffusely distributed nodules in various sizes. Most nodules are large（blue arrow）, and the fibrous septa are widened （yellow arrow）. Please distinguish macronodular cirrhosis from micronodular cirrhosis in morphology.

3. 3　Varices of esophagus（Fig.7-7）

The submucosa veins of the lower esophagus are congested, dilated, crooked like earthworms with dark red in morphology and protrude into the mucosal surface（blue arrows）.

3. 4　Chronic congestion of spleen（congestive splenomegaly）（Fig.7-8）

The spleen is obviously enlarged and the splenic tissue on the cut section is dark red. The white pulps are atrophic, or even disappeared. There are scattered dark brown siderotic nodules（blue arrow）.

4. Carcinoma of alimentary tract

Carcinomas of alimentary tract usually occur at the sites of physiological stenosis or food retention. For example, esophagus cancer commonly occurs in the middle third of esophagus, while gastric carcinoma is in the lesser curvature of pyloric antrum, and carcinoma of the colon is mostly in rectum, secondly in sigmoid colon or ascending colon.

4. 1　Early gastric carcinoma（Fig.7-9）

This is a subtotal gastrectomy specimen and the neoplasm locates in the lesser curvature. There is a shallow ulcer in the mucosa, cancerous erosion（blue arrow）. The ulcer margin is slightly irregular. What's the definition of early gastric carcinoma in morphology?

According to growth patterns, interstitial amount, and secondary ulceration of cancer tissues, advanced carcinoma（late carcinoma）is grossly divided into the following types:

4. 2　Polypoid or mushroom type（Fig.7-10～7-12）

When extending into the lumens, the tumors are considered as polypoid, or fungating masses by exophytic growth, and the tumor surfaces commonly shed from the mass due to necrosis（blue arrows）. The tumor tissues usually infiltrate superficial zones of the alimentary walls, and involve certain part of the circumference.

4. 3   Ulcerative type（Fig.7-13～7-15）

An ulcerative cancer in the esophagus, stomach or colon mainly grows into deep zones of the wall and involves a part of circumference (blue arrows). The tumor surface is apt to necrosis, and appears as ulcers, and the tumor base is rough.

4. 4   Diffusely infiltrating or narrowing type（Fig.7-16～7-18）

This type of tumor infiltrates all the layer of digestive tracts with or without fibrous connective tissue hyperplasia. When fibrous connective tissue obviously proliferates, the involved wall of alimentary tract becomes so thickened and hard as to make annular stricture (blue arrows). If the tumor widely spreads and permeates gastric wall, the stomach is named as leather-bottle stomach.

5. The tumors of liver

5. 1   Primary hepatocellular carcinoma（unifocal mass type）（Fig.7-19）

The whole liver is obviously enlarged, and a large mass is noticeable in the right lobe of the liver (blue circle), with hemorrhage and necrosis in the center. Multiple satellite cancerous nodules are around the tumor mass.

5. 2   Primary hepatocellular carcinoma（multinodular type）（Fig.7-20）

Multiple irregular cancer nodules (blue arrows) scatter in the liver, and the liver becomes stiff and irregular.

5. 3   Primary hepatocellular carcinoma（diffuse type）（Fig.7-21）

The cancer tissues are dispersed in the whole liver which is rough. There are scattered hemorrhage and necroses without visible nodules on the cut surface.

Ⅲ. Tissue sections

1. Non neoplastic diseases

1. 1   Gastritis

1. 1. 1   Acute gastritis（Fig. 7-22）

This is a gastric biopsy specimen from clinical gastroscopy. Some epithelial cells are degenerative and necrotic with focal bleeding in the gastric superficial mucosal tissue. Blood vessels within the lamina propria are dilated and congested. A large number of inflammatory cells, mainly neutrophils (yellow arrows), are notable.

1. 1. 2   Chronic superficial gastritis（Fig. 7-23）

This is a piece of mucosal tissue from gastric biopsy. Some inflammatory cells (mainly lymphocytes and plasma cells) infiltrate into the lamina propria.

1. 1. 3   Chronic atrophic gastritis（Fig. 7-24）

The mucosal inherent glands are atrophic and lamina propria is edematous. There are some inflammatory cells infiltration and lymphocyte follicle formation in the mucosa. The local gland epithelial cells present intestinal metaplasia (blue arrows).

1. 2　Chronic gastric ulcer (Fig.7-25)

On the center of the section, there is a mucosal defect showing the ulcerative tissue, which involves gastric mucosa, submucosa and part of muscularis. It can be roughly divided into four layers from superficiality to depth: inflammatory exudate, necrotic tissue, fresh granulation tissue (green arrows), and old scar tissue. Vessels trapped within the scar tissue present proliferative endoarteritis with thickened walls (blue asterisks). Nerve fibers often show degeneration, rupture, and spherical proliferation (blue arrow). At the edge of the ulcer, mucosa epithelium hyperplasia and chronic inflammatory cells infiltration are obvious.

1. 3　Viral hepatitis

1. 3. 1　Acute fulminant hepatitis (Fig. 7-26)

The liver show extensive massive necrosis (blue asterisks), and hepatocytes in the lobules almost disappear, with a small number of lymphocytes infiltration (blue arrow).

1. 3. 2　Chronic hepatitis (Fig. 7-27)

There are significant bridge necroses in the liver (blue arrow) with numerous inflammatory cells infiltration. The inflammatory cells are mainly lymphocytes, macrophages and plasma cells. Fibrous connective tissue hyperplasia is observed in the portal areas (yellow arrow). Some liver cells having eosinophilic, granular, glassy cytoplasm are defined as ground-glass hepatocytes (black arrow), which is closely associated with hepatitis B positive infection.

1. 4　Liver cirrhosis

1. 4. 1　Micronodular cirrhosis (Fig. 7-28)

Hyperplastic fibrous connective tissues are diffuse, which has destroyed normal structure of the liver. The injured area is replaced by regenerative hepatocyte nodules, pseudolobules (blue asterisks). The pseudolobules are characterized by irregular arrangement of hepatic cells and loss of normal distribution of central and portal tracts. Hepatocytes in the pseudolobule may be normal, degenerative, regenerative, and necrotic. The fibrous septa (green asterisks) contain fine collagen fibers with proliferative small bile ducts, pseudobiliary ducts and infiltrating lymphocytes and monocytes.

1. 4. 2　Macronodular cirrhosis (Fig. 7-29)

Pathological changes in macronodular cirrhosis are similar to micronodular cirrhosis which includes extensive hyperplastic fibrous connective tissues (green asterisks) and pseudolobules (blue asterisks). But the hepatocytes degeneration and necrosis in the pseudolobules is more serious, and the width of fibrous septa is broader with severe inflammatory cell infiltration and bile duct hyperplasia.

1. 5   Inflammatory bowel disease

1. 5. 1   Ulcerative colitis (Fig. 7-30)

There is an extensive ulcer in the intestinal mucosa (blue arrow). Neutrophils, lymphocytes, plasma cells and eosinophils infiltrate into the mucosa and submucosa. Minimal abscesses can be observed in the intestinal fossae (yellow arrow).

1. 5. 2   Crohn's disease (Fig. 7-31)

The deep ulcer reaching to the muscle layer is observed in the intestinal wall. It presents lamina propria edema, lymphatic vessels dilation and lymphatic tissue hyperplasia (yellow asterisks), as well as local noncaseating granulomas.

2.   The malignant tumors of digestive system

2. 1   Early gastric carcinoma (Fig.7-32)

The neoplastic cells are confined to the mucosal layer, and the mucosal muscle layer is intact. The neoplastic cells appear as irregular adenoid structures, with lots of red-stained unstructured necrotic materials in the cavities (blue asterisks).

2. 2   Esophageal squamous cell carcinoma (Fig.7-33)

The neoplastic cells appear as irregular cancer nests (black arrows), which involve the whole esophageal wall. The blue arrow indicates squamous epithelium.

2. 3   Gastric adenocarcinoma (Fig.7-34)

The neoplastic tissue has involved the gastric mucosa, submucosa and muscle layers. Tumor cells arrange irregularly as glandular tubes, and some neoplastic glandular cavities contain dislodged neoplastic cells (black asterisks). The blue arrow shows non-tumor gastric mucosa.

2. 4   Colonic adenocarcinoma (Fig.7-35)

The tumor tissues have infiltrated the colonic submucosa by infiltrating growth. The tumor cells appear as irregular glandular structures, and some glands have mucoid substances in the lumens.

2. 5   Hepatocellular carcinoma (Fig.7-36)

The neoplastic tissue displays variable differentiation. In the well differentiated areas, tumor cells arrange in cords with rich sinusoids (blue asterisks). The neoplastic cells have enlarged nuclei with prominent nucleoli and hyperchromatism, and some contain bile pigments in the cytoplasm. The poorly differentiated regions present sheets of anaplastic cells with weak basophilic cytoplasm. Cancer tissues compress the surrounding liver tissue, but showing a relatively clear boundary between them.

2. 6   Metastatic adenocarcinoma of liver (Fig.7-37)

The liver architecture is mostly disrupted and occupied by cancerous tissue. Cancerous cells derive from glandular epithelial cells and form irregular adenoid structures with different sizes and shapes (blue asterisks). The black asterisks indicate incompletely injured liver tissue.

IV. Clinic pathologic discussion

Cases 1

A 35-year-old woman has experienced epigastric dull pain for more than 3 years. The abdominal pain has increased with vomiting since last year. During the latest two months, her face, hands and feet began to swell, especially in the left upper limb, with decreased urine volume and poor appetite. Half an hour ago, she excreted black stool and vomited a lot of blood, then suddenly fainted. Therefore, she was admitted to emergency. Physical examination: she is thin with pale face and cold limbs. Her blood pressure is 60/40 mmHg, and heart sound was fast and weak. Bilateral cervical, left supraclavicular, and axillary lymph nodes were significantly enlarged. Laboratory testing: Hemoglobin: 90g/L, plasma total protein: 42 g/L, albumin: 14 g/L. The rescue was ineffective.

Autopsy: Severe edema was examined in the left upper limb as well both lower limbs and the back. There was 1 000 mL and 500 mL yellowish clear effusion in the thoracic and abdominal cavities, respectively. A hard mass with the size of 4 cm×5 cm×5 cm was found in the lesser curvature of gastric pylorus, and ulcer and bleeding were present on the surface of the tumor. She was pathologically diagnosed as adenocarcinoma (Fig. 7-38 A, B). Adenocarcinoma tissue was also found in peripheral gastric lymph nodes as well as cervical and axillary lymph nodes (Fig.7-38 C, D). The liver was swollen, pale yellow, and soft. The liver cells were filled with round vacuoles, and the nuclei were pushed aside (Fig.7-38 E, F). The renal tubular epithelial cells were filled with pink particles in the cytoplasm.

(1) How to explain clinical manifestations of this patient at the time of admission, and try to analyze the possible causes.

(2) What results in edema and hydrops in this case?

(3) What are pathological diagnoses of the liver and kidney?

(4) According to pathological developing process, list the pathological diagnoses of the involved tissues.

Case 2

A 26 years old man was hospitalized because of fever, upper abdominal fullness, and fatigue for 6 days. The patient felt fatigue, cold, and had a fever with upper abdominal fullness 6 days ago. The next day, these symptoms became worsened and the urine was yellow. On the third day, the overall skin got yellow, and he felt more fatigue with nausea and vomiting.

Physical examination: the liver lower margin was not be touched under the rib, and the upper margin was at the sixth intercostal. Laboratory examination: serum total bilirubin:

330 μmol/L (normal < 34 μmol/L), ALT: 1 050 U/L (normal < 100 U/L). HBsAg($+$), prothrombin time: 148 seconds (normal: 13 seconds).

Hospitalization: The jaundice was gradually deepened after admission. There were neuropsychiatric symptoms in the next afternoon. He was unconscious on the third day, the liver was progressively shrunk, and large amount of bleeding occurred continuously from the digestive tract. On the 5th day, his temperature suddenly increased up to 40℃, and he died of continuous convulsions with liver and kidney failure.

Autopsy: His sclera and systemic skin presented highly yellow. The liver was obviously shrunken, the right lobe was within the rib arch, the left lobe was above the xiphoid process, and the weight was 730 g (normal 1 500 g). The hepatic capsule was crumpled, the surface was dark red and yellow, and the liver was soft and curled, especially in the left lobe. The cut section was yellowish-green and the lobule structure was unclear. Microscopic examination: the liver presented massive necrosis, only a small number of hepatocytes around the residual portal area still remained, with extensive bleeding (Fig.7-39). Renal tubular epithelial cells were alterative, especially in the distal tubules. Renal tubular lumens were filled with casts. Lung tissues presented extensive hemorrhage. The epicardium was also hemorrhagic.

(1) Which type of hepatitis is for this case?

(2) The patient is a young man with good resistance, why is the hepatitis so severe?

(3) Why did the patient present systemic bleeding?

(4) Why did renal failure occur?

V. Questions

1. Compare the macroscopic features of benign gastric ulcer with malignant gastric ulcer in morphology.

2. Try to explain why chronic gastric ulcer is not easy to be healed, and list the common complications.

3. What are pathological characteristics of acute fulminant viral hepatitis? Try to discuss the pathological basis of clinic manifestations.

4. What are the causes and pathological features of liver cirrhosis?

5. Describe the main collateral circulation and complications caused by cirrhosis.

6. Describe the mutual relationship among hepatitis, cirrhosis, and primary hepatocellular carcinoma.

7. Summarize the common morphological features of carcinomas of digestive tract.

8. Terms: Acidophilic body (Councilman body), Spotty necrosis, Piecemeal necrosis, Bridging necrosis, Liver cirrhosis, Pseudolobule, Ground-glass hepatocyte, Early gastric carcinoma, Leather-bottle stomach.

Ⅵ. 附图 (Figures)

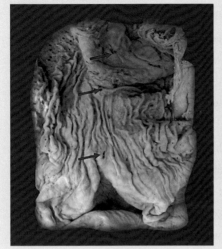

图 7-1 急性胃溃疡

Fig.7-1 Acute gastric ulcer

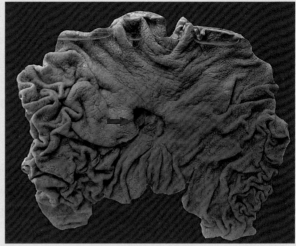

图 7-2 慢性胃溃疡

Fig.7-2 Chronic gastric ulcer

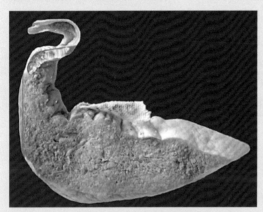

图 7-3 急性重型肝炎

Fig.7-3 Acute fulminant hepatitis

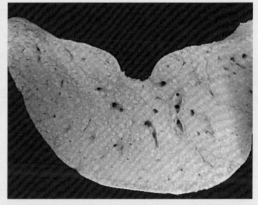

图 7-4 亚急性重型肝炎

Fig.7-4 Subacute fulminant hepatitis

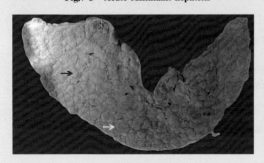

图 7-5 小结节性肝硬化

Fig.7-5 Micronodular cirrhosis

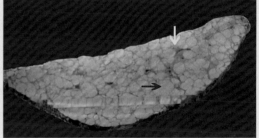

图 7-6 大结节性肝硬化

Fig.7-6 Macronodular cirrhosis

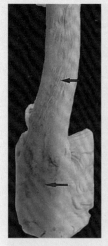
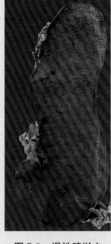
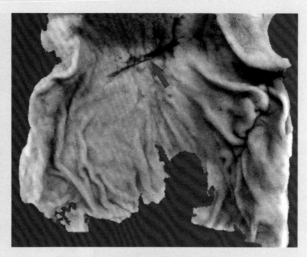

图 7-7 食管
静脉曲张
Fig.7-7 Varices
of esophagus

图 7-8 慢性脾淤血
Fig.7-8 Chronic
congestion of spleen

图 7-9 早期胃癌
Fig.7-9 Early gastric carcinoma

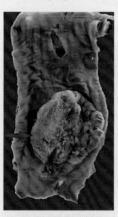
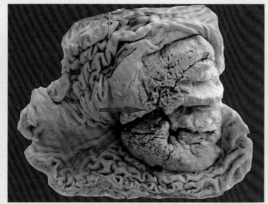
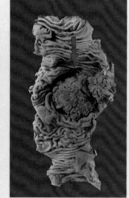

图 7-10 食管癌
（蕈伞型）
Fig.7-10 Esophageal
carcinoma（mushroom type）

图 7-11 胃癌（息肉型）
Fig.7-11 Gastric carcinoma（polypoid type）

图 7-12 结肠癌
（息肉型）
Fig.7-12 Colonic
carcinoma（polypoid type）

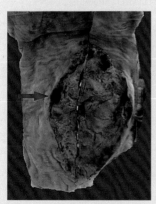
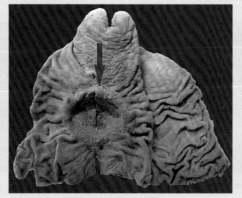
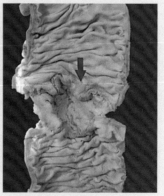

图 7-13 食管癌（溃疡型）
Fig.7-13 Esophageal
carcinoma（ulcerative type）

图 7-14 胃癌（溃疡型）
Fig.7-14 Gastric carcinoma（ulcerative type）

图 7-15 结肠癌（溃疡型）
Fig.7-15 Colonic carcinoma
（ulcerative type）

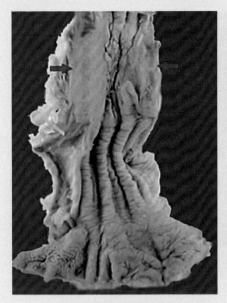

图 7-16　食管癌（缩窄型）
Fig.7-16　Esophageal carcinoma
（narrowing type）

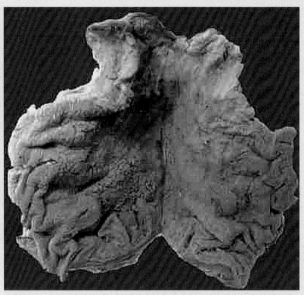

图 7-17　胃癌（浸润型）
Fig.7-17　Gastric carcinoma（infiltrating type）

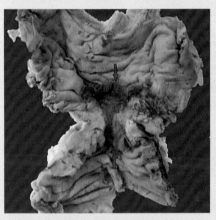

图 7-18　结肠癌（浸润型）
Fig.7-18　Colonic carcinoma
（infiltrating type）

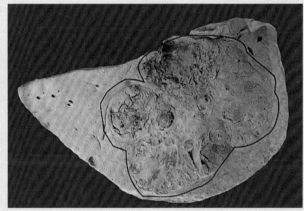

图 7-19　原发性肝癌（巨块型）
Fig.7-19　Primary hepatocellular carcinoma（unifocal mass type）

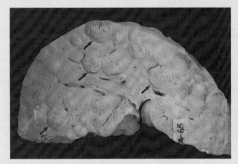

图 7-20　原发性肝癌（多结节型）
Fig.7-20　Primary hepatocellular carcinoma
（multinodular type）

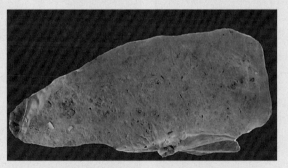

图 7-21　原发性肝癌（弥漫型）
Fig.7-21　Primary hepatocellular carcinoma（diffuse type）

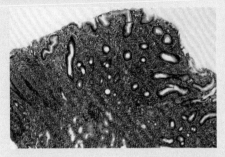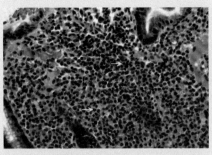

图 7-22　急性胃炎（×100；×400）
Fig.7-22　Acute gastritis（×100；×400）

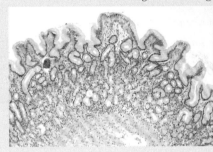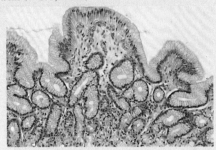

图 7-23　慢性浅表性胃炎（×100；×200）
Fig.7-23　Chronic superficial gastritis（×100；×200）

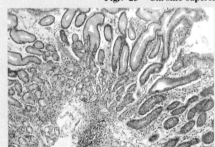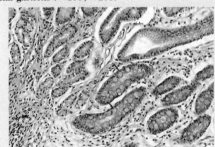

图 7-24　慢性萎缩性胃炎（×100；×200）
Fig.7-24　Chronic atrophic gastritis（×100；×200）

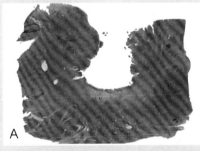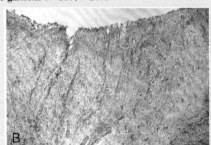
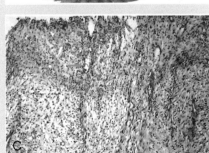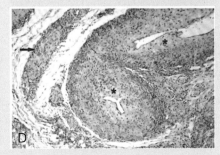

图 7-25　慢性胃溃疡（A：×2；B：×40；C，D：×100）
Fig.7-25　Chronic gastric ulcer（A：×2；B：×40；C，D：×100）

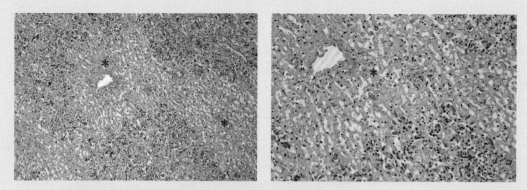

图 7-26　急性重型肝炎（×100；×200）
Fig.7-26　Acute fulminant hepatitis（×100；×200）

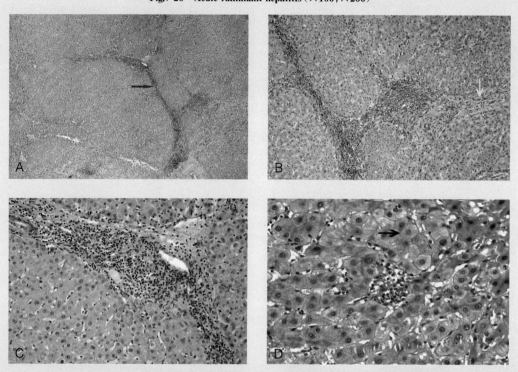

图 7-27　慢性肝炎（A：×40；B：×100；C，D：×200）
Fig.7-27　Chronic hepatitis（A：×40；B：×100；C，D：×200）

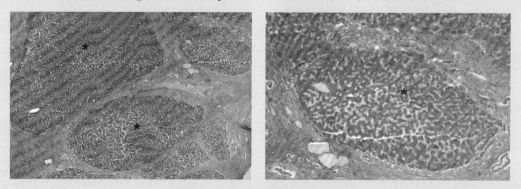

图 7-28　小结节性肝硬化（×40；×100）
Fig.7-28　Micronodular cirrhosis（×40；×100）

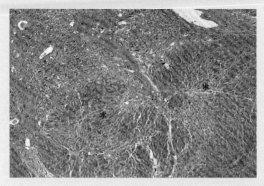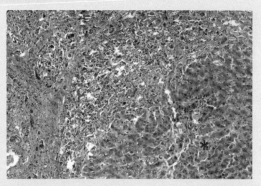

图 7-29　大结节性肝硬化（×40；×100）
Fig.7-29　Macronodular cirrhosis（×40；×100）

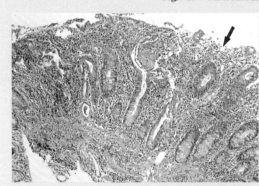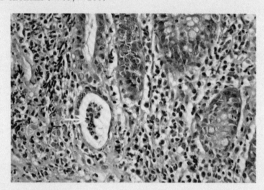

图 7-30　溃疡性结肠炎（×40；×200）
Fig.7-30　Ulcerative colitis（×40；×200）

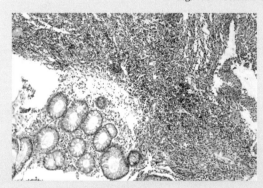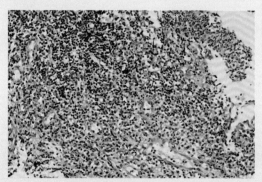

图 7-31　克罗恩病（×40；×200）
Fig.7-31　Crohn's disease（×40；×200）

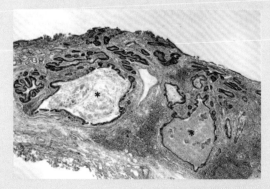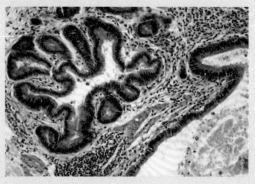

图 7-32　早期胃癌（×40；×200）
Fig.7-32　Early gastric carcinoma（×40；×200）

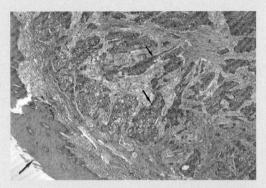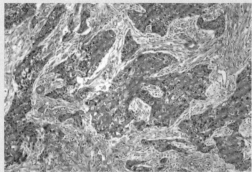

图 7-33　食管鳞状细胞癌（×40；×100）

Fig.7-33　Esophageal squamous cell carcinoma（×40；×100）

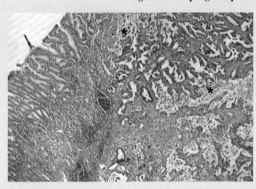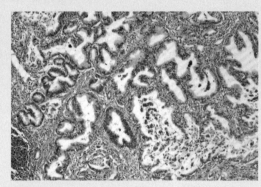

图 7-34　胃腺癌（×40；×100）

Fig.7-34　Gastric adenocarcinoma（×40；×100）

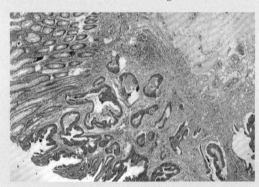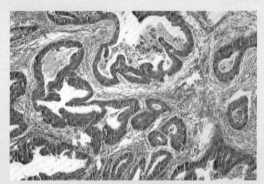

图 7-35　结肠腺癌（×40；×100）

Fig.7-35　Colonic adenocarcinoma（×40；×100）

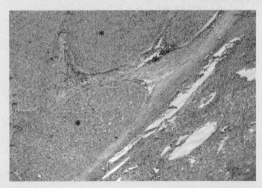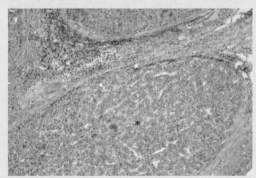

图 7-36　肝细胞性肝癌（×40；×100）

Fig.7-36　Hepatocellular carcinoma（×40；×100）

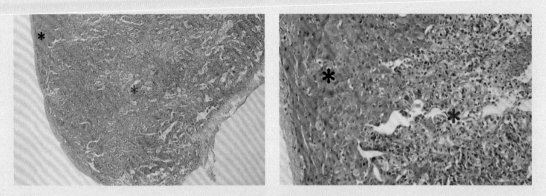

图 7-37　肝转移性腺癌（×40；×100）

Fig.7-37　Metastatic adenocarcinoma of liver（×40；×100）

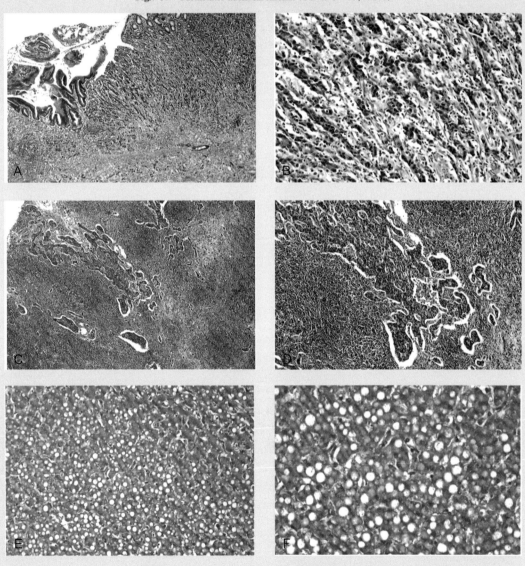

图 7-38　案例 1（A,C；×40；E；×100；B,D,F；×200）

Fig.7-38　Case1（A,C；×40；E；×100；B,D,F；×200）

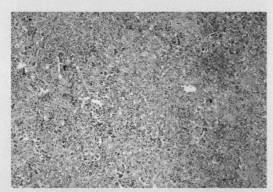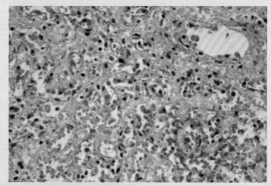

图 7-39　案例 2（×40；×200）
Fig.7-39　Case 2（×40；×200）

张爱凤（Aifeng Zhang）

第八章
淋巴造血系统疾病

一、目的要求

1. 掌握淋巴瘤的概念、霍奇金淋巴瘤的分型和病理特点。
2. 熟悉非霍奇金淋巴瘤的常见类型和病变特点。
3. 了解白血病的基本概念、分类和病变特点。

导学

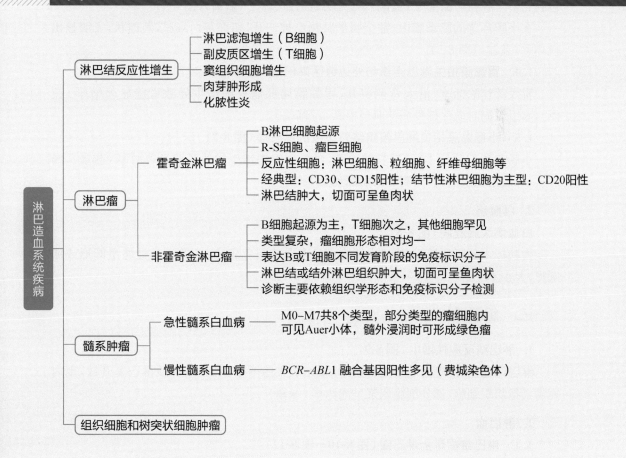

二、大体标本

1. 淋巴瘤

1.1 脾脏霍奇金淋巴瘤（图 8-1）

标本为荷瘤脾脏，被切成片状。表面呈不规则结节状隆起（蓝箭），包膜完整、欠光滑，有纤维素附着。脾脏切面大部分区域被淡红色肿瘤组织占据，和周围组织分界清楚。肿瘤质软、细腻，纤维组织增生，分割包绕肿瘤组织，但不完整。肿瘤内可见出血坏死。

1.2 淋巴结非霍奇金淋巴瘤（图 8-2）

非霍奇金淋巴瘤累及纵隔淋巴结、腰淋巴结、髂淋巴结等。可见淋巴结（蓝圈）肿大、粘连，切面灰红色、细腻，鱼肉状，无明显出血、坏死。图中尚见食管（已剪开）和双肾。

1.3 肠系膜淋巴结非霍奇金淋巴瘤（图 8-3～图 8-5）

不整形灰黄色脂肪组织中多个灰白色、不规则或略呈球形肿物（蓝星）。有些肿物和周围组织界限清楚，包膜完整；有些肿物相互融合，与周围组织分界不清。肿物切面细腻，有明显出血、坏死（图 8-3）。

与图 8-3 类似的不整形组织中有多个大小不等球形肿物，和周围组织界限较清楚，包膜完整。肿物切面细腻（蓝圈），可见明显出血、坏死（蓝箭）（图 8-4）。

在小肠环绕的肠系膜内，数个圆形肿物已被切开，切面灰白细腻，鱼肉状，无明显出血坏死（蓝星）（图 8-5）。

1.4 胃黏膜相关淋巴组织结外边缘区淋巴瘤（图 8-6）

胃大部切除标本，沿大弯侧剪开，胃黏膜局部瘤组织增生导致胃壁显著增厚（蓝圈），瘤组织同时向深部浸润使肌层中断（绿箭头）。

1.5 小肠黏膜相关淋巴组织结外边缘区淋巴瘤（图 8-7）

小肠节段切除标本，已沿长轴剪开，可见瘤组织增生导致肠壁显著增厚（蓝星），肠腔狭窄，瘤组织灰白色，无明显出血坏死。

2. 白血病

白血病大脑浸润（图 8-8）

大脑标本的冠状切面，浅层白质内可见多个暗灰色病灶（蓝箭），病灶略呈圆形或卵圆形，大小不一。

三、组织切片

1. 淋巴结反应性增生（图 8-9）

淋巴结充血，淋巴滤泡增生（绿星）、窦组织细胞增生（蓝星）；髓质淋巴窦开放，窦内充满大量组织细胞，部分细胞胞浆呈泡沫样（绿箭）。

2. 淋巴瘤

2.1 淋巴结霍奇金淋巴瘤（图 8-10～图 8-12）

淋巴结的正常结构消失，被瘤组织取代，瘤组织内可见散在大细胞（蓝箭头，

图 8-11A,C)。瘤细胞圆形或椭圆形,体积大,胞浆丰富,略嗜酸或嗜碱性;单核、双核、多核或分叶核,核大,常呈圆形或椭圆形,染色质粗,沿核膜聚集呈块状,核膜厚;核内有大的嗜酸性核仁,直径常超过红细胞,形似包涵体,周围常常有空晕,是诊断性 R-S 细胞(红箭,图 8-11B;黑箭,图 8-11D),对霍奇金淋巴瘤具有诊断意义。还有一些大细胞形状不规则,胞浆丰富、强嗜酸性染色,核嗜碱性染色增强,细节观察不清,是凋亡的肿瘤细胞,又称为干尸细胞(绿箭,图 8-11B)。肿瘤细胞分布于多种反应性细胞成分混合组成的背景下,这些细胞包括组织细胞、淋巴细胞、嗜酸性粒细胞、嗜中性粒细胞和浆细胞(蓝圈)。间质纤维组织显著增生,毛细血管增生。图 8-11D 见典型双核 R-S 细胞,双核面对面排列,彼此对称,称为镜影细胞(黑箭),蓝箭示其他 R-S 细胞。经典型霍奇金淋巴瘤免疫组化染色显示瘤细胞 CD30、CD15 阳性(图 8-11E,F)。

图 8-10,8-12 示霍奇金淋巴瘤和非霍奇金淋巴瘤细胞的各种形态。

2.2　弥漫性大 B 细胞淋巴瘤(图 8-13)

此型非霍奇金淋巴瘤常见,瘤细胞的直径为小淋巴细胞的 4～5 倍,细胞形态多样,类似中心母细胞,免疫母细胞,或者伴有浆细胞分化。本切片高倍视野下见单一形态的大淋巴细胞样肿瘤细胞弥漫性浸润,瘤细胞核呈圆形、较空亮,有清楚的核仁,核分裂象多见(蓝箭头)。免疫组化染色显示瘤细胞 CD20 阳性。

2.3　滤泡性淋巴瘤(图 8-14)

肿瘤细胞呈明显的结节状生长,主要由中心细胞所构成,大小较一致。免疫组化染色显示瘤细胞 BCL2 阳性。

3. 白血病

3.1　急性髓系白血病小脑浸润(图 8-15)

小脑分子层见 3 个卵圆形肿瘤侵犯病灶,局部脑组织被破坏,瘤细胞密集成团(蓝星)。绝大部分瘤细胞幼稚,核呈圆形、较空亮,有核仁,胞浆量少,淡伊红染;偶见成熟粒细胞;蓝箭头所示为不同分化程度的瘤细胞。黑星示邻近的小脑非肿瘤组织。

3.2　急性髓系白血病脾脏浸润(图 8-16)

低倍镜下,脾脏红髓见瘤细胞密集浸润。高倍镜下,瘤细胞核呈圆形、较空亮,有核仁,偶见成熟粒细胞;蓝箭头所示为部分幼稚瘤细胞。

3.3　慢性髓系白血病肝脏浸润(图 8-17)

瘤细胞主要在肝窦和汇管区浸润(蓝箭头),可见不同发育阶段的瘤细胞(蓝箭),幼稚细胞核呈圆形、较空亮,有核仁,可见杆状核及分叶核粒细胞。

四、临床病理讨论

案例　患者,男,10 岁。左下颌角肿大半年,乏力、低热 1 个月,右下腹隐痛 10 天。体检发现左下颌鸡蛋大肿块,质地中等,固定。腹部 CT 显示盲肠下端球形肿物,直径 4.5 cm。左下颌肿物活检,分别做细胞遗传学分析和病理检查,发现瘤细胞 MYC 基因易位,病理组织形态如图 8-18。

该病最可能的诊断是什么?请列出诊断依据。

五、 思考题

1. 淋巴瘤的组织起源有何特点?

2. 淋巴瘤发病率升高的原因有哪些?

3. 淋巴瘤常见临床表现是什么? 其分期的标准是什么?

4. 临床上如何诊断淋巴瘤?

5. 试述霍奇金淋巴瘤病理分型及其病变特点。

6. 简述滤泡性淋巴瘤和 Burkitt 淋巴瘤的形态特征及分子标志。

7. 试述白血病的常见临床表现。

8. 名词解释:R-S 细胞,镜影细胞,满天星现象,费城染色体,绿色瘤,类白血病反应,Auer 小体。

Chapter 8

Diseases of Lymphoid and Hematopoietic Systems

I . Aims

1. To grasp the concept of lymphoma, classification and pathological characteristics of Hodgkin lymphoma.

2. To familiarize with the common types and pathological features of non-Hodgkin lymphoma.

3. To understand the basic concept, classification and pathological characteristics of leukemia.

Guidance to study

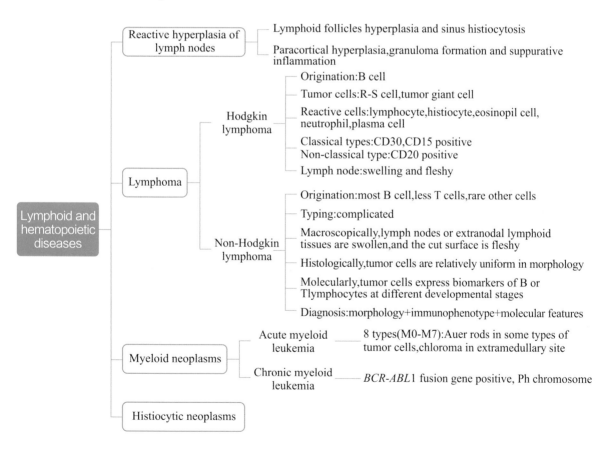

II. Gross specimens

1. Lymphoma

1.1　Hodgkin lymphoma of spleen（Fig.8-1）

The specimen is a cut surface of tumor-bearing spleen. The surface is elevated with irregular nodules (blue arrow). The capsule is complete and not smooth with fibrinous exudate. Most of the spleen is occupied by light-red, soft and fine tumor tissue which is clearly separated from the surrounding tissue. The tumor tissue is surrounded by hyperplastic fibrous tissue incompletely. Hemorrhage and necrosis can be seen within the tumor.

1.2　Non-Hodgkin lymphoma of lymph nodes（Fig.8-2）

The mediastinal lymph nodes, lumbar lymph nodes, iliac lymph nodes are involved by non-Hodgkin lymphoma. The lymph nodes (blue circles) are swollen and blended, the cut surface is gray-red and fleshy, and no obvious bleeding and necrosis are observed. The cut esophagus and bilateral kidneys are seen in the picture.

1.3　Non-Hodgkin lymphoma of mesenteric lymph nodes（Fig.8-3～Fig.8-5）

There are many gray-white, irregular or spherical tumors (blue stars) in the irregular gray-yellow adipose tissue. Some tumors have clear boundaries with surrounding tissues by complete capsules. Other tumors become aggregated into the neighbouring ones, and the borders are unclear. The section of the tumor is fine with distinct bleeding and necrosis (Fig.8-3).

There are many spherical tumors with different sizes (blue circles) in the irregular tissue, which is similar to the specimen shown in the Fig.8-3, On the section, the tumors display delicate texture with obvious hemorrhage and necrosis (blue arrow), which are clearly circumscribed from the surrounding tissues due to complete fibrous capsules (Fig.8-4).

In the mesenteric tissue surrounded by small intestine, several round masses (blue stars) have been cut. The sections are gray-white and fine without visible bleeding and necrosis (Fig.8-5).

1.4　Gastric extranodal marginal zone lymphoma of mucosa-associated lymphoid tissue（Fig.8-6）

The specimen of subtotal gastrectomy was cut along the greater curvature. The involved gastric wall was thickened by the local hyperplastic tumor tissue (blue circles). The tumor tissue has infiltrated into the deep part of gastric wall and splitted the muscular layer (green arrowhead).

1. 5   Small intestinal extranodal marginal zone lymphoma of mucosa-associated lymphoid tissue (Fig.8-7)

The small intestinal specimen has been cut along the long axis. The intestinal wall becomes thickened due to the hyperplasia of tumor tissue (blue stars), and the intestinal cavity is narrow. The tumor tissue is gray-white and shows no bleeding and necrosis.

2. Leukemia

Brain involvement by leukemia (Fig.8-8)

On the coronal section of brain specimen, multiple dark gray lesions (blue arrows) can be observed in the superficial white matter, and the neoplastic foci are round or oval in shape and different in size.

Ⅲ. Tissue sections

1. Reactive hyperplasia of lymph nodes (Fig.8-9)

Lymphoid follicles hyperplasia (green stars) and sinus histiocytosis (blue stars) are apparent in the lymph nodes. Medullary lymphatic sinuses are dilated and filled with a large number of histiocytic cells. Among of histiocytic cells, some present foam-like cytoplasm (green arrows).

2. Lymphoma

2. 1   Hodgkin lymphoma of lymph node (Fig.8-10~Fig.8-12)

The normal structure of lymph nodes is replaced by tumor tissue, and some large tumor cells are noticed with abundant cytoplasm (blue arrowheads, Fig.8-11 A, C). The tumor cells are round or oval with slightly eosinophilic or basophilic cytoplasm. Their nuclei are large in size and mononuclear, binuclear, polynuclear or lobulated in morphology, and round or oval in shape. The chromatin is dense and aggregated along nuclear membrane, which leads to thick nuclear membrane. There is a large eosinophilic nucleolus, which is often larger than a red blood cell in diameter, and appears as an inclusion body with empty halo. The large cells with the above-mentioned morphological characteristics are diagnostic R-S cells (red arrows in Fig.8-11B, blue and black arrows in Fig.8-11D), which is of diagnostic significance for Hodgkin lymphoma. Some large cells display irregular shape, rich cytoplasm, strong eosinophilic staining, enhanced nuclear basophilic staining and unclear details, and the cells are apoptotic tumor cells which are also known as mummified cells (green arrows, Fig.8-11B). Tumor cells distribute in the background of reactive cells composed of multiple components, histiocytes, lymphocytes, eosinophils, neutrophils and plasma cells (blue circles). Interstitial fibrous tissue and capillaries are significantly hyperplastic. Figure 8-11D shows typical binuclear R-S cells, and the two nuclei are symmetric and stand face to face, thus to be defined as mirror-image cells(black arrow). Classical Hodgkin lymphoma presents positive tumor cells after labelled by CD30 and CD15 antibodies(Fig.8-11E and F).

Fig.8-10 and 8-12 demonstrate various types of tumor cells in Hodgkin lymphoma and non-Hodgkin lymphoma respectively.

2. 2　Diffuse large B-cell lymphoma(Fig.8-13)

The subtype of non-Hodgkin lymphoma is common in clinic. The diameter of tumor cells is uniform, appearing as big as 4～5 times of a small lymphocyte. The cells are diverse in morphology, which are similar to centroblasts, immunoblasts, and differentiating plasma cells. Their nuclei are round, empty and bright, with clear nucleoli, and mitotic images are easily observed(blue arrows). Immunohistochemical findings demonstrate that the tumor cells are positive for CD20.

2. 3　Follicular lymphoma(Fig.8-14)

The tissue presents nodular aggregates of lymphoma cells which is mainly composed of centrocytes with uniform size. Immunohistochemical stained tissues show that the tumor cells are BCL2 positive.

3.　Leukemia

3. 1　Cerebellum involvement by acute myeloid leukemia(Fig.8-15)

Three oval tumor lesions have invaded the cerebellar molecular layer, and destroyed the normal structure of cerebellum tissue. Most of the clustered tumor cells (blue stars) are immature with round, empty and bright nuclei as well as scant cytoplasm. Mature granulocytes are seldom seen. The blue arrows show tumor cells at various stages of differentiation. The black star displays the adjacent non-neoplastic area of the cerebellum.

3. 2　Spleen involvement by acute myeloid leukemia(Fig.8-16)

The tumor cells have broken into the red medullary of the spleen with round or slightly indented nuclei. Mature granulocytes are occasionally observed. The blue arrows show some immature tumor cells.

3. 3　Liver involvement by chronic myeloid leukemia(Fig.8-17)

The tumor cells have mainly infiltrated into hepatic sinuses and portal areas(blue arrowheads). They(blue arrows)are at different developmental stages with immature round or slightly indented nuclei. Some granulocyte-like tumor cells show either rod or lobulated nuclei.

IV. Clinical pathological discussion

Case

A 10-year-old boy has been noticed to have swollen left mandibular angle for half a year, fatigue and low-grade fever for 1 month, and dull pain in the right lower abdomen for 10 days. The physical examination found that the egg-sized left mandibular mass could not be moved with medium hardness. Abdominal CT revealed a spherical mass at the lower end of the cecum, with a diameter of 4.5 cm. The left mandibular nodule biopsy was sent for cytogenetic analysis and pathological examination. MYC gene translocation was detected in the tumor cells. The pathological findings are shown in Fig.8-18.

What is the most likely diagnosis of the left mandibular mass? Please list the diagnostic key points.

V. Questions

1. What are the characteristics of the tissue origin of lymphoma?

2. Why is the morbidity of lymphoma increasing?

3. What are the common clinical manifestations of lymphoma? What is the standard of staging?

4. What indicators are required to make a diagnosis of lymphoma clinically?

5. To describe the classification and pathological characteristics of Hodgkin lymphoma.

6. Please describe briefly the morphology and molecular markers of both follicular lymphoma and Burkitt lymphoma.

7. What are the common clinical manifestations of leukemia?

8. Terms: R-S cell, Mirror image cell, "Starry sky" appearance, Philadelphia chromosome, Chloroma, Leukemoid reaction, Auer rods.

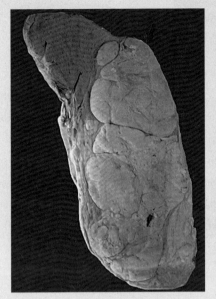

图 8-1　脾脏霍奇金淋巴瘤
Fig.8-1　Hodgkin lymphoma of spleen

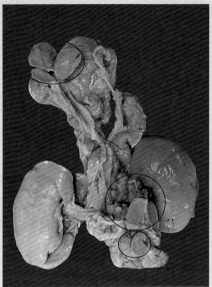

图 8-2　淋巴结非霍奇金淋巴瘤
Fig.8-2　Non-Hodgkin lymphoma
of lymph nodes

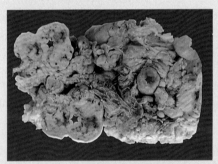

图 8-3　肠系膜淋巴结非霍奇金淋巴瘤
Fig.8-3　Non-Hodgkin lymphoma
of mesenteric lymph nodes

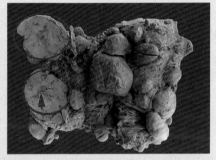

图 8-4　肠系膜淋巴结非霍奇金淋巴瘤
Fig.8-4　Non-Hodgkin lymphoma
of mesenteric lymph nodes

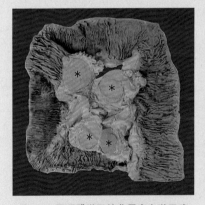

图 8-5　肠系膜淋巴结非霍奇金淋巴瘤
Fig.8-5　Non-Hodgkin lymphoma
of mesenteric lymph nodes

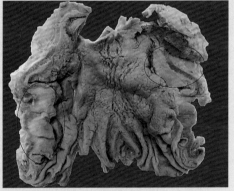

图 8-6　胃结外边缘区淋巴瘤，MALT 型
Fig.8-6　Gastric extranodal marginal
zone lymphoma（MALT type）

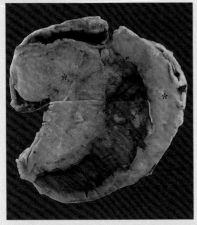

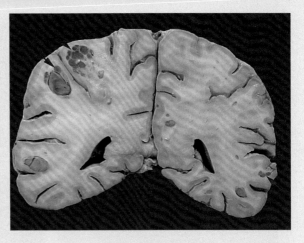

图 8-7　小肠结外边缘区淋巴瘤，MALT 型
Fig.8-7　Intestinal extranodal marginal zone lymphoma（MALT type）

图 8-8　白血病大脑浸润
Fig.8-8　Brain involvement by leukemia

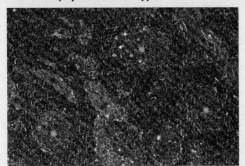

图 8-9　淋巴结反应性增生（×100；×400）
Fig.8-9　Reactive hyperplasia of lymph nodes（×100；×400）

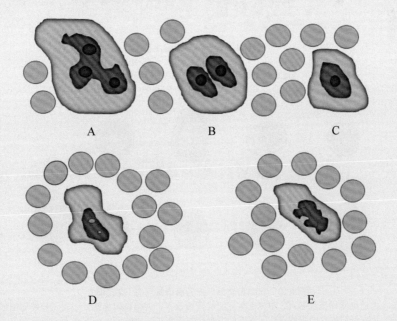

图 8-10　霍奇金淋巴瘤的瘤细胞形态（模式图）
A. 多形性 R-S 细胞；B. 镜影细胞；C. 单核 R-S 细胞；D. 腔隙型 R-S 细胞；E. 爆米花样 R-S 细胞
Fig.8-10　Diagrammatic representation of neoplastic cells in Hodgkin lymphoma
A. Pleomorphic R-S cell；B. Classical R-S cell（mirror image cell）；C. Mononuclear R-S cell；
D. Lacunar R-S cell；E. Popcorn R-S cell

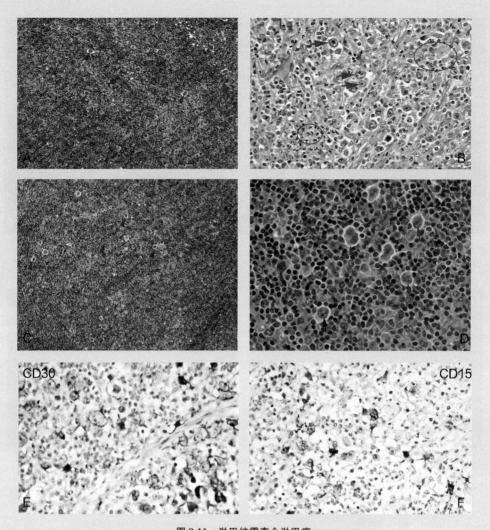

图 8-11　淋巴结霍奇金淋巴瘤
（A,C:×100；B,D:×400；E,F:×400，免疫组织化学染色）
Fig.8-11　Hodgkin lymphoma of lymph nodes
（**A,C:×100；B,D:×400；E,F:×400,immunohistochemistry staining**）

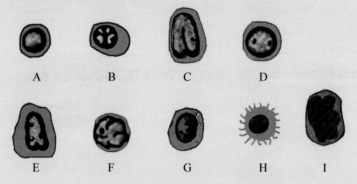

图 8-12　非霍奇金淋巴瘤的瘤细胞形态（模式图）
A. 小淋巴细胞样瘤细胞；B. 小淋巴浆细胞样瘤细胞；C. 大核裂瘤细胞；D. 大无核裂瘤细胞；
E. 免疫母细胞样瘤细胞；F. T 淋巴母细胞样瘤细胞；G. 小淋巴母细胞样无核裂瘤细胞；
H. 毛细胞样瘤细胞；I. T 核裂瘤细胞（蕈样霉菌病）
Fig.8-12　Diagrammatic presentation of neoplastic cells in non-Hodgkin lymphoma
A. Small lymphocytic；B. Small lymphocytic, plasmacytoid；C. Large cleaved；D. Large non-cleaved；
E. Immunoblastic；F. Lymphoblastic（T cell）；G. Small lymphoblastic non-cleaved（Burkitt）；
H. Hairy cell；I. Cleaved T cell（mycosis fungoides）

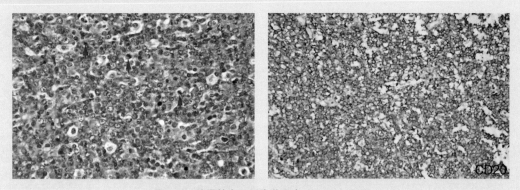

图 8-13　弥漫性大 B 细胞淋巴瘤（×400；×100）
Fig.8-13　Diffuse large B-cell lymphoma（×400；×100）

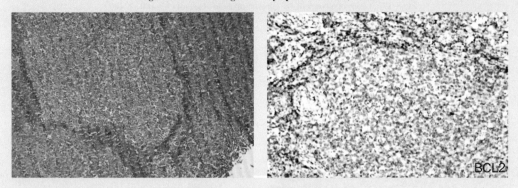

图 8-14　滤泡性淋巴瘤（×100）
Fig.8-14　Follicular lymphoma（×100）

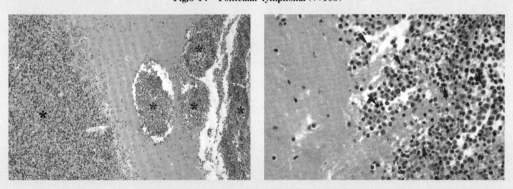

图 8-15　急性髓性白血病小脑浸润（×100；×400）
Fig.8-15　Cerebellum involvement by acute myeloid leukemia（×100；×400）

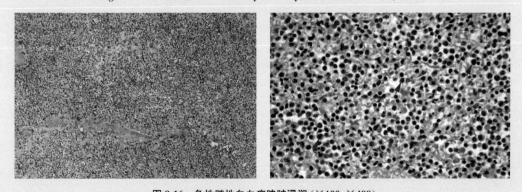

图 8-16　急性髓性白血病脾脏浸润（×100；×400）
Fig.8-16　Spleen involvement by acute myeloid leukemia（×100；×400）

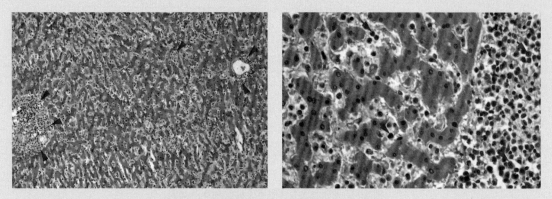

图 8-17 慢性髓性白血病肝脏浸润（×100；×400）
Fig.8-17 Liver involvement by chronic myeloid leukemia（×100；×400）

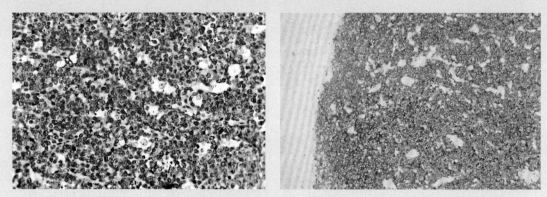

图 8-18 案例（HE，×400；CD20 免疫组化阳性，×100）
Fig.8-18 Case（H.E.，×400；positive immunohistochemistry staining of CD20，×100）

陈平圣（Pingsheng Chen）

第九章

泌尿系统疾病

一、目的要求

1. 掌握膜性肾小球病、IgA 肾病、慢性肾小球肾炎的形态特征。

2. 掌握急性、慢性肾盂肾炎的形态特征。

3. 掌握肾癌、膀胱癌的形态特征。

4. 熟悉急性弥漫性增生性肾小球肾炎、新月体性肾小球肾炎和微小病变性肾小球病的形态特征。

5. 了解其他类型的肾小球肾炎的病理特征。

导学

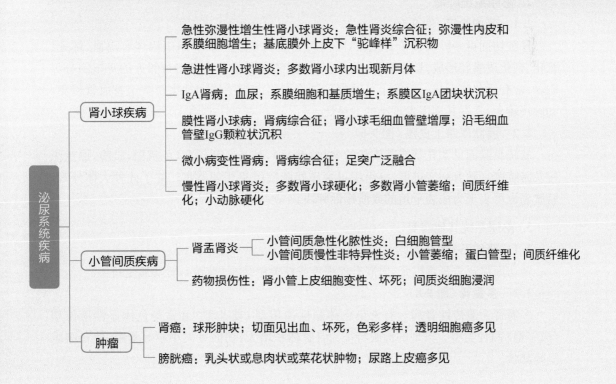

二、 大体标本

1. 肾小球肾炎

1.1　急性弥漫性增生性肾小球肾炎（图9-1）

又称毛细血管内增生性肾小球肾炎、感染后肾小球肾炎。肾脏体积增大，包膜已剥离，表面光滑、充血，故称为"大红肾"（若见弥漫性分布的小出血点则称为"蚤咬肾"）。切面见皮质增厚，皮髓质分界尚清楚，髓质呈红褐色（高度淤血所致）。

1.2　急进性肾小球肾炎（图9-2）

又称新月体性肾小球肾炎。肾脏体积增大，色苍白，质软，表面光滑，包膜已剥离。切面见皮质增厚，色白略带黄色。

1.3　微小病变性肾小球病（图9-3）

又称微小病变肾病、脂性肾病或足突病。肾脏外观呈分叶状，体积增大，颜色变浅。切面隐约可见黄色细线（蓝箭头），为脂质在肾小管上皮细胞沉积所致。

1.4　慢性肾小球肾炎（图9-4）

又称慢性硬化性肾小球肾炎。肾脏体积明显缩小，重量减轻，颜色苍白，表面呈弥漫性颗粒状，亦称继发性颗粒性固缩肾。包膜与皮质表面粘连，不易剥离。切面皮质变薄，皮髓质分界不清。请结合理论知识判断对侧肾脏是否会出现同样的病理改变，这种外观的肾脏还可出现于哪些疾病？

2. 泌尿系统肿瘤

2.1　肾细胞癌（图9-5）

肾脏切面见一肿块位于肾上极，略向表面隆起（蓝星）。癌组织因伴有出血、坏死、软化、钙化或囊腔形成，切面呈红、黄、灰白相间的多彩状。癌组织与邻近的肾组织分界明显，常有假包膜形成。但镜下可观察到肿瘤细胞向周围浸润性生长甚至有血管侵犯。如肿块较大，常在其周围发现小的卫星灶。

2.2　膀胱尿路上皮癌（图9-6）

膀胱黏膜面见菜花状或乳头状的突起（蓝星），其基底部较宽，色灰白，质脆，癌组织侵及膀胱壁。随着病变进展，癌组织可穿破膀胱壁侵犯相邻器官。除了此种大体外观，膀胱癌也可表现为浅表平坦的或溃疡性肿块。

3. 泌尿系统其他病变

3.1　肾结石（图9-7）

肾切面见肾盂肾盏扩张，内嵌有棕褐色或棕黄色结石（蓝箭），肾实质受挤压。

3.2　多囊肾（图9-8）

多囊肾为遗传性肾病。有常染色体隐性遗传型（婴儿型）和常染色体显性遗传型（成年型）两种类型。典型的肉眼特征为肾脏体积增大，切面见大小不等囊腔，使肾组织呈蜂窝状。

三、组织切片

1. 肾小球肾炎

1.1 急性弥漫性增生性肾小球肾炎（图 9-9）

弥漫性病变,镜下见几乎所有肾小球体积增大,表现为:① 肾小球的细胞数目增多（图 9-9A,B）,具体包括 A. 毛细血管内皮细胞和系膜细胞的增生和肿胀（这两种细胞在光学显微镜下不易区分）,B. 单核细胞及中性粒细胞浸润。② 鲍曼囊囊腔变窄,有的囊内可见有伊红色、结构模糊、似纤维素样物质。③ 肾小管上皮细胞肿胀,胞浆内可见伊红染细颗粒,管腔内有管型。④ 肾间质充血及中性粒细胞浸润。免疫荧光观察到肾小球内沿毛细血管袢分布的 IgG 颗粒状荧光（图 9-9C）。电镜下（图 9-9D）见肾小球毛细血管基底膜与足细胞（P）间"驼峰状"电子致密物沉积（黄星）。

1.2 急进性肾小球肾炎（图 9-10）

病变弥漫,累及切片中全部肾小球。低倍镜下可见肾小球体积增大,多数肾小球囊壁上皮细胞及成纤维细胞增生以及单核细胞浸润形成新月体（蓝箭,图 9-10A）,少数肾小球已纤维化、透明变;高倍镜下可清楚观察到新月体的成分（蓝星,图 9-10B）。另见肾小管上皮细胞低平,部分肾小管上皮细胞萎缩甚至消失,管腔内有蛋白管型（图 9-10A）。肾间质水肿,伴有炎细胞浸润,纤维化。请思考:① 新月体成分的演变过程。② 该病变可能导致的严重后果有哪些? ③ 是否见到新月体即可诊断此型肾炎?

1.3 膜性肾小球病（图 9-11）

本病早期光镜下肾小球病变不明显,随后毛细血管壁逐渐增厚僵硬;大量免疫复合物沉积在上皮细胞和基底膜之间。镜下主要表现为肾小球毛细血管壁弥漫性增厚（图 9-11A）;PASM 染色将基底膜染成黑色后,可显示增厚的基底膜及与之垂直的钉突（绿箭头,图 9-11B,C）。免疫荧光表现为典型的沿毛细血管壁分布的 IgG 颗粒状荧光（图 9-11D）。电镜显示上皮细胞下团块状电子致密物（绿星,图 9-11E）,沉积物随后可逐渐被基质包绕（绿星,图 9-11F）,继而被溶解吸收,形成虫蚀状空隙。

1.4 微小病变性肾小球病（图 9-12）

光镜下肾小球病变不明显（图 9-12A,B）,肾小管上皮细胞内有重吸收的红色蛋白颗粒及圆形脂质空泡（图 9-12C）。免疫荧光检测显示抗体、补体阴性。电镜显示足细胞突起广泛融合（图 9-12D）。

1.5 局灶性节段性肾小球硬化（图 9-13）

光镜下可见病变肾小球比例不超过一半。对于单个病变的肾小球,部分毛细血管袢发生塌陷、玻璃样变或硬化,硬化区可在门部（绿星,图 9-13A）、顶部（绿星,黑箭头,图 9-13B-D）或其他区域。免疫荧光检查显示病变的节段内有 IgM 和 C3 沉积。电镜显示足细胞突起广泛融合。注意:由于病变呈局灶、节段性分布,偶见穿刺活检的肾小球均正常,这种情况下不要误诊为微小病变性肾小球病。

1.6 膜增生性肾小球肾炎（图 9-14）

光镜下,肾小球体积增大,肾小球细胞增生、系膜基质增多,毛细血管袢呈分叶状外观（图 9-14A，B）。PASM 染色示肾小球毛细血管基底膜明显增厚，节段呈双轨状（绿箭），偶见内皮下嗜复红蛋白（免疫复合物）沉积（蓝箭，图 9-14C）。电镜示内皮下电子致密物沉积（绿星，图 9-14D）。

1.7　IgA 肾病（图 9-15）

光镜下的典型表现是弥漫性肾小球系膜细胞增生和系膜基质增多，系膜区不同程度增宽（蓝星，图 9-15A，B）；毛细血管祥偶见节段纤维素样坏死（蓝箭，图 9-15B），系膜区嗜复红蛋白沉积（红箭，图 9-15B）。免疫荧光检查可见系膜区高强度 IgA（图 9-15C）和 C3 补体沉积。电镜显示系膜区团块状电子致密物沉积（红星，图 9-15D）。

1.8　慢性肾小球肾炎（图 9-16）

肾组织中大量肾小球纤维化及玻璃样变（绿星，图 9-16A，B）、互相靠近集中，小部分肾小球体积代偿性增大。大部分肾小管萎缩、基底膜增厚（蓝箭头）、消失，少数肾小管代偿性扩张，有些甚至扩张呈囊状，肾小管腔内常见各种管型（图 9-16B，C）。间质纤维结缔组织增生，有多量淋巴细胞和浆细胞浸润。小动脉管壁增厚、透明变、管腔狭窄（绿箭），有的动脉内膜明显纤维性增厚（图 9-16D）。

2. 肾小管-间质性肾炎

2.1　急性肾盂肾炎（图 9-17）

肾间质内大量中性粒细胞浸润，肾小管上皮细胞变性坏死，腔内充满中性粒细胞和细胞碎片（绿箭头，图 9-17A，B）。肾小球一般正常。思考：按照炎症性质划分，急性肾盂肾炎属于哪一类炎症？

2.2　慢性肾盂肾炎（图 9-18）

病变呈灶性分布，因反复发作病变形态较复杂。镜下见肾盂黏膜上皮增生，层次增加（绿星），上皮下慢性炎细胞浸润（图 9-18A）。病灶内多数小管萎缩或消失，部分肾小管扩张，其内充满胶样管型（蓝箭），因其类似甲状腺的组织形态，又称为肾小管的甲状腺化；肾小球呈现球周纤维化或玻璃样变（蓝星）；肾间质内伴有大量炎细胞浸润（图 9-18B）。急性发作期可见肾组织内中性粒细胞浸润，甚至脓肿形成。

3. 泌尿系统肿瘤

3.1　肾透明细胞癌（图 9-19）

低倍镜下见肿瘤组织（蓝星）和受挤压的肾组织（绿星），瘤组织伴出血，瘤细胞向肾组织内浸润性生长（图 9-19A）。瘤细胞呈圆形或多边形，胞质透明或颗粒状，细胞核小且圆，染色质分布均匀，可见大小不等的核仁（图 9-19B）。间质毛细血管和血窦丰富。请注意，有些肿瘤细胞非透明，胞浆红染，内含颗粒状物质（细胞是否透明取决于胞浆内脂质和糖原的含量）。

3.2　膀胱尿路上皮癌（图 9-20）

低倍镜图显示高级别浸润性乳头状尿路上皮癌局部，乳头表面癌细胞层次多，排列紧密，乳头中轴为血管和少量结缔组织（图 9-20A）。高倍镜下见癌细胞在肌层浸润性生长，细胞大小、形态差异较大，异型性明显；细胞核浓染，核浆比升高，偶见病理性核分裂象（绿箭，图 9-20B）。

四、临床病理讨论

案例 1 患者,女性,23 岁,尿泡沫增多 10 天。临床检查:全身水肿。实验室检查:蛋白尿(++++),血清白蛋白 28 g/L(正常值:40~55 g/L)。临床印象:肾病综合征。病理学检查:组织学、特殊染色、电镜及免疫荧光典型视野见图 9-21。

(1)请描述病理学检查结果,并结合临床资料给出患者的病理诊断。

(2)请解释患者蛋白尿和水肿的机制。

(3)请讨论诊断该病时需注意的鉴别诊断。

案例 2 患者,男性,30 岁,常规体检发现"血尿、蛋白尿"。实验室检查:蛋白尿(++),血尿(+++),尿蛋白 2.2g/24h,血清白蛋白 42g/L,尿沉渣红细胞 100 个/高倍视野,肾功能检查无异常。病理学检查:组织学、特殊染色及免疫荧光典型视野和电镜见图 9-22。

(1)请给出该患者的病理诊断,并说明理由。

(2)尝试解释该病理学变化如何导致患者出现相应体征及实验室检查结果。

五、思考题

1. 请阐述肾小球的结构和功能。

2. 请回答血尿、蛋白尿、少尿、无尿、多尿、管型尿的判断标准。

3. 请以急性增生性肾小球肾炎为例,分析病理变化如何导致患者的临床表现。

4. 导致成人肾病综合征最常见的是哪一类肾小球肾病?有何病理形态特征?

5. 请描述膀胱尿路上皮癌的好发部位、最常见的大体类型和镜下特征。

6. 名词解释:肾病综合征,肾炎综合征,新月体,局灶性节段性肾小球硬化。

Chapter 9

Diseases of Urinary System

Ⅰ. Aims

1. To grasp the pathologic characteristics of membranous nephropathy, IgA nephropathy and chronic sclerosing glomerulonephritis.

2. To grasp the pathologic characteristics of acute and chronic pyelonephritis.

3. To grasp the pathologic characteristics of kidney cancer and bladder cancer.

4. To familiarize with the pathologic characteristics of acute diffuse proliferative glomerulonephritis, rapidly progressive glomerulonephritis, and minimal change glomerulopathy.

5. To understand the pathologic characteristics of other kinds of glomerulonephritis.

Guidance to study

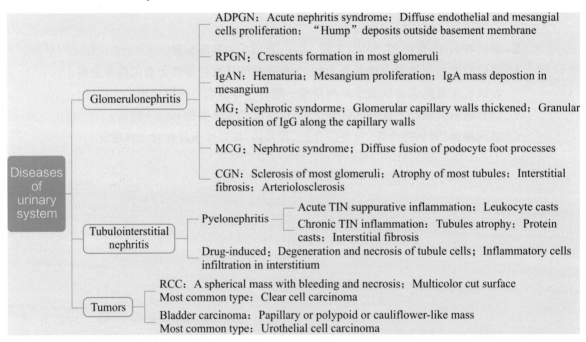

ADPGN: Acute nephritis syndrome; Diffuse endothelial and mesangial cells proliferation; "Hump" deposits outside basement membrane

RPGN: Crescents formation in most glomeruli

IgAN: Hematuria; Mesangium proliferation; IgA mass depostion in mesangium

MG: Nephrotic syndorme; Glomerular capillary walls thickened; Granular deposition of IgG along the capillary walls

MCG: Nephrotic syndrome; Diffuse fusion of podocyte foot processes

CGN: Sclerosis of most glomeruli; Atrophy of most tubules; Interstitial fibrosis; Arteriolosclerosis

Acute TIN suppurative inflammation: Leukocyte casts

Chronic TIN inflammation: Tubules atrophy; Protein casts; Interstitial fibrosis

Drug-induced: Degeneration and necrosis of tubule cells; Inflammatory cells infiltration in interstitium

RCC: A spherical mass with bleeding and necrosis; Multicolor cut surface
Most common type: Clear cell carcinoma

Bladder carcinoma: Papillary or polypoid or cauliflower-like mass
Most common type: Urothelial cell carcinoma

Glomerulonephritis / Tubulointerstitial nephritis / Pyelonephritis / Tumors — Diseases of urinary system

Abbreviation: ADPGN, acute diffuse proliferative glomerulonephritis; RPGN, rapidly progressive glomerulonephritis (or CrGN, crescentic glomerulonephritis); IgAN, IgA nephropathy; MG, membranous glomerulonephritis (or MN, membranous nephropathy); MCG, minimal change glomerulopathy (or MCD, minimal change disease); CGN, chronic glomerulonephritis (or CSGN, chronic sclerosing glomerulonephritis); TIN: tubulointerstitial nephritis; RCC, renal cell carcinoma

Ⅱ. Gross specimens

1. Glomerulonephritis

1.1   Acute diffuse proliferative glomerulonephritis (Fig.9-1)

It is also called endocapillary proliferative glomerulonephritis or postinfectious glomerulonephritis. The kidney is slightly enlarged, and the surface is smooth and congested. It will be called flea-bite kidney when there are diffuse hemorrhagic petechiae. The cut surface shows that there is a clear boundary between thick cortex and from congested medulla.

1.2   Rapidly progressive glomerulonephritis (Fig.9-2)

It is also called crescentic glomerulonephritis. The kidney is enlarged and pale with smooth surface. The capsule has been removed. The cut surface reveals a broad cortex which is pale with yellowish.

1.3   Minimal change glomerulopathy (Fig.9-3)

It is also called minimal change glomerulonephritis, lipoid nephrosis, or foot process disease. Grossly, the kidney is slightly lobulated, large and pale. The cut surface reveals a broad cortex with thin yellowish-white stripes (blue arrowheads), which are caused by lipid deposition in renal tubular epithelial cells.

1.4   Chronic glomerulonephritis (Fig.9-4)

The kidney is small with low weight, pale-red or gray-yellow, and firm with finely granular surface. It is also called secondary granular and contracted kidney. The capsule has adhered the cortex too tight to be removed. The cortex is symmetrically thin. There is no clear boundary between the cortex and the medulla. Please consider whether the contralateral kidney has the same pathological changes, and other possible diseases presenting the same morphological changes as the kidney.

2. Tumors of urinary system

2.1   Renal cell carcinoma (Fig.9-5)

The cross section of the kidney shows a mass at the upper pole (blue asterisk). The cut section of the tumor is variegated due to hemorrhage, necrosis, softening, calcification, and cyst formation. The tumor is often surrounded with a pseudo-capsule. Despite the sharp delineation from the normal kidney, the tumor infiltration (including venous invasion) can be checked by microscopic examination. Sometimes small satellite nodules can be found in the surrounding parenchyma, indicating metastases.

2.2   Bladder urothelial carcinoma (Fig.9-6)

As shown in the specimen, these broadly based, cauliflower-like or papillary tumors (blue asterisk) have developed in the trigonum. It is gray-white in color and fragile. As the disease progresses, the cancerous tissue may penetrate the bladder wall and invade adjacent organs. Bladder carcinoma can also appear as a plaque-like or ulcerated friable mass involving the entire mucosa.

3. Other diseases of urinary system

3.1　Renal calculi（Fig.9-7）

The cut surface of the kidney shows renal pelvis and calyx expanded with dark brown or yellow brown calculi (blue arrows), and the parenchyma becomes thin.

3.2　Polycystic kidney（Fig.9-8）

Polycystic kidney disease (PKD) is a kind of hereditary kidney disease. The disease has two forms: autosomal recessive disorder (infantile type) and autosomal dominant disease (adult type). The typical gross features include large size of the kidney and "honeycomb" appearance of the cut surface which is the result of multiple cysts with varying sizes.

Ⅲ. Tissue sections

1. Glomerulonephritis

1.1　Acute diffuse proliferative glomerulonephritis（Fig.9-9）

Almost all the glomeruli are enlarged in the examined slice. The glomerular tufts are distended and hypercellular (Fig.9-9A, B). The hypercellularity of the glomerulus is due to swelling and proliferation of mesangial and endothelial cells, together with a variable infiltration of monocytes and neutrophils. Sometimes, epithelial proliferation of Bowman's capsule and fibrinoid exudate in the space can be observed. The tubules contain red cell casts and the tubular cells show degenerative changes (swelling and granular). The interstitium is usually hyperemic with neutrophils infiltration. Immunofluorescence staining demonstrates that granular IgG fluorescence distributes along capillary loops in the glomerulus (Fig.9-9C). Electron microscopy shows the "humped" electron dense deposits between the basement membrane of glomerular capillary and podocyte (P) (yellow asterisks, Fig.9-9D).

1.2　Rapidly progressive glomerulonephritis（Fig.9-10）

All the glomeruli in the section become enlarged. The histologic picture is dominated by the formation of so-called crescents within Bowman's spaces in most of the glomeruli (blue arrows, Fig.9-10A). These crescents are composed of parietal cells, fibroblasts and monocytes infiltrating into Bowman's space. Some glomeruli undergo fibrosis or hyaline degeneration. The composition of crescents can be clearly observed at high magnification (blue asterisk, Fig.9-10B). In addition, the tubular epithelial cells become flattened showing an appearance of atrophy, or even disappeared. There are protein casts in the lumens (Fig.9-10A). Renal interstitial edema with inflammatory cells and fibrosis is also distinct in the picture. Please think: (1) What is the developing process of crescents related to histological components? (2) What clinical manifestations can these pathological changes lead to? (3) Can you make a diagnosis of crescent glomerulonephritis if you have found crescent formation?

1. 3   Membranous nephropathy (Fig.9-11)

In the early stage of this disease, the glomeruli may appear normal. However, accompanying with the disease development, diffuse thickening of the capillary walls become typical morphological features due to the formation of more and more immune complexes between the epithelial cells and GBM(Fig.9-11A). By PASM staining, the thickened GBM and the spikes perpendicular to it are shown (green arrowhead; Fig.9-11B; Fig.9-11C). Immunofluorescence microscopy displays typical granular IgG fluorescence along the capillary loops (Fig.9-11D). Electron microscopy reveals subepithelial deposits of immune complexes (green asterisks, Fig.9-11E). As the disease progresses, the proliferating matrix gradually envelops the deposits (green asterisks, Fig.9-11F), incorporating them into the GBM. Later, the trapped deposits become degraded, and eventually disappear, leaving cavities within the GBM.

1. 4   Minimal change glomerulopathy (Fig.9-12)

Under light microscope, there is no apparent abnormality in the glomeruli (Fig.9-12A, B). Reabsorbed red protein particles and round lipid vacuoles are often observed in the tubular epithelial cells (Fig.9-12C). Immunofluorescence test shows no deposits of immunoglobulins and complements. The morphological hallmark of this disease is the diffuse fusion of podocyte processes under electron microscopy (Fig.9-12D).

1. 5   Focal segmental glomerulosclerosis (FSGS) (Fig.9-13)

Less than 50% of glomeruli are involved, furthermore lesions occur in only partial capillary loops within an affected glomerulus. These tufts undergo collapse, hyaline change, and sclerosis. As shown in the picture, sclerosis areas can be observed in the hila (green asterisk, Fig.9-13A), poles(green asterisk and black arrowheads, Fig.9-13B-D), and other areas of capillary loops. Immunoflurorescence microscopy reveals deposits including IgM and C3 in the involved segment. Electron microscopy demonstrates effacement including foot processes that can also be observed in minimal change glomerulopathy. Because of the focal and segmental lesions, sometimes, all the glomeruli from the biopsy appear normal, which should be differentiated from minimal change glomerulopathy.

1. 6   Membranoproliferative glomerulonephritis (Fig.9-14)

The glomeruli are large with more mesangial matrix. The number of glomerular cells increases because of the proliferation of mesangial cells and infiltration of leukocytes. The capillary loops display a lobular architecture (Fig. 9-14A, B). With PASM staining, the thickened GBM with a double-tracked appearance is clearly observed (green arrows, Fig.9-14C). Occasionally, subendothelial fuchsinophilic deposits (immune complexes) can be found (blue arrow, Fig.9-14C). By electron microscopy, subendothelial deposits are visible (green asterisk, Fig.9-14D).

1.7　IgA nephropathy（Fig.9-15）

The histological feature is diffuse proliferation of glomerular mesangial cells and mesangial matrix, resulting in widened mesangial areas (blue asterisks, Fig. 9-15A, B). Segmental fibrinoid necrosis of capillary loops (blue arrow, Fig.9-15B) and deposition of fuchsinophilic proteins in the mesangium (red arrow, Fig.9-15B) are occasionally found. Immunoflurorescence microscopy shows apparent deposition of IgA (Fig.9-15C) and C3 in the mesangium. Some massive electron-dense deposits are detected in the mesangium by electron microscopy (red asterisks, Fig.9-15D).

1.8　Chronic glomerulonephritis（Fig.9-16）

Lots of the glomeruli observed in the tissue section have congregated, which showing atrophic changes with fibrosis and hyalinization (green asterisks, Fig. 9-16A, B), and the surrounding renal tubules are atrophic with thickened basement membrane (blue arrow, Fig.9-16B), or even completely disappeared. Close to the atrophic nephrons, a small number of glomeruli present compensatory hypertrophy, and the neighbouring tubules display cystic dilation with casts (Fig.9-16B, C). Marked fibrosis and infiltration of numerous lymphocytes and plasma cells are present in the interstitium. The small arteries present thickened walls with hyalinization, and narrow lumina, and some arterial intima are fibrotic (green arrows, Fig.9-16D).

2.　Tubulointerstitial nephritis

2.1　Acute pyelonephritis（Fig.9-17）

There are a large number of neutrophils in the interstitium. The renal tubules display alterative epithelial cells with neutrophils and cellular debris in the lumens (green arrowheads, Fig.9-17A, B). The glomeruli are generally normal. According to pathological nature of inflammation, which type of inflammation is considered for acute pyelonephritis?

2.2　Chronic pyelonephritis（Fig.9-18）

Because of the repeated attacks, the pathological changes are complicated containing diverse types of injuries. Hyperplasia of the renal pelvis mucosa (green asterisks) and infiltration of chronic inflammatory cells are shown in the subepithelial layer and renal interstitium. Most of the renal tubules are atrophic, or even disappeared. Others are often dilated and filled with pink casts (blue arrows), presenting an appearance of "thyroidization". The glomerulus shows periglomerular fibrosis or hyalinization (blue asterisk). Neutrophils infiltration and even abscess formation may be observed in the acute episode.

3. Tumors of urinary system

3.1　Renal clear cell carcinoma（Fig.9-19）

At low magnification, the tumor tissue (blue asterisk) and adjacent compressed normal tissue (green asterisk) are identified. The cancerous area shows local hemorrhage and tumor cells have infiltrated into the surrounding normal tissue (Fig.9-19A). The neoplastic cells are round or polygon with vacuolated or granular cytoplasm. The nuclei are usually small and round with evenly distributed chromatin, and nucleoli in varied sizes (Fig.9-19B). There are abundant capillaries and blood sinuses in the stroma. Sometimes, the tumor cells may be solid with granular pink cytoplasm, which depends on the amounts of lipid and glycogen.

3.2　Bladder urothelial carcinoma（Fig.9-20）

The low magnification view represents part of high grade infiltrating papillary urothelial carcinoma. The typical papillary epithelia with fibrovascular core are observed. The number of cell layers of epithelium dramatically increase and these tumor cells arrange closely (Fig.9-20A). The malignant cells have infiltrated into the muscular layer. These cells have marked pleomorphism showing varied size and shape, hyperchromatic, high ratio of nucleus to cytoplasm. Mitotic figures are occasionally found (green arrow, Fig.9-20B).

IV. Clinical pathological discussion

Case 1

Female, 23 years old, with a 10-day history of "increased foamy urine".

Physical examination: systemic edema.

Lab tests: proteinuria (++++), serum albumin 28 g/L (normal reference value, 40~55 g/L).

Clinical impression: nephrotic syndrome.

Pathological examination: typical figures of H.E. staining, special staining, electron microscopy, and immunofluorescence test are shown as follows (Fig.9-21).

(1) Please describe the pathological changes and make a pathological diagnosis.

(2) Please illustrate the mechanism of the patient's proteinuria and edema.

(3) Please discuss differential diagnoses of this disease.

Case 2

Male, 30 years old, "hematuria and proteinuria" were found during his regular medical examinations.

Lab tests: proteinuria (++), hematuria (+++), urine protein 2.2g/24hr, serum albumin 42g/L, erythrocytes in urine sediment analysis 100/HPF, normal renal function.

Pathological examination: typical figures of H.E. staining, special staining, electron microscopy, and immunofluorescence test are shown as follows (Fig.9-22).

(1) Please make a pathological diagnosis and give your reasons.

(2) Please try to explain how these pathological changes lead to the patient's clinical manifestations.

Ⅴ. Questions

1. Please describe the structure and function of glomeruli.

2. Please give the diagnostic criterions of hematuria, proteinuria, oliguria, anuria, polyuria and urine casts.

3. In acute diffuse proliferative glomerulonephritis, how do the morphological changes cause the clinical manifestations?

4. Which kind of the glomerulonephritis is the most frequent cause of nephrotic syndrome in adults? What are the pathological characteristics?

5. Please describe the predilection site, the most common gross type and the typical microscopic features of bladder urothelial carcinoma.

7. Terms: Nephrotic syndrome, Nephritic syndrome, Crescent, Focal and segmental glomerulosclerosis.

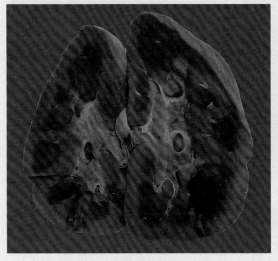

图 9-1　急性弥漫性增生性肾小球肾炎
Fig.9-1　Acute diffuse proliferative glomerulonephritis

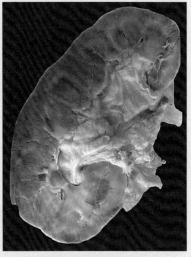

图 9-2　急进性肾小球肾炎
Fig.9-2　Rapidly progressive glomerulonephritis

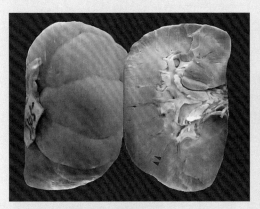

图 9-3　微小病变性肾小球病
Fig.9-3　Minimal change glomerulopathy

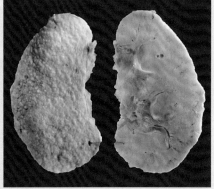

图 9-4　慢性肾小球肾炎
Fig.9-4　Chronic glomerulonephritis

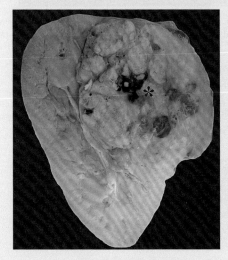

图 9-5　肾细胞癌
Fig.9-5　Renal cell carcinoma

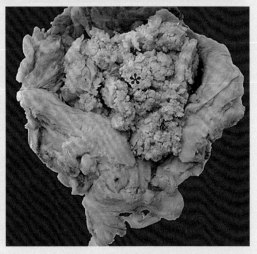

图 9-6　膀胱尿路上皮癌
Fig.9-6　Bladder urothelial carcinoma

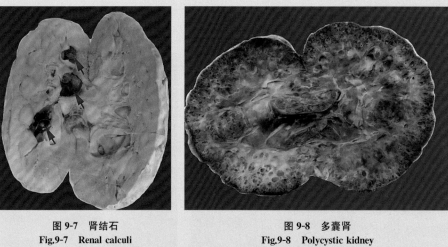

图 9-7 肾结石
Fig.9-7 Renal calculi

图 9-8 多囊肾
Fig.9-8 Polycystic kidney

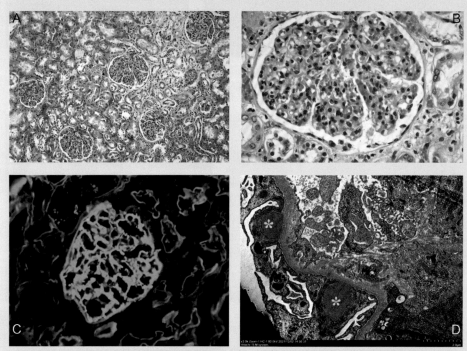

图 9-9 急性弥漫性增生性肾小球肾炎
Fig.9-9 Acute diffuse proliferative glomerulonephritis
P：足突细胞（podocyte）。A，B：HE（×100；×400）；C：IgG IF（×200）；D：TEM（×3000）

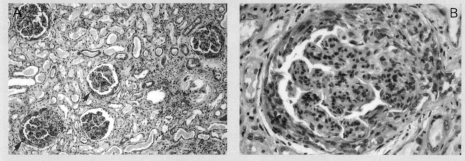

图 9-10 急进性肾小球肾炎
Fig.9-10 Rapidly progressive glomerulonephritis
A. ×100；B. ×400

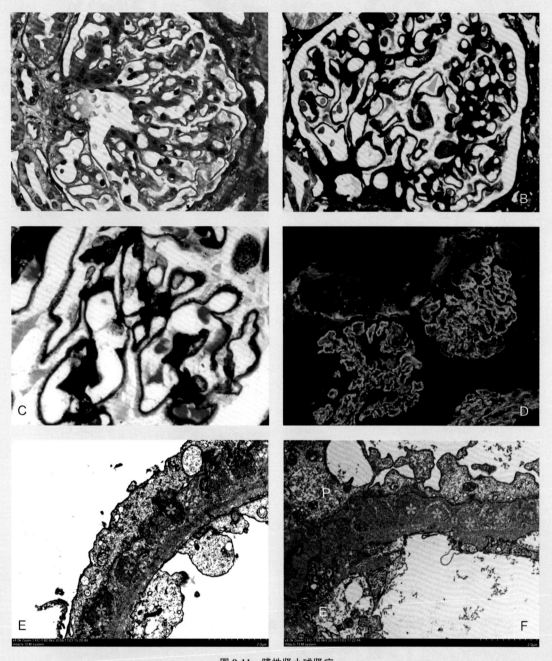

图 9-11　膜性肾小球肾病

Fig.9-11　Membranous nephropathy

P：足突细胞（podocyte），E：内皮细胞（endothelial cell）。

A：PAS（×400）；B：PASM（×400）；C：PASM（×1000）；D：IgG IF（×200）；E，F：TEM（×4000）

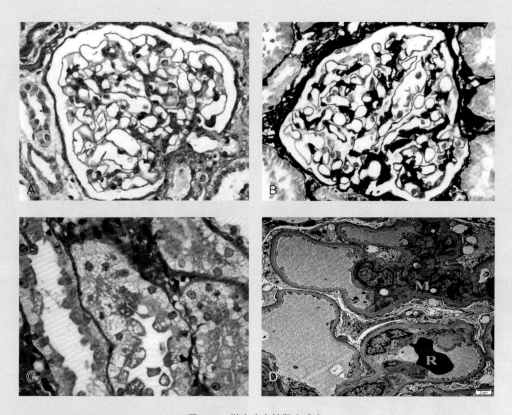

图 9-12　微小病变性肾小球病

Fig.9-12　Minimal change glomerulopathy

P：足突细胞（podocyte）；E：内皮细胞（endothelial cell）；R：红细胞（erythrocyte）；M：系膜细胞（Mesangial cell）。

A：PAS（×400）；B：PASM（×400）；C：PAS（×400）；D：TEM（×4000）

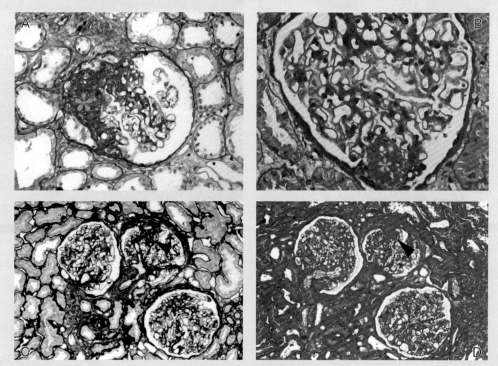

图 9-13　局灶节段性肾小球硬化

Fig.9-13　Focal segmental glomerulosclerosis

A，B：PAS（×200；×400）；C：GMS（×200）；D：MASSON（×200）

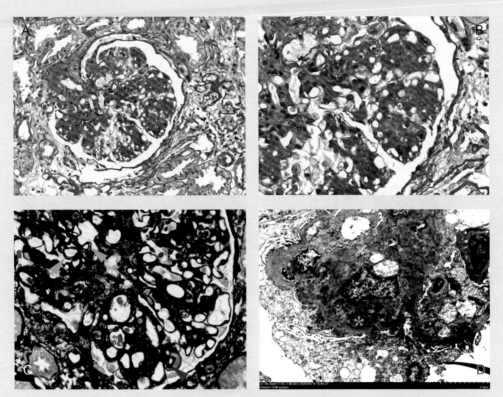

图 9-14　膜增生性肾小球肾炎
Fig.9-14　Membranoproliferative glomerulonephritis
A，B：PAS（×200；×400）；C：PASM（×400）；D：TEM（×1500）

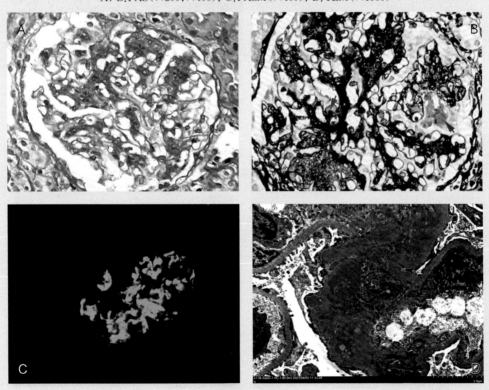

图 9-15　IgA 肾病
Fig.9-15　IgA nephropathy
A：PAS（×400）；B：PASM（×400）；C：IgA IF（×400）；D：TEM（×1500）

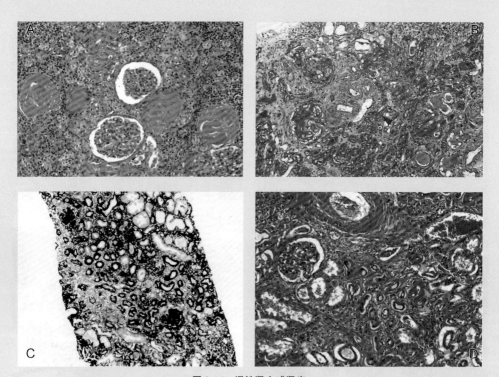

图 9-16　慢性肾小球肾炎

Fig.9-16　Chronic glomerulonephritis

A：H.E.（×200），B：PAS（×200），C：PASM（×100），D：H.E.（×200）

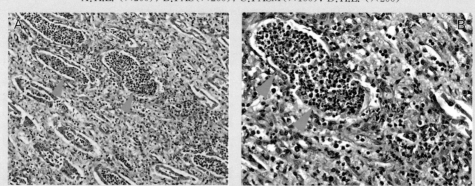

图 9-17　急性肾盂肾炎（×200；×400）

Fig.9-17　Acute pyelonephritis（×200；×400）

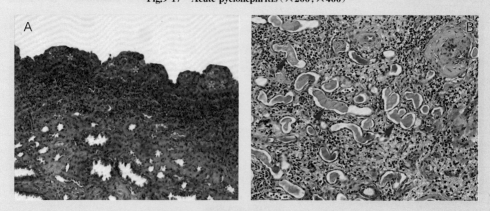

图 9-18　慢性肾盂肾炎（×100；×200）

Fig.9-18　Chronic pyelonephritis（×100；×200）

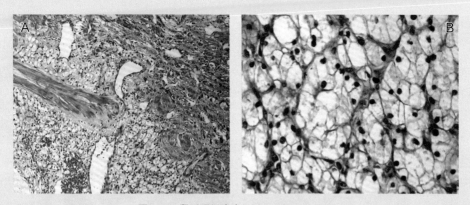

图 9-19　肾透明细胞癌（H.E.，×100；×400）

Fig.9-19　Renal clear cell carcinoma（H.E.，×100；×400）

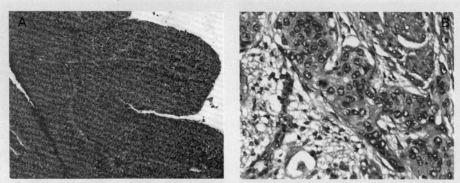

图 9-20　膀胱尿路上皮癌（H.E.，×100；×400）

Fig.9-20　Bladder urothelial carcinoma（H.E.，×100；×400）

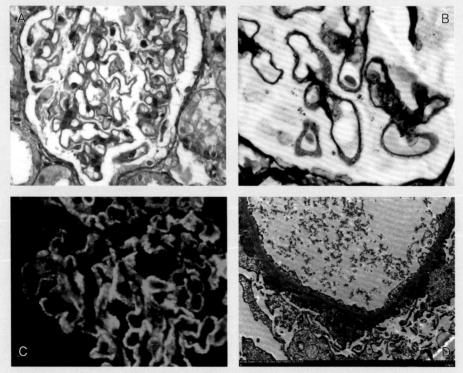

图 9-21　案例 1

Fig.9-21　Case 1

A：PAS（×400），B：PASM（×1000），C：IgG IF（×400），D：TEM（×2500）

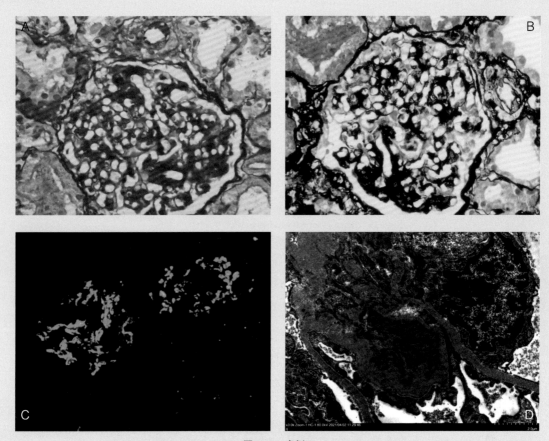

图 9-22　案例 2

Fig.9-22　Case 2

A:PAS(×400)，B:PASM(×400)，C:IgA IF(×200)，D:TEM(×3000)

许纯,陈平圣 (Chun Xu, Pingsheng Chen)

第十章

生殖系统和乳腺疾病

一、目的要求

1. 掌握子宫颈癌、乳腺癌的病理变化和扩散转移方式。

2. 熟悉葡萄胎、侵袭性葡萄胎和绒毛膜癌的基本病理特征。

3. 了解卵巢浆液性和黏液性肿瘤、前列腺疾病的形态特征。

导学

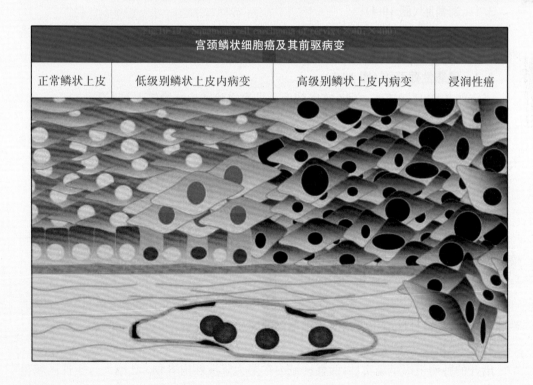

宫颈鳞状细胞癌及其前驱病变			
正常鳞状上皮	低级别鳞状上皮内病变	高级别鳞状上皮内病变	浸润性癌

二、 大体标本

1. 子宫颈疾病

子宫颈鳞状细胞癌（图 10-1）

宫颈部位见灰白色肿瘤组织（蓝星）浸润，沿内膜面向上延伸至子宫体（黑星），部分肿瘤组织坏死脱落，形成溃疡（蓝箭）。请思考：子宫颈癌直接蔓延可能累及的器官有哪些？

2. 子宫体疾病

2.1　子宫内膜腺癌（图 10-2）

子宫腔内膜增厚，肿瘤组织粗糙不平，呈乳头状生长突向宫腔（蓝圈），肿瘤内可见局灶性出血（蓝星）。

2.2　子宫平滑肌瘤（图 10-3）

子宫腔内可见一境界清晰、表面光滑、灰白色、质地坚韧的平滑肌源性肿瘤（蓝圈），局部伴有出血灶（蓝星）。黑箭示患者宫内放置的节育器，嵌顿于部分肿瘤组织。

3. 滋养层细胞疾病

3.1　葡萄胎（图 10-4）

子宫体积增大，宫腔扩张，其内充满葡萄状水泡（蓝星），水泡壁薄，其内液体清亮透明，子宫壁结构尚完好（黑星），未见水泡状组织侵及。

3.2　侵袭性葡萄胎（图 10-5）

子宫体积增大，宫腔略扩张，宫壁切面可见水泡状绒毛结构侵入（蓝圈）。

3.3　绒毛膜癌（图 10-6）

子宫腔内见一灰黑色的结节状肿块（蓝圈），切面粗糙，已侵入子宫肌壁，肿瘤组织内有广泛出血坏死，新鲜标本中呈暗红或紫蓝色。请思考：肿瘤内为何出血坏死明显？

4. 卵巢肿瘤

4.1　卵巢浆液性乳头状囊腺瘤（图 10-7）

所示为一剖开的囊性肿瘤，浆液性囊内容物已流失，残留的囊壁上可见部分区域肿瘤组织增生，呈乳头状向囊内突起（蓝圈）。

4.2　卵巢黏液性囊腺瘤（图 10-8）

肿瘤组织剖面可见大小不等的囊腔，腔内充满胶冻样黏液性物质（蓝星）。与浆液性肿瘤相比，黏液性肿瘤中囊内富于糖蛋白的物质较易保留。

4.3　卵巢粒层细胞瘤（图 10-9）

剖开的肿瘤组织呈囊实性，囊性区域内主要为浆液性内容物（已流失），实性区域呈灰白或灰黄色，明显呈黄色的实性区域（蓝圈）主要由富含脂质的黄素化的粒层细胞构成。

4.4　卵巢成熟性囊性畸胎瘤（图 10-10）

肿瘤整体呈囊状，囊壁（黑星）较薄，剖开的囊内可见大量毛发，混杂的皮脂样物质大部分已流失,囊壁上可见一明显的结节状突起(头节,蓝星)。

5. 前列腺疾病

前列腺增生症(图 10-11)

前列腺体积增大,质地较韧,切面可见多个大小不等的结节状病灶(蓝圈),结节内可见蜂窝状腔隙(腺体增生)或实性区域(纤维、平滑肌增生)。

6. 阴茎肿瘤

阴茎鳞状细胞癌(图 10-12)

多个灰白色、菜花状或结节状肿瘤组织(蓝星)已占据阴茎龟头,肿瘤团块相互融合,蔓延至阴茎体,黑星示残留的皮肤及阴囊组织。

7. 乳腺疾病

7.1 乳腺导管内乳头状瘤(图 10-13)

扩张的乳腺导管内可见明显的息肉样肿块(蓝圈),质地较软,易碎,部分区域有小灶性出血。

7.2 乳腺纤维腺瘤(图 10-14)

乳腺组织内有一卵圆形、境界清晰的结节状肿块(蓝圈),切面灰白色,质韧,呈分叶状,可见裂隙状区域。蓝箭示皮肤。

7.3 乳腺癌(图 10-15)

经乳头(黑星)的乳腺组织矢状切面内可见一质硬、形状不规则的灰白色肿块(蓝星),其边缘呈蟹足状向周围组织浸润(蓝箭),乳头已明显内陷。

7.4 肝转移性乳腺癌(图 10-16)

患者有乳腺癌病史,肝内可见多个大小不等、境界较清晰的圆形结节(蓝箭),镜检证实为乳腺浸润性导管癌肝内转移灶。

三、组织切片

1. 子宫颈疾病

1.1 子宫颈纳博特囊肿(图 10-17)

子宫颈阴道部被覆的鳞状上皮(黑星)略有增生,上皮下可见一扩张呈囊状的腺体(蓝圈),内衬分泌黏液的柱状上皮细胞(蓝箭),囊内有大量黏液潴留(蓝星)。

1.2 子宫颈息肉(图 10-18)

息肉样肿物内可见宫颈黏膜上皮、腺体(蓝箭)和间质结缔组织(黑圈)增生明显,混杂有数量不等的炎细胞浸润(蓝圈),间质水肿,小血管扩张充血(蓝星)。

1.3 子宫颈鳞状细胞癌(图 10-19)

肿瘤组织(蓝星)呈相互融合的巢片状浸润于宫颈组织内,表面可见残留的鳞状上皮(黑星),部分被覆上皮已坏死脱落(绿星)。高倍镜下,可见肿瘤细胞异型性明显,核分裂象多见(蓝箭)。

1.4　子宫颈腺癌（图 10-20）

与略呈反应性增生的腺体（黑箭）相比较，肿瘤性的腺样结构（蓝圈）排列紊乱，可见核大、深染，多形性的癌细胞，部分肿瘤性腺腔内有少量黏液分泌物，近腔面可见核分裂象（绿箭）。

2. 子宫体疾病

腹壁子宫内膜异位症（图 10-21）

腹壁软组织内查见异位的子宫内膜腺体（蓝箭）和间质（蓝星），部分区域陈旧性出血（蓝圈），含铁血黄素沉积明显。该患者有剖宫产手术史。

3. 滋养层细胞疾病

3.1　葡萄胎（图 10-22）

葡萄胎中绒毛结构因间质高度水肿而增大，间质内血管消失，滋养层细胞大量增生（蓝星）。蓝箭示细胞滋养层细胞，绿箭示合体滋养层细胞，黑星示绒毛间质，请注意与正常绒毛形态比较。

3.2　侵袭性葡萄胎（图 10-23）

子宫肌层（黑星）内大量巢片状的滋养层细胞（蓝圈）侵袭，与周围的平滑肌组织界限不清，其中可见水泡状绒毛结构（蓝星）。与葡萄胎相比较，明显增生的细胞滋养层细胞（蓝箭）和合体滋养层细胞（绿箭）均具有一定程度的异型性。

3.3　侵袭性葡萄胎肺栓塞（图 10-24）

侵袭性葡萄胎的绒毛组织经血管栓塞至肺。肺组织被破坏，有明显的出血坏死（绿星），并查见水泡状绒毛（蓝星）。蓝箭和绿箭分别示具有异型性的细胞滋养层细胞和合体滋养层细胞，黑星示残留肺组织。

3.4　绒毛膜癌（图 10-25）

癌组织（蓝星）主要由分化不良的似细胞滋养层细胞（蓝箭）和似合体滋养层细胞（绿箭）构成，呈团块状或条索状，广泛浸润于子宫肌层（黑星）中，可见癌细胞坏死。请思考：该肿瘤组织内是否可查见绒毛结构？

4. 卵巢肿瘤

4.1　卵巢浆液性囊腺瘤（图 10-26）

肿瘤的纤维性囊壁（黑星）内有单层立方或矮柱状上皮衬覆（蓝箭），可见较宽的乳头状结构（蓝圈），衬覆细胞形态较一致，无异型性。

4.2　卵巢黏液性囊腺瘤（图 10-27）

肿瘤囊腔（蓝星）衬覆单层高柱状上皮（蓝箭），细胞核位于基底部，胞浆内充满黏液。黑星示囊壁纤维间质成分。

5. 前列腺疾病

5.1　慢性前列腺炎（图 10-28）

前列腺部分腺泡或导管内可见混杂有炎细胞的分泌物（绿星），上皮细胞鳞状化生（蓝箭），注意与正常的上皮细胞（黑箭）形态比较。间质中可见灶性单核细胞、淋巴细胞和浆细胞浸润（蓝星）。

5.2　前列腺增生症（图 10-29）

多个结节状病灶（蓝星）内可见增生的纤维平滑肌穿插于众多腺体之间，腺腔大小不一，部分腔内可见淀粉样小体，增生的腺体上皮由两层细胞构成，内层细胞呈柱状（蓝箭），外层基底细胞呈立方或扁平状（绿箭），部分上皮细胞似乳头状凸向腔内（蓝圈）。黑星示结节状病灶之间明显增生的纤维平滑肌间质。

5.3　前列腺癌（图 10-30）

癌组织（蓝星）呈弥漫浸润，注意与残留的正常腺泡（黑星）相比较。肿瘤细胞可围成排列紧密的小腺泡或呈条索状结构（蓝圈），小腺泡由单层癌细胞构成，外层的基底细胞缺如，癌细胞核体积增大，核仁明显（蓝箭）。

6. 乳腺疾病

6.1　乳腺导管内乳头状瘤（图 10-31）

扩张的导管内可见复杂分支的乳头状病变（蓝圈），乳头状结构（绿圈）具有明显的纤维血管轴心（绿星），表面被覆增生的两层细胞，导管上皮细胞（蓝箭）和肌上皮细胞（黑箭）。

6.2　乳腺纤维腺瘤（图 10-32）

肿瘤主要由增生的纤维间质（绿星）和腺体（蓝星）组成，包膜完整（黑星），部分腺体被周围纤维结缔组织挤压成裂隙状。腺体由两层细胞构成，腔面的上皮细胞（蓝箭）和外侧的肌上皮细胞（黑箭）。

6.3　乳腺导管原位癌（图 10-33）

乳腺多个导管内可见呈实性或筛状结构的肿瘤细胞团（蓝星），瘤细胞增生活跃，排列紊乱，核大而多形（蓝箭），局限于导管内，导管外层的肌上皮细胞（黑箭）可见。黑星示乳腺小叶结构无明显受累。

6.4　乳腺浸润性导管癌（图 10-34）

癌组织（蓝圈）呈条索状或不规则团块弥漫浸润于纤维间质内，临近的乳腺小叶（黑星）结构部分受累，癌细胞（蓝箭）大小不一，异型性明显。周围间质内纤维组织增生显著，部分区域见黏液样变（绿星）。

6.5　乳腺黏液癌（图 10-35）

小簇状的癌细胞团块（蓝箭）漂浮在黏液湖（绿星）中，黏液湖之间可见宽窄不等的纤维间隔（黑星）完全或不全分隔。

四、临床病理讨论

案例　患者，女性，58 岁，右侧乳腺外上象限可触及一大小约 2 cm 的非活动性肿块，BI-RADS：5 类。术后大体标本见病灶呈灰白色，质地较韧，与周围组织分界欠清，镜下形态如图 10-36 所示。

（1）该患者最可能的病理诊断是什么？

（2）如果患者未行治疗，该病变可能会有哪些不良进展？

五、 思考题

1. 宫颈鳞状上皮癌前病变如何分类?

2. 从形态学角度,如何区分葡萄胎、侵袭性葡萄胎和绒毛膜癌?

3. 常见的卵巢生殖细胞肿瘤有哪些?

4. 名词解释:高级别鳞状上皮内病变,宫颈微浸润鳞状细胞癌,Call-Exner 小体,乳腺粉刺癌,乳腺佩吉特病(Paget 病)。

Chapter 10

Diseases of Genital System and Breast

I . Aims

1. To grasp the morphological changes, invasion and metastasis of cervical carcinoma and breast cancer.

2. To familiarize with the pathological characteristics of hydatidiform mole, invasive mole and choriocarcinoma.

3. To understand the common types and their morphological features of ovarian tumors and prostatic diseases.

Guidance to study

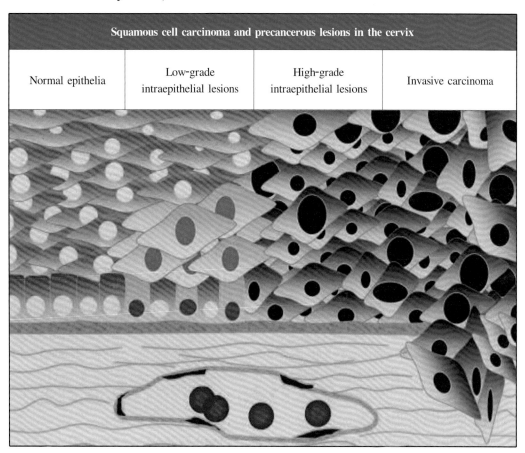

Squamous cell carcinoma and precancerous lesions in the cervix			
Normal epithelia	Low-grade intraepithelial lesions	High-grade intraepithelial lesions	Invasive carcinoma

II. Gross specimens

1. Diseases of uterine cervix

Squamous cell carcinoma of cervix (Fig. 10-1)

The specimen shows gray-white cancerous invasion (blue asterisks) in the cervix, consisting ulcerative changes (blue arrow). The cancerous lesion spreads up to the uterine corpus (black asterisk). Please consider the vulnerably involved organs related to direct spread of cervical carcinoma.

2. Diseases of uterine corpus

2. 1　Endometrial adenocarcinoma (Fig.10-2)

The endometrium is significantly thickened with tumor involvement. The cancerous lesion presents papillary protrusions toward the uterus cavity (blue circle), with focal hemorrhage (blue asterisks).

2. 2　Uterine leiomyoma (Fig.10-3)

The blue circle shows one gray-white and firm mass derived from smooth muscle cells, with smooth surface and sharp demarcation, and hemorrhage can be observed (blue asterisk). It is worth noting that an intrauterine device (black arrow) was embedded in the tumor tissue.

3. Gestational trophoblastic diseases

3. 1　Hydatidiform mole (Fig.10-4)

The uterus is markedly enlarged, and the cavity is dilated and filled with grape-like, translucent and friable clusters of chorionic villi (blue asterisk). The uterus wall remains intact (black asterisk), with no invasion of chorionic villi.

3. 2　Invasive mole (Fig.10-5)

The uterus is mildly enlarged and the cavity is expanded slightly. The hydropic villi can be found in the uterus wall (blue circles).

3. 3　Choriocarcinoma (Fig.10-6)

A dark gray large and friable mass (blue circle) is observed in the uterus cavity. On cut section, it is rough, hemorrhagic and necrotic, and the myometrium has been invaded. Please think about why hemorrhage and necrosis are so distinct in cancer tissues with choriocarcinoma?

4. Ovarian tumors

4. 1　Serous papillary cystadenoma of ovary (Fig.10-7)

The specimen is opened to show cystic tumor lined by papillary projections (blue circles).

The clear serous fluid in the cyst has flowed away.

4. 2　Mucinous cystadenoma of ovary（Fig.10-8）

On the cut surface of ovary tumor, there are some cysts filled with jelly-like mucinous substance (blue asterisks) in various sizes. Compared to serous tumor, the glycoprotein-rich gelatinous mucus is easy to be retained after the cysts are cut.

4. 3　Granulosa cell tumor of ovary（Fig.10-9）

The cut tumor tissue presents cystic and solid areas. Nothing is observed in the cysts because the serous content has run off. The solid areas (blue circle) are gray-white or gray-yellow, and the yellow areas are mainly composed of lipid-rich luteinized granular cells.

4. 4　Mature cystic teratoma of ovary（Fig.10-10）

The tumor presents a large cyst with thin wall (black asterisk). On the cut cyst, matted hair is obvious, and the mixed sebaceous substance has almost flowed away. A prominent nodular projection (Rokitansky's protuberance, blue asterisk) can be observed on the inner cyst wall.

5. Prostatic diseases

Benign prostatic hyperplasia（Fig. 10-11）

The prostate is enlarged, solid, and tensile. On cut section, there are some nodules in various sizes (blue circles) with honey-comb cystic spaces (hyperplastic glands) and solid areas (hyperplastic fibromuscular tissue).

6. Tumors of penis

Squamous cell carcinoma of penis（Fig. 10-12）

The glans has been infiltrated by multiple gray-white, cauliflower-like or nodular masses (blue asterisks). The masses are confluent, and spread to the body of penis. The black asterisk indicates remained skin and scrotum tissue.

7. Breast diseases

7. 1　Intraductal papilloma of breast（Fig.10-13）

A prominent polypoid mass is soft and friable in the dilated duct (blue circle), and some areas present focal hemorrhage.

7. 2　Breast fibroadenoma（Fig.10-14）

In the resected breast tissue, there is a well-circumscribed, gray-white oval mass. On cut section, it is multilobular firm and elastic with slit-like spaces. The blue arrow indicates the skin.

7. 3　Breast carcinoma（Fig.10-15）

The breast tissue is cut along the ripple (black asterisk), and the section displays a gray-white, irregular hard mass (blue asterisk) which shows crab-like invasion (blue arrows) into the surrounding tissue, and the ripple is obviously retracted.

7. 4 Metastatic breast carcinoma in liver (Fig.10-16)

The liver tissue is removed from the patient with breast carcinoma. Multiple round nodules (blue arrows) are observed to be well-circumscribed, and different in size, which are histologically proved to be metastatic tumors from breast invasive ductal carcinoma.

Ⅲ. Tissue sections

1. Diseases of uterine cervix

1. 1 Nabothian cyst of cervix (Fig.10-17)

The ectocervix is covered by proliferative squamous epithelium (black asterisk). There is a dilated cystic gland (blue circle) lined by mucin-secreting columnar epithelial cells (blue arrows), and abundant mucus (blue asterisks) exists in the cystic cavity.

1. 2 Cervical polyp (Fig.10-18)

The polypoid mass is composed of proliferative cervical mucinous epithelial cells, glands (blue arrows), and interstitial connective tissues (black circle) with infiltrating inflammatory cells (blue circle), edematous stroma, dilated and congested small blood vessels (blue asterisks).

1. 3 Squamous cell carcinoma of cervix (Fig.10-19)

The tumor tissue (blue asterisks) shows confluent nests infiltrating into the cervical tissue, and the remained squamous epithelium (black asterisk) on the surface has partly desquamated due to necrosis (green asterisk). At high magnification, cancer cells present obvious atypia with easily observed pathological mitoses (blue arrows).

1. 4 Adenocarcinoma of cervix (Fig.10-20)

Compared to responsively hyperplastic glands (black arrows), neoplastic gland-like structures (blue circle) arrange disorderly, and tumor cells (blue arrow) appear as pleomorphic shapes with large deep-stained nuclei. A little mucous secretion is present in the lumens of neoplastic glands, and mitotic figures (green arrow) can be observed in the cancer cells close to the lumens.

2. Diseases of uterine corpus

Endometriosis of abdominal wall (Fig.10-21)

The soft tissue is from abdominal wall, and the patient has had a caesarean delivery. The tissue contains some ectopic endometrial glands (blue arrows) and stroma (blue asterisk). Old focal hemorrhage (blue circle) with obvious hemosiderin deposition is also observed.

3. Gestational trophoblastic diseases

3. 1　Hydatidiform mole (Fig.10-22)

The chorionic villi are covered by apparently hyperplastic trophoblastic cells (blue asterisks), with less vascularized, loose, and edematous stroma (black asterisks). The blue and green arrows indicate cytotrophoblast and syncytiotrophoblast cells, respectively. Please compare the villi in this tissue with the normal villi in morphology.

3. 2　Invasive mole (Fig.10-23)

Abundant nest-like trophoblastic cells (blue circle) have penetrated into the myometrium (black asterisk). A hydropic villus (blue asterisk) is noticed within the myometrium. Compared to the trophoblastic cells of hydatidiform mole, both hyperplastic cytotrophoblasts (blue arrow) and syncytiotrophoblasts (green arrow) present atypia, to a certain extent.

3. 3　Pulmonary embolism involved by invasive mole (Fig.10-24)

The invasive villi have invaded into the pulmonary tissue through blood vessels, and remarkable hemorrhage and necrosis (green asterisks) as well hydropic villi (blue asterisks) are observed in the lung. The blue and green arrows indicate atypical cytotrophoblast and syncytiotrophoblast cells, respectively. The black asterisk shows remained lung tissue.

3. 4　Choriocarcinoma (Fig.10-25)

The cancerous tissue (blue asterisks) consists of pleomorphic masses or cords of poorly differentiated cytotrophoblast-like (blue arrow) and syncytiotrophoblast-like cells (green arrow), which has extensively invaded the myometrium (black asterisks). Therefore, necrotic and hemorrhagic tissues are easily observed. Please consider whether chorionic villi are examined in the choriocarcinoma tissue.

4. Ovarian tumors

4. 1　Serous cystadenoma of ovary (Fig.10-26)

The tumor tissue displays fibrous cystic wall (black asterisks) which is lined by single layer of cuboidal or low columnar epithelia (blue arrows). The epithelia may appear as broad papillary structures (blue circle), and the epithelial cells show uniform without marked atypia in morphology.

4. 2　Mucinous cystadenoma of ovary (Fig.10-27)

The cysts (blue asterisks) of the tumor are covered by single layer of tall columnar epithelium (blue arrows), and the nuclei of epithelial cells are located at the base part of the cells, with rich mucus in the cytoplasm. The black asterisks indicate fibrous interstitium.

5. Prostatic diseases

5. 1　Chronic prostatitis（Fig.10-28）

Some prostatic acini and ducts are lined by metaplastic squamous epithelial cells（blue arrows）, and display inflammatory secretory materials（green asterisks）. Please notice the difference between the metaplastic epithelia and normal epithelia（black arrow）. There are focal monocytes, lymphocytes, and plasma cells（blue asterisks）infiltration in the stroma.

5. 2　Benign prostatic hyperplasia（Fig.10-29）

Multiple nodular lesions（blue asterisks）display hyperplastic fibromuscular stroma mixed with numerous vary-sized glands. Some lumens show corpora amylacea, and the hyperplastic glandular epithelial cells consist of two-layer cells, inner columnar cells（blue arrow）and outer cuboidal or flattened basal cells（green arrow）. Some of the proliferative epithelial cells develop into papillary structures and protrude into the lumens（blue circle）. The black asterisk presents marked hyperplasia of fibromuscular stroma between the nodular lesions.

5. 3　Prostatic carcinoma（Fig.10-30）

The diffusely infiltrating cancerous tissues (blue asterisks) show different morphology compared to the remained normal acini (black asterisks). The tumor cells arrange in crowded small acini or cords（blue circles）, and small acini are composed of monolayer large cells with distinct nucleoli（blue arrows）. The outer basal cells are absent.

6. Breast diseases

6. 1　Intraductal papilloma of breast（Fig.10-31）

The papillary infoldings with complicated branches (blue circle) are examined in the dilated ducts. The papillary structures (green circles) display prominent fibrovascular cores (green asterisks) covered by two-layer cells, ductal epithelial cells (blue arrow) and myoepithelial cells（black arrow）.

6. 2　Fibroadenoma of breast（Fig.10-32）

The tumor is composed of proliferative fibrous stroma（green asterisks）and glands（blue asterisks）, with an intact capsule（black asterisk）. Some glands appear as slit-like structures squeezed by surrounding fibrous connective tissues. The glands consist of two-layer of cells, inner epithelial cells（blue arrow）and outer myoepithelial cells（black arrow）.

6. 3　Ductal carcinoma in situ of breast（Fig.10-33）

Multiple mammary ducts present solid or cribriform tumor cell clusters（blue asterisks）, and the actively proliferative tumor cells are disorganized and confined to the ducts. The tumor cells have large and pleomorphic nuclei (blue arrow), and outer myoepithelial cells (black arrow)of the ducts can be observed. The black asterisk indicates uninvolved lobules.

6. 4　Invasive ductal carcinoma of breast（Fig.10-34）

The cords-like or irregular nests-like cancerous tissues (blue circle) have diffusely infiltrated into the fibrous stroma, and the adjacent breast lobules (black asterisks) are locally involved. The cancer cells (blue arrows) are different in size with prominent atypia. The surrounding stroma displays desmoplastic and mucoid degeneration (green asterisk).

6. 5　Mucinous carcinoma of breast（Fig.10-35）

The cancerous cell clusters (blue arrows) float in the mucin-rich pools (green asterisks), and the mucinous pools are partitioned by fibrous septa (black asterisks) with different width.

Ⅳ. Clinical pathological discussion

Case

A 58-year-old woman has a palpable immobile mass with the diameter of about 2 cm in the superior lateral quadrant of her right breast, and BI‐RADS is category Ⅴ. The surgical specimen appears as gray white and flexible, with unclear boundary. Microscopic examination is shown as Fig.10-36.

(1) What is the most likely pathological diagnosis of the breast?

(2) Please list the possible consequences of the lesion if the patient has refused any medical intervention.

Ⅴ. Questions

1. What can cervical squamous epithelial precancerous lesions be classified into?

2. Please distinguish hydatidiform mole from invasive mole and choriocarcinoma in morphology.

3. What are the common ovarian germ cell derived tumors?

4. Terms: High-grade intraepithelial lesion (HSIL), Cervical microinvasive squamous cell carcinoma, Call-Exner body, Comedocarcinoma of breast, Paget disease of breast.

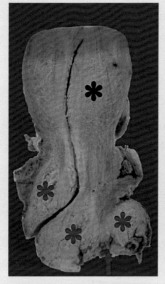

图 10-1　子宫颈鳞状细胞癌

Fig.10-1　Squamous cell
carcinoma of cervix

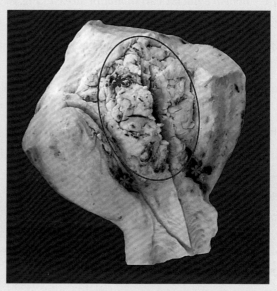

图 10-2　子宫内膜腺癌

Fig.10-2　Endometrial adenocarcinoma

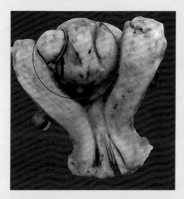

图 10-3　子宫平滑肌瘤

Fig.10-3　Uterine leiomyoma

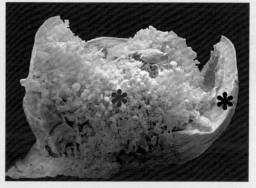

图 10-4　葡萄胎

Fig.10-4　Hydatidiform mole

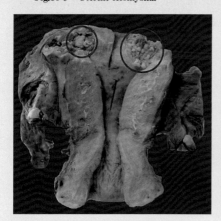

图 10-5　侵袭性葡萄胎

Fig.10-5　Invasive mole

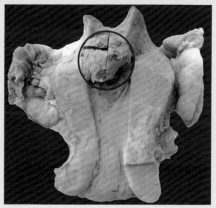

图 10-6　绒毛膜癌

Fig.10-6　Choriocarcinoma

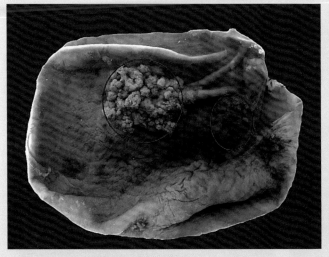

图 10-7 卵巢浆液性乳头状囊腺瘤
Fig.10-7 Serous papillary cystadenoma of ovary

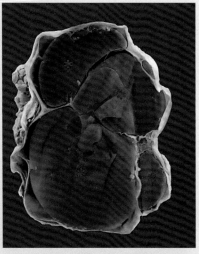

图 10-8 卵巢黏液性囊腺瘤
Fig.10-8 Mucinous cystadenoma
of ovary

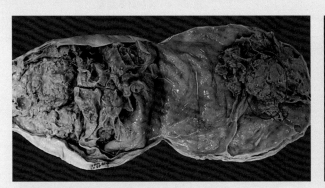

图 10-9 卵巢粒层细胞瘤
Fig.10-9 Granulosa cell tumor of ovary

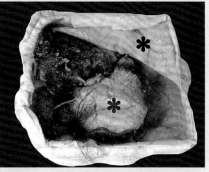

图 10-10 卵巢成熟性囊性畸胎瘤
Fig.10-10 Mature cystic teratoma of ovary

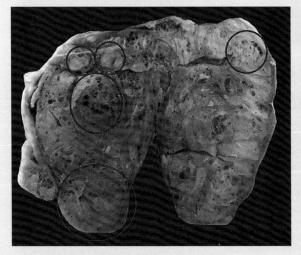

图 10-11 前列腺增生症
Fig.10-11 Benign prostatic hyperplasia

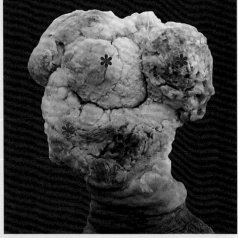

图 10-12 阴茎鳞状细胞癌
Fig.10-12 Squamous cell carcinoma of penis

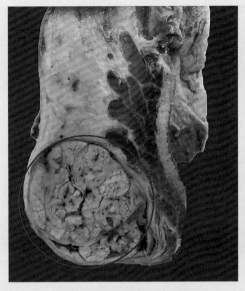

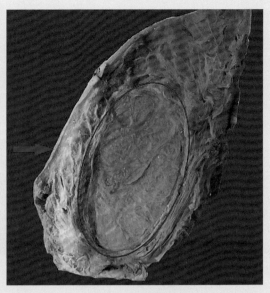

图 10-13 乳腺导管内乳头状瘤
Fig.10-13 Intraductal papilloma of breast

图 10-14 乳腺纤维腺瘤
Fig.10-14 Breast fibroadenoma

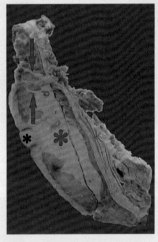

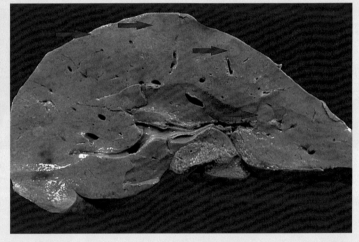

图 10-15 乳腺癌
Fig.10-15 Breast carcinoma

图 10-16 肝转移性乳腺癌
Fig.10-16 Metastatic breast carcinoma in liver

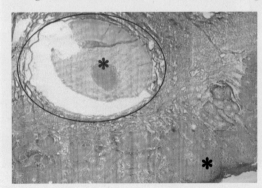

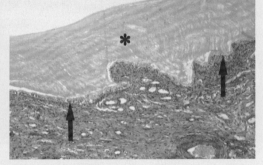

图 10-17 子宫颈纳博特囊肿（×40；×100）
Fig.10-17 Nabothian cyst of cervix（×40；×100）

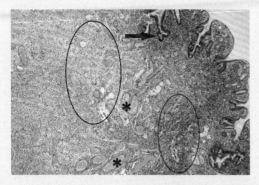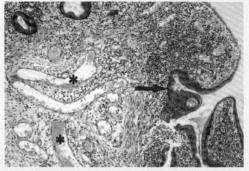

图 10-18　子宫颈息肉（×40；×100）
Fig.10-18　Cervical polyp（×40；×100）

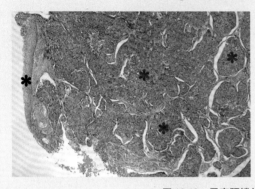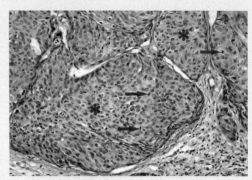

图 10-19　子宫颈鳞状细胞癌（×40；×400）
Fig.10-19　Squamous cell carcinoma of cervix（×40；×400）

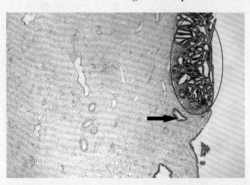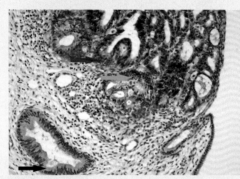

图 10-20　子宫颈腺癌（×40；×200）
Fig.10-20　Adenocarcinoma of cervix（×40；×200）

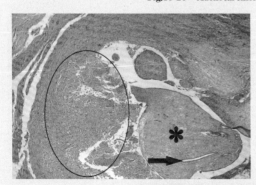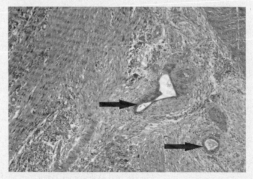

图 10-21　腹壁子宫内膜异位症（×40；×100）
Fig.10-21　Endometriosis of abdominal wall（×40；×100）

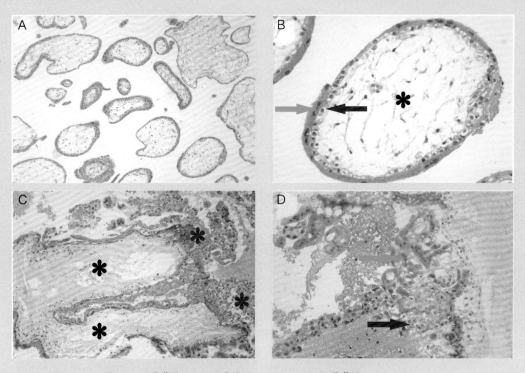

图 10-22　葡萄胎（A，B：正常绒毛×40；×400；C，D：葡萄胎×100；×200）
Fig.10-22　Hydatidiform mole（A，B：Normal villi×40；×400；C，D：Hydatidiform mole×100；×200）

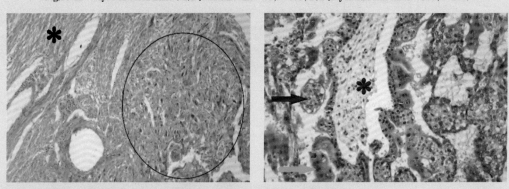

图 10-23　侵袭性葡萄胎（×100；×200）
Fig.10-23　Invasive mole（×100；×200）

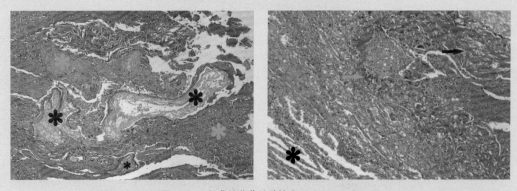

图 10-24　侵袭性葡萄胎肺栓塞（×40；×100）
Fig.10-24　Pulmonary embolism involved by invasive mole（×40；×100）

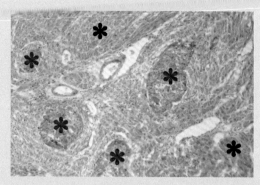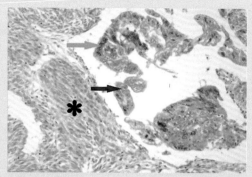

图 10-25　绒毛膜癌（×100；×200）
Fig.10-25　Choriocarcinoma（×100；×200）

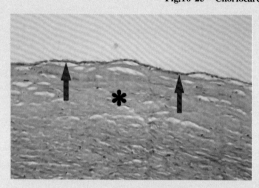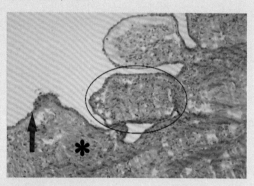

图 10-26　卵巢浆液性囊腺瘤（×200）
Fig.10-26　Serious cystadenoma of ovary（×200）

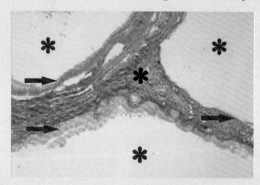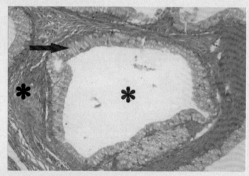

图 10-27　卵巢黏液性囊腺瘤（×100；×200）
Fig.10-27　Mucinous cystadenoma of ovary（×100；×200）

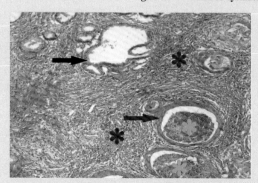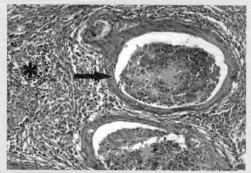

图 10-28　慢性前列腺炎（×100；×200）
Fig.10-28　Chronic prostatitis（×100；×200）

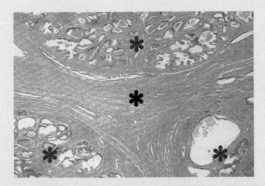
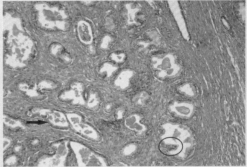

图 10-29　前列腺增生症（×40；×100）

Fig.10-29　Benign prostatic hyperplasia（×40；×100）

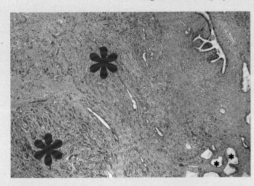
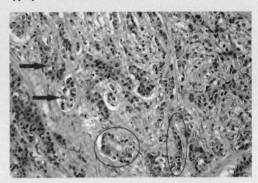

图 10-30　前列腺癌（×40；×200）

Fig.10-30　Prostatic carcinoma（×40；×200）

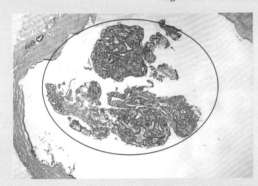
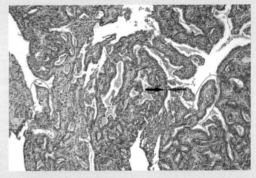

图 10-31　乳腺导管内乳头状瘤（×40；×100）

Fig.10-31　Intraductal papilloma of breast（×40；×100）

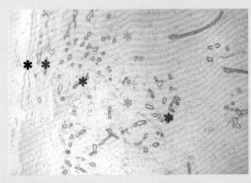
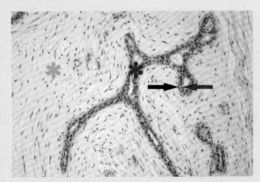

图 10-32　乳腺纤维腺瘤（×40；×200）

Fig.10-32　Fibroadenoma of breast（×40；×200）

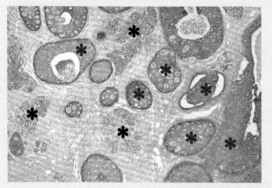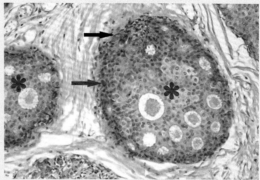

图 10-33 乳腺导管原位癌（×40；×200）

Fig.10-33 Ductal carcinoma in situ of breast（×40；×200）

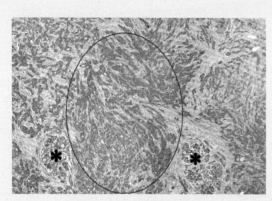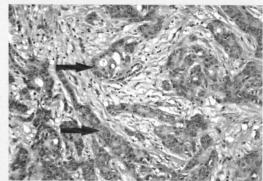

图 10-34 乳腺浸润性导管癌（×40；×200）

Fig.10-34 Invasive ductal carcinoma of breast（×40；×200）

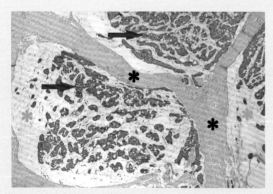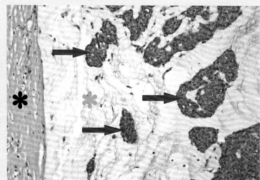

图 10-35 乳腺黏液癌（×40；×200）

Fig.10-35 Mucinous carcinoma of breast（×40；×200）

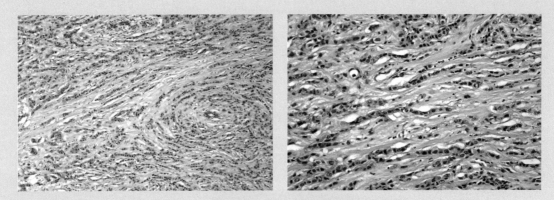

图 10-36　案例（×100；×200）
Fig.10-36　Case（×100；×200）

潘旻，卜晓东（Min Pan，Xiaodong Bu）

第十一章

内分泌系统疾病

一、目的要求

1. 掌握弥漫性非毒性甲状腺肿及三个病变阶段的形态特征。
2. 掌握弥漫性毒性甲状腺肿的病变特征。
3. 掌握甲状腺乳头状癌的大体和组织学形态特征。
4. 熟悉结节性甲状腺肿、甲状腺腺瘤和甲状腺滤泡癌的形态鉴别。
5. 了解桥本甲状腺炎、肾上腺嗜铬细胞瘤的病变特征。

导学

	结节性甲状腺肿	甲状腺腺瘤	甲状腺滤泡癌
大体形态	常为大小不等的多发结节	常为孤立性单发结节	常为孤立性单发结节
包膜	无完整包膜	厚薄不等的纤维包膜	厚包膜,常伴有包膜侵犯
血管侵犯	无	无	可以有
滤泡大小	常为正常或者巨滤泡	常为小滤泡或者正常	常为小滤泡或者正常
衬覆细胞	常为单层平坦到低立方形	常为单层,形态一致的多边形细胞	多边形细胞,有密集细胞区域,可形成筛状或者小梁状结构
细胞核	圆形或卵圆形,大小一致	圆形或卵圆形,大小一致	可以有核分裂象,核多形性,可见核仁
与临近组织的关系	临近组织与结节内滤泡有类似形态,无明显压迫	临近组织多为正常滤泡,有明显受压现象	肿瘤常突破包膜进入临近组织或广泛侵犯

二、 大体标本

1. 甲状腺疾病

1.1　甲状腺囊肿（图11-1）

甲状腺组织切面可见一边界清晰的囊性病变（蓝圈），其内为血性内容物，黑星示周围残存的正常甲状腺组织。

1.2　弥漫性非毒性甲状腺肿（图11-2）

甲状腺弥漫性对称性增大，包膜完整，切面呈棕褐色，可见大量胶冻状物质，无明显结节状结构。请思考：此标本对应的是弥漫性非毒性甲状腺肿的哪一期肉眼形态？

1.3　弥漫性毒性甲状腺肿（图11-3）

该标本为切开的甲状腺，呈弥漫性对称性增大，表面光滑，切面灰红色，胶质少，质地似肌肉，无明显结节形成。

1.4　甲状腺乳头状癌（图11-4）

呈书页状剖开的甲状腺组织切面中可见一质地较硬的灰白色病灶（蓝圈），肿瘤部分区域与周围组织的界限欠清晰，黑星示正常的甲状腺组织。

2. 肾上腺疾病

2.1　肾上腺出血（图11-5）

标本为沿冠状面剖开的一侧肾脏以及肾上腺。肾上腺内可见一弥漫性出血灶（蓝星），下方的肾脏组织略有挤压（黑星）。肾上腺出血多见于婴儿，可表现为腹膜后肿块或肾上腺功能不全，可能与胎儿缺氧、败血症等疾病有关。

2.2　肾上腺皮质腺瘤（图11-6）

肾上腺皮质内可见一淡黄或金黄色，境界较清晰的占位性病灶（蓝圈）。黑星示残留的正常肾上腺组织。

2.3　肾上腺嗜铬细胞瘤（图11-7）

肿瘤组织呈球形，质地较软，切面呈黄白色，部分肿瘤组织出血、坏死及囊性变（蓝星）。

2.4　肾上腺转移性肺癌（图11-8）

标本为一原发性肺癌转移至肾上腺。肾上腺体积明显增大（蓝星），切面呈灰白色，边界不清，下方可见剖开的同侧肾脏（黑星）。

三、 组织切片

1. 甲状腺疾病

1.1　弥漫性非毒性甲状腺肿（图11-9）

切片中可见大小不一的滤泡结构，滤泡腔内为大量均质伊红染的胶质（蓝星）。大部分滤泡上皮细胞呈扁平或立方状（蓝箭），伴有小滤泡形成（黑星）。

1.2　弥漫性毒性甲状腺肿（图11-10）

切片组织内见不同大小的滤泡形成（蓝星），滤泡上皮细胞增生呈高柱状或复层（蓝箭),有的呈乳头样增生(蓝圈)。滤泡腔内胶质较稀薄,周边的胶质可见大小不一的吸收空泡(黑箭),间质内血管较丰富,部分区域淋巴组织增生(黑星)。

1.3 桥本甲状腺炎(图 11-11)

甲状腺组织受损萎缩,部分滤泡上皮细胞被破坏,呈嗜酸性变(蓝箭),间质内大量淋巴细胞浸润(黑星),伴有淋巴滤泡形成(蓝星)。

1.4 甲状腺腺瘤(图 11-12)

黑星示正常甲状腺组织,肿瘤包膜完整(绿星)。瘤组织由大小较一致、排列拥挤的滤泡构成(蓝星),部分滤泡内可见胶质。蓝箭示肿瘤性的滤泡上皮细胞,可形成微滤泡结构。

1.5 甲状腺乳头状癌(图 11-13)

黑星示正常甲状腺组织。肿瘤细胞呈复杂乳头状分支结构排列(蓝星),乳头结构中轴为纤维和血管组织,高倍镜下可见癌细胞核呈毛玻璃样外观(蓝箭),核增大、重叠,部分癌细胞可见核沟(黑箭)及核内假包涵体(绿箭)。

1.6 甲状腺滤泡癌(图 11-14)

肿瘤组织(蓝星)周围包裹有较厚的纤维包膜(绿星),部分肿瘤组织已侵犯至包膜外(蓝圈),包膜内外的肿瘤组织形态类似,黑星示正常甲状腺组织。高倍镜下可见肿瘤性的滤泡结构(蓝箭),部分滤泡腔内尚有胶质残余。

1.7 淋巴结转移性甲状腺髓样癌(图 11-15)

受累淋巴结的大部分区域已被实体巢片状分布的肿瘤组织(蓝星)占据,其间为宽窄不等的纤维性间质分隔(蓝箭),黑星示残留的周边淋巴组织。瘤细胞(黑箭)呈圆形、梭形或多角形,核仁不明显,核分裂象罕见。

2. 肾上腺疾病

2.1 肾上腺出血(图 11-16)

肾上腺皮质内可见明显的出血灶,各带分界不清,黑星示残余的肾上腺皮质结构。

2.2 肾上腺皮质腺瘤(图 11-17)

肿瘤组织(蓝星)具有完整的包膜(绿星),与周围的正常肾上腺组织(黑星)之间分界清晰。富含类脂质的肿瘤细胞(蓝箭)胞浆透明或微嗜酸性,核较小,排列成团,由内含毛细血管的少量间质分隔。

2.3 肾上腺嗜铬细胞瘤(图 11-18)

肿瘤细胞排列成界限清楚的细胞球(蓝圈),边缘有纤细的纤维血管间质(蓝箭),血窦丰富(蓝星)。瘤细胞呈多角形或梭形,具有细颗粒状嗜碱性胞浆,核圆形或卵圆形。

四、临床病理讨论

案例 1 患者,女性,63 岁,家住北方农村,颈部肿物已多年。近几年肿物体积逐渐增大,出现吞咽困难、声音嘶哑等症状而入院就诊。体检发现甲状腺明显肿大,其内可触及多结节,甲状腺功能无明显变化。行甲状腺切除术,术后标本(图 11-19)送病理检查。

（1）试描述该手术标本的形态特征，该患者最可能的病理诊断是什么？

（2）试绘制该标本在镜下可能的组织学形态特征。

案例 **2**　男性，65 岁，口渴多饮 5 年，尿液中泡沫增多半年。空腹血糖 8.1 mmol/L，糖化血红蛋白 7.8%，24 小时尿蛋白 2.1 g。肾脏穿刺活组织检查结果如图 11-20 所示。该患者肾脏病变最可能的病理诊断是什么？依据何在？

五、 思考题

1. 弥漫性非毒性甲状腺肿的病理变化可分为哪三个时期？

2. 桥本甲状腺炎和纤维性甲状腺炎有何病理形态区别？

3. 甲状腺癌常见的病理类型有哪些？

4. 肾上腺嗜铬细胞瘤是良性肿瘤吗？

5. 糖尿病的病理变化主要表现在哪些方面？

6. 名词解释：黏液水肿，砂粒体，甲状腺髓样癌，库欣（Cushing）综合征，非胰岛素依赖型糖尿病。

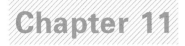

Chapter 11

Diseases of Endocrine System

Ⅰ. Aims

1. To grasp the morphological characteristics of diffuse nontoxic goiter and its three phases.

2. To grasp the morphological characteristics of diffuse toxic goiter.

3. To grasp the morphology of papillary thyroid carcinoma.

4. To familiarize with the morphological differences among nodular goiter, thyroid adenoma, and follicular thyroid carcinoma.

5. To understand the morphological features of Hashimoto thyroiditis and adrenal pheochromocytoma.

Guidance to study

	Nodular goiter	Thyroid adenoma	Follicular thyroid carcinoma
Macroscopic appearance	Usually vary-sized multiple nodules	Usually solitary nodule	Usually solitary nodule
Capsule	Not intact	Fibrous capsule in different thickness	Thick, with capsular invasion
Vascular invasion	No	No	Sometimes
Follicle size	Normal or big follicles	Small follicles or normal	Small follicles or normal
Lining cells	Flat or cubic cells in single layer	Single layer, polygonal cells in uniform morphology	Polygonal cells, hypercellularity, might form cribriform or trabecular structure
Nuclei	Round or oval, equal-size	Round or oval, equal-size	Mitosis, nuclear pleomorphism, prominent nucleoli
Correlation with surrounding tissue	Similar morphology in surrounding tissue, no compression	Normal follicles in surrounding tissue, with compression	Capsular invasion or widely invasion

Ⅱ. Gross specimenss

1. Thyroid diseases

1.1　Thyroid cyst（Fig.11-1）

A sharply marginated cyst is shown on the cut section of thyroid（blue circle）, in which diffuse hemorrhage could be observed. The black asterisk shows the remaining normal thyroid.

1.2　Diffuse nontoxic goiter（Fig.11-2）

The goiter is symmetrically and diffusely enlarged, with smooth surface and intact capsule. The cut section is brown. Large amount of colloid is visible, but it shows no nodular structure. Please think about which stage of simple goiter this specimen indicates.

1.3　Diffuse toxic goiter（Fig.11-3）

This is a cut thyroid. It is symmetrically and diffusely enlarged with smooth surface. The cut section is gray-red, and shows lobulated structure, few colloid, and muscle-like texture, but no obvious nodules are developed.

1.4　Papillary thyroid carcinoma（Fig.11-4）

On the cut section of the thyroid, there is a gray-white and solid mass（blue circles）. The boundary between the tumor and surrounding tissue is unclear. The black asterisks show normal thyroid.

2. Adrenal gland diseases

2.1　Hemorrhage in adrenal gland（Fig.11-5）

This is a kidney with adrenal gland. On the cut section, diffuse hemorrhage（blue asterisks）is obvious in the adrenal gland. The kidney beneath is slightly compressed（black asterisk）. Hemorrhage in adrenal gland is usually seen in fetus, with manifestations as retroperitoneal mass or adrenal insufficiency. And it's possibly associated with fetal anoxia, sepsis, etc.

2.2　Adrenal cortical adenoma（Fig.11-6）

There is a light yellow or golden space-occupying lesion with clear boundary（blue circles）in the cortex of adrenal gland. The black asterisks show the remaining normal adrenal gland.

2.3　Adrenal pheochromocytoma（Fig.11-7）

On the cut section, the spherical tumor is yellow-white and soft with hemorrhage, necrosis and cystic degeneration（blue asterisks）.

2. 4   Adrenal metastatic lung carcinoma（Fig.11-8）

It is a metastatic tumor from primary lung carcinoma. The adrenal gland increases in size (blue asterisks). The cut section of the tumor is gray-white, with poorly-defined boundary, and a cut kidney is beneath the tumor on the same side (black asterisks).

Ⅲ. Tissue sectionss

1. Thyroid diseases

1. 1   Diffuse nontoxic goiter（Fig.11-9）

In the slice, there are follicles in various sizes, and they are filled by homogeneous pink colloid (blue asterisks). Majority of the proliferative follicular epithelial cells are flat or cubic (blue arrows), with small follicles (black asterisks).

1. 2   Diffuse toxic goiter（Fig.11-10）

The tissue presents some follicles in various sizes (blue asterisks). The proliferated follicular epithelial cells are columnar or stratified (blue arrows), and some of them show papillary proliferation (blue circle). The colloids in the follicular lumens are thin, and absorptive vacuoles (black arrow) are visible in the peripheral areas next to epithelium. There are abundant blood vessels, and hyperplastic lymphoid tissue (black asterisk) in the stroma.

1. 3   Hashimoto thyroiditis（Fig.11-11）

The thyroid is atrophic with eosinophilic degeneration (blue arrows) of follicular epithelial cells which has been injured partially. There are large number of lymphocytes infiltrating the stroma (black asterisks), with lymphoid follicles (blue asterisk).

1. 4   Thyroid adenoma（Fig.11-12）

The tumor with intact capsule (green asterisks) is composed of relatively uniform and densely arranged follicles (blue asterisk), and some of which present colloid. The blue arrows point at neoplastic follicular epithelial cells with microfollicles formation. The black asterisk shows normal thyroid tissue.

1. 5   Papillary thyroid carcinoma（Fig.11-13）

The normal thyroid tissue is shown with black asterisks, and the tumor is indicated by blue asterisks. The tumor cells arrange in complicated papillary branches with fibrovascular core. At high magnification, tumor cell nuclei show ground glass appearance (blue arrows). The cell nuclei are big in size and overlapping, and some of them have nuclear groove (black arrow) or pseudoinclusion (green arrow).

1. 6   Follicular thyroid carcinoma（Fig.11-14）

The tumor (blue asterisks) are surrounded by thick fibrous capsule (green asterisks) . The tumor presents cancerous follicles (blue arrows), and some of which has remaining colloid. Some tumor cells have invaded outside the capsule (blue circle), with the same histologic morphology as the tumor cells inside the capsule. The black asterisk indicates normal thyroid tissue.

1. 7　Metastatic medullary thyroid carcinoma in lymph nodes（Fig.11-15）

The majority of the lymph node has been occupied by the cancer tissue (blue asterisks), and the cancer cells appear as solid nests divided by fibrous stroma (blue arrows) in various thicknesses. The tumor cells are round, fusiform, or polygon (black arrows) without obvious nucleoli, and mitoses are rarely observed. The remaining lymphatic tissue is indicated by black asterisks.

2.　Adrenal gland diseases

2. 1　Adrenal hemorrhage（Fig.11-16）

Obvious hemorrhage can be found in the adrenal cortex, without clear boundary. The black asterisks show the remaining adrenal cortex tissues.

2. 2　Adrenal cortical adenoma（Fig.11-17）

The tumor (blue asterisk) has intact capsule (green asterisks), thus, it is demarcated from the surrounding normal tissues (black asterisks). The tumor is composed of cells containing lipids (blue arrows). The tumor cells display transparent or eosinophilic cytoplasm and small nuclei, arrange as cell clusters, and are separated by stroma containing capillaries.

2. 3　Adrenal pheochromocytoma（Fig.11-18）

The tumor cells arrange in well-defined nests (Zellballen) (blue circles), and are separated by delicate fibrovascular stroma (blue arrows) containing rich blood sinuses (blue asterisks). The tumor cells are polygon or fusiform, having granulated basophilic cytoplasm, and oval or round nuclei.

Ⅳ. Clinical pathological discussion

Case 1

A 63-year-old female who lives in rural areas in northern China has had a lump in her neck for years, and lately the mass gradually has being increased in size. The patient complains difficulty in swallowing and hoarseness. Physical examination detects obviously swollen goiter, with multiple nodules, but the thyroid function remains normal. The pathological change of the removed thyroid is examined, and the representative images are shown in Fig.11-19.

(1) Please describe the morphological characteristics of the specimen. And what is the mostly pathological diagnosis of the excised tissue?

(2) Please try to draw the likely histological morphological changes of the specimen.

Case 2

A 65-year-old man has been thirsty and polydipsia for 5 years, and has suffered increasing urine foams in the recent half a year. Laboratory tests show fast blood glucose of 8. 1 mmol/L, glycosylated hemoglobin of 7. 8%, and 24 hr urine protein of 2. 1g. The histological figures from kidney biopsy are shown in Fig.11-20.

What is the most likely diagnosis of the patient? And list the diagnostic points.

V. Questions

1. Which three stages can pathological changes of diffuse nontoxic goiter be divided into?

2. What is the pathological difference between Hashimoto thyroiditis and fibrous thyroiditis?

3. What are the common pathological types of thyroid carcinoma?

4. Is adrenal pheochromocytoma benign tumor?

5. What are the main pathological changes of diabetes mellitus?

6. Terms: Myxoedema, Psammoma body, Medullary thyroid carcinoma, Cushing syndrome, Non-insulin-dependent diabetes mellitus.

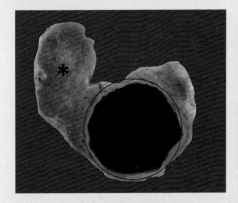

图 11-1　甲状腺囊肿
Fig.11-1　Thyroid cyst

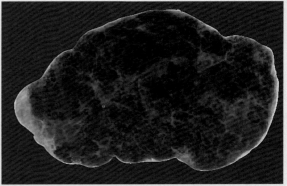

图 11-2　弥漫性非毒性甲状腺肿
Fig.11-2　Diffuse nontoxic goiter

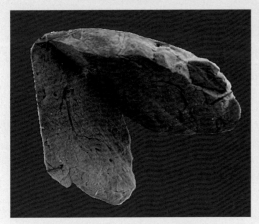

图 11-3　弥漫性毒性甲状腺肿
Fig.11-3　Diffuse toxic goiter

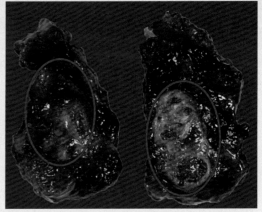

图 11-4　甲状腺乳头状癌
Fig.11-4　Papillary thyroid carcinoma

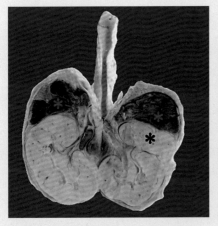

图 11-5　肾上腺出血
Fig.11-5　Hemorrhage in adrenal gland

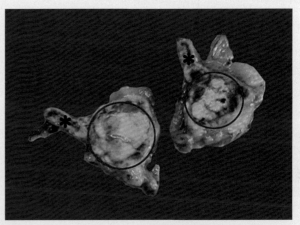

图 11-6　肾上腺皮质腺瘤
Fig.11-6　Adrenal cortical adenoma

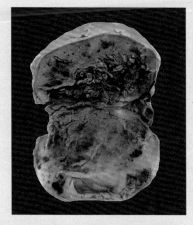
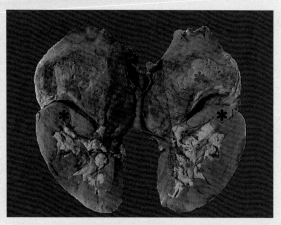

图 11-7　肾上腺嗜铬细胞瘤
Fig.11-7　Adrenal pheochromocytoma

图 11-8　肾上腺转移性肺癌
Fig.11-8　Adrenal metastatic lung carcinoma

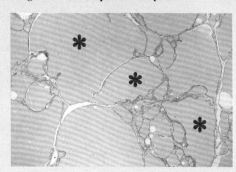
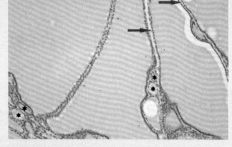

图 11-9　弥漫性非毒性甲状腺肿（×40；×200）
Fig.11-9　Diffuse nontoxic goiter（×40；×200）

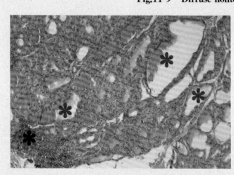
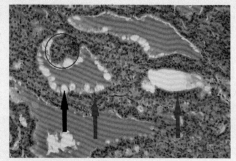

图 11-10　弥漫性毒性甲状腺肿（×100；×200）
Fig.11-10　Diffuse toxic goiter（×100；×200）

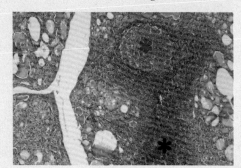
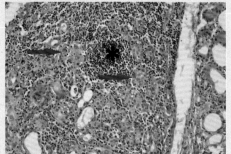

图 11-11　桥本甲状腺炎（×100；×200）
Fig.11-11　Hashimoto thyroiditis（×100；×200）

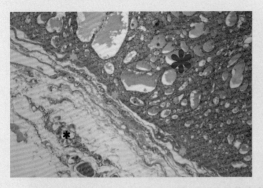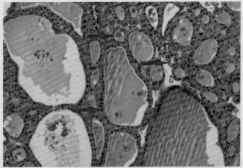

图 11-12　甲状腺腺瘤（×40；×200）

Fig.11-12　Thyroid adenoma（×40；×200）

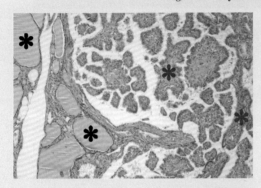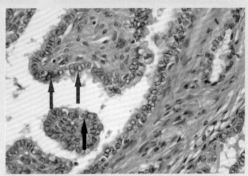

图 11-13　甲状腺乳头状癌（×100；×400）

Fig.11-13　Papillary thyroid carcinoma（×100；×400）

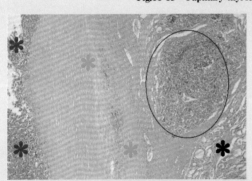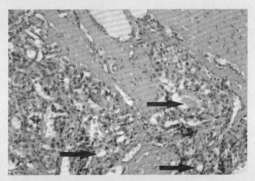

图 11-14　甲状腺滤泡癌（×40；×200）

Fig.11-14　Follicular thyroid carcinoma（×40；×200）

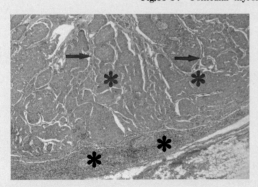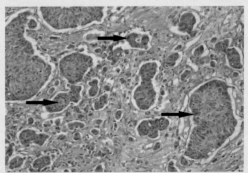

图 11-15　淋巴结转移性甲状腺髓样癌（×40；×200）

Fig.11-15　Metastatic medullary thyroid carcinoma in lymph nodes（×40；×200）

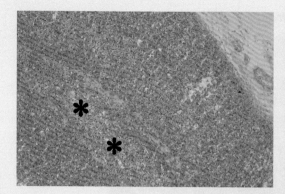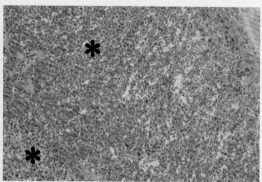

图 11-16 肾上腺出血（×100；×200）
Fig.11-16 Adrenal hemorrhage（×100；×200）

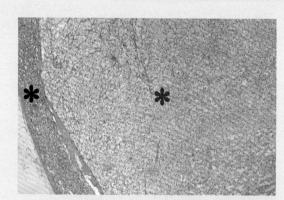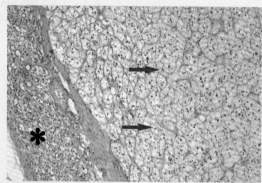

图 11-17 肾上腺皮质腺瘤（×40；×100）
Fig.11-17 Adrenal cortical adenoma（×40；×100）

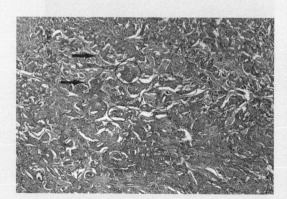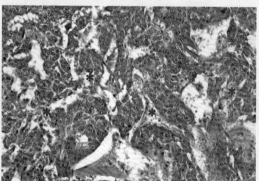

图 11-18 肾上腺嗜铬细胞瘤（×40；×200）
Fig.11-18 Adrenal pheochromocytoma（×40；×200）

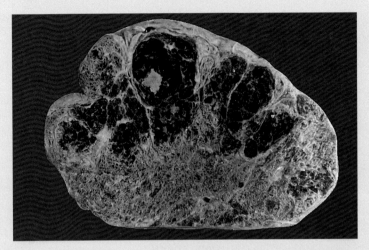

图 11-19　案例 1
Fig.11-19　Case 1

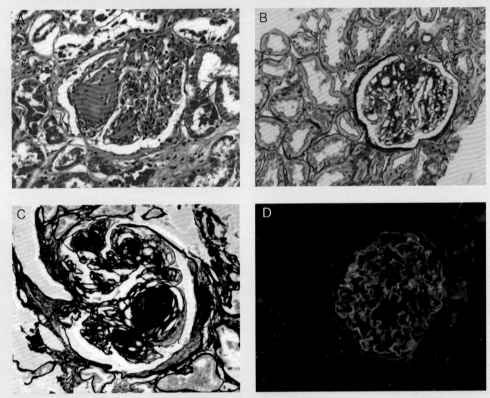

图 11-20　案例 2：肾脏穿刺活检组织
（A：H.E. 染色×200；B：PAS 染色×200；C：PASM 染色×200；D：IgG 免疫荧光×200）
Fig.11-20　Case 2：Biopsy of kidney tissue
（A：H.E. ×200；B：PAS×200；C：PASM×200；D：IgG immunofluorescence×200）

潘旻，卜晓东（Min Pan，Xiaodong Bu）

第十二章

神经系统疾病

一、目的要求

1. 掌握流行性脑脊髓膜炎和流行性乙型脑炎的病理特点并熟悉临床病理联系。
2. 掌握脑出血常见部位及特点。
3. 了解神经系统肿瘤的常见类型和病理特征。
4. 了解中枢神经系统疾病常见的并发症。

导学

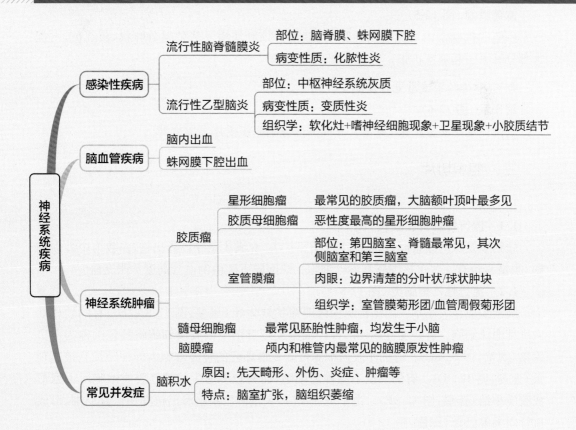

二、 大体标本

1. 感染性疾病

1.1　流行性脑脊髓膜炎（图 12-1）

大脑表面血管扩张充血,脑膜混浊,部分血管由于周围有多量灰黄色脓性渗出物积聚而变得模糊不清,脑回变宽,脑沟变窄。

1.2　流行性乙型脑炎（图 12-2）

大脑冠状切面,脑回变宽,脑沟变窄,左右侧大脑不对称,大脑皮髓质交界处与基底核区域有少量稀疏散在或密集的针头大小的灰色略透明的点状软化灶（蓝箭）。

2. 脑血管疾病

2.1　脑出血（图 12-3）

大脑的水平切面,经过内囊。一侧内囊基底核处大量出血（蓝箭）,已将内囊破坏,血液涌入两侧脑室,侧脑室扩大并出现明显积血。

2.2　蛛网膜下腔出血（图 12-4）

大脑冠状切面,大脑沟回处可见弥漫红色出血灶（蓝箭）。

3. 神经系统肿瘤

室管膜瘤（图 12-5）

一侧的侧脑室内可见一实性肿块（蓝箭）,该肿块境界清楚呈分叶状,灰红色,占据大部分脑室引起脑室扩张。

4. 中枢神经系统常见并发症

脑积水（图 12-6）

双侧侧脑室明显扩张（蓝箭）,其周围部分脑组织受压萎缩变薄。

三、 组织切片

1. 感染性疾病

1.1　流行性脑脊髓膜炎（图 12-7）

软脑膜及蛛网膜增厚,蛛网膜下腔明显扩大,充满大量脓性渗出物,多数为中性粒细胞（黑箭）,也有一些单核细胞和淋巴细胞。蛛网膜下腔内的血管高度扩张充血。

1.2　流行性乙型脑炎（图 12-8）

脑组织散在大小不一的结构疏松区即筛状软化灶（黑星,图 12-8A,B）,有的软化灶内可见泡沫细胞。有些变性坏死的神经细胞周围有增生的胶质细胞将其包围称为卫星现象（黄箭,图 12-8C）。有的小胶质细胞侵入变性坏死的神经细胞内即神经细胞被噬现象（蓝箭,图 12-8D）。有的部位不见神经细胞,而为较多增生的神经胶质细胞所占据形成胶质小结（蓝星,图 12-8E）。由于炎症反应,大量淋巴细胞渗出包围在血管周围,形成血管周围淋巴套（绿箭,图 12-8F）。

2. 脑血管病变

蛛网膜下腔出血（图 12-9）

软脑膜及蛛网膜增厚,蛛网膜下腔明显扩大,充满红细胞。邻近的皮层脑组织轻度水肿,神经元周围的间隙变宽(蓝箭)。

3. 中枢神经系统肿瘤

3.1　弥漫性星形细胞瘤（图 12-10）

肿瘤组织内可见神经原纤维背景,肿瘤细胞弥漫性分布,细胞分化良好,大小一致,细胞核呈圆形、卵圆形,无核分裂象。间质有少量毛细血管增生,无明显出血坏死。

3.2　胶质母细胞瘤（图 12-11）

肿瘤细胞密集,异型性明显,细胞境界不清,胞浆及胞核明显多形性,小的肿瘤细胞呈梭形,还可见怪异的单核或多核瘤巨细胞;瘤组织坏死明显,可见假栅栏状坏死灶及坏死周围栅栏状排列的瘤细胞(蓝星);间质血管增生明显,可见肾小球样血管,其中有大量增生的周细胞(黄星)。

3.3　室管膜瘤（图 12-12）

肿瘤细胞密度中等,形态较一致呈梭形,胞浆丰富,细胞核呈圆形或椭圆形,呈一致性。瘤细胞围绕血管排列形成假菊形团(黄星)。血管周围假菊形团中的细胞以细长胞体突起与血管壁相连,在血管周围形成红染的无核区(蓝箭)。

3.4　髓母细胞瘤（图 12-13）

肿瘤由相对较小的原始细胞组成,细胞核深染,胞质少而边界不清。细胞密集,间质有纤细的纤维,瘤细胞围绕纤维轴心放射状排列形成 Homer-Wright 菊形团(蓝星),具有一定诊断意义。

3.5　脑膜瘤（图 12-14）

肿瘤细胞分化良好,无核分裂象,呈大小不等同心圆状或漩涡状排列,其中央的血管壁常可见玻璃样变性,并可见钙化的砂粒体(蓝箭)。

四、 临床病理讨论

案例　患儿,女性,5 岁,因持续性头痛及高热 24 小时入院。查体显示体温 38.4℃,脉搏 85 次/分,呼吸 18 次/分,血压 125/85 mmHg,头部 CT 检查未见肿块及中线移位。继而进行腰椎穿刺行脑脊液检查。检查结果显示脑脊液混浊呈脓样;白细胞总数显著增多,为 $1\ 000 \times 10^6$/L,以中性粒细胞为主,葡萄糖含量为 0.9 mmol/L(正常 2.5～4.5 mmol/L),蛋白质含量为 1.3 g/L(正常 0.2～0.4 g/L)。

(1) 依据临床表现及脑脊液检查结果首先考虑什么疾病?

(2) 该病的可能病因是什么? 如何确诊?

五、 思考题

1. 流行性脑脊髓膜炎的临床表现有哪些?

2. 流行性脑脊髓膜炎和流行性乙型脑炎有哪些不同特点?

3. 中枢神经系统常见的肿瘤有哪些类型?

4. 某成人在大脑额叶白质出现一球型占位性病变,请问可能的病变有哪些? 如何从病理形态学进行鉴别?

5. 名词解释:流行性脑脊髓膜炎,神经细胞卫星现象,胶质小结,嗜神经细胞现象。

Chapter 12

Diseases of Nervous System

Ⅰ. Aims

1. To grasp the pathological characteristics of epidemic cerebrospinal meningitis and epidemic encephalitis B, and understand their clinico-pathological relationship.

2. To grasp the common sites and characteristics of intracerebral hemorrhage.

3. To understand the common types and pathologic features of neurologic tumors.

4. To understand the common complications of diseases of nervous system.

Guidance to study

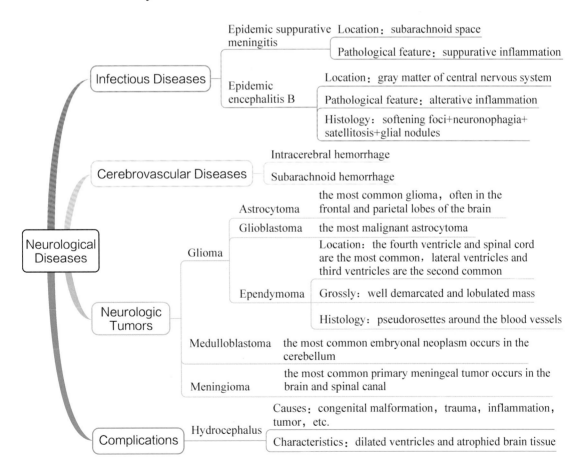

Ⅱ. Gross specimens

1. Infectious diseases

1.1 Epidemic cerebrospinal meningitis（Fig.12-1）

The blood vessels on the surface of the brain are dilated and congested, and the meninge is cloudy. Some blood vessels become blurred due to the accumulation of yellow purulent exudate around them, and the brain shows broad gyri and narrow sulci.

1.2 Epidemic encephalitis B（Fig.12-2）

The coronal section of the brain shows that the gyri have become wide with narrow sulci. The left and right cerebral hemispheres are asymmetric in size, and there are a few scattered pinhead-sized softening foci at the cortical medulla junction and the basal ganglia in the left hemisphere（blue arrows）.

2. Cerebrovascular diseases

2.1 Cerebral hemorrhage（Fig.12-3）

This is a horizontal section of the brain, passing through the internal capsule. There is massive hemorrhage in the internal capsule and the basal ganglia（blue arrows）, which has destroyed the internal capsule, and a large amount of blood breaks into the bilateral ventricles. As a result, the lateral ventricles are enlarged with obvious hematocele.

2.2 Subarachnoid hemorrhage（Fig.12-4）

This is the coronal section of the brain. Diffuse red hemorrhagic foci are observed in the cerebral sulci（blue arrows）.

3. Neurologic tumors

Ependymoma（Fig.12-5）

There is a solid mass（blue arrow）in the lateral ventricle. This grayish-red mass is well demarcated and lobulated, and it has occupied most of the ventricle, leading to ventricular dilation.

4. Complications of nervous system

Hydrocephalus（Fig.12-6）

The bilateral ventricles are markedly dilated（blue arrows）, and the surrounding brain tissues are compressed and atrophied.

Ⅲ. Tissue sections

1. Infectious diseases

1. 1   Epidemic cerebrospinal meningitis（Fig.12-7）

The pia mater and arachnoid membrane are thickened. Subarachnoid space is significantly enlarged and filled with purulent exudate containing a large number of neutrophils（black arrow）and a small amount of fibrins, monocytes and lymphocytes. Among of them, fibrins interweave into a mesh. The blood vessels in the subarachnoid space are dilated and congested.

1. 2   Epidemic encephalitis B（Fig.12-8）

In the section of the brain, the whole brain tissue presents scattered liquefactive necrotic tissue, namely sieve-like softening foci（black stars, Fig.12-8A, B）, and foam cells can be seen in some softening foci. Some degenerated and necrotic neurons are surrounded by proliferating glial cells, and referred to as satellitosis（yellow arrows, Fig. 12-8C）. Some microglial cells have invaded into the degenerated or necrotic neurons, which are defined as neuronophagias（blue arrow, Fig.12-8D）. Some areas present no nerve cells, but are occupied by more glial cells, and such aggregation of glial cells is known as glial nodule（blue stars, Fig.12-8E）. As a result of inflammatory response, a large number of lymphocytes exude and surround the blood vessels, forming a perivascular sheath（green arrows, Fig.12-8F）.

2. Cerebrovascular diseases

Subarachnoid hemorrhage（Fig.12-9）

The pia mater and arachnoid membrane are thickened, and the subarachnoid cavity is enlarged and filled with red blood cells. There is mild edema of the adjacent cerebral cortex, and the spaces around neurons become widened（blue arrows）.

3. Neurologic tumors

3. 1   Diffuse astrocytoma（Fig.12-10）

The well differentiated tumor cells diffusely distribute in the fibrillary background with uniform size. The nuclei are round or oval without mitotic figures. A few capillaries display hyperplasia in the stroma, but no hemorrhage and necrosis are visible.

3. 2   Glioblastoma（Fig.12-11）

The tumor cells are densely distributed with obvious atypia, the pleomorphism of cytoplasm and nucleus is apparent with undefined cell boundary. Not only small fusiform tumor cells but also weird mononuclear or multinucleated giant tumor cells can be observed.

There are palisaded tumor cells centering serpiginous bands of necrosis (blue asterisk). Microvascular proliferation is prominent, and glomeruloid vessels containing a large number of pericytes (yellow asterisk) can be observed.

3.3　Ependymoma (Fig.12-12)

The density of tumor cells is moderate, and the morphology is relatively uniform showing spindle in shape with abundant cytoplasm and round or oval nuclei. They arrange around the blood vessels and form pseudorosettes (yellow asterisks). The cells in the pseudorosettes are contiguous with the blood vessel wall by elongating their cell bodies, which forms a red-stained nuclear-free zone around the blood vessel (blue arrows).

3.4　Medulloblastoma (Fig.12-13)

The neoplasm consists of relatively small primitive cells, and these small cells have hyperchromatic nuclei and little cytoplasm. The neoplastic cells are dense with fine fibers in the stroma. The tumor cells arrange radially around the fiber core, which appears as Homer-Wright rosette (blue asterisks), a morphological change with diagnostic significance.

3.5　Meningioma (Fig.12-14)

The tumor cells are well differentiated without mitoses. They arrange in whorled or concentric pattern with different sizes. In the center, the vascular wall is commonly hyaline degenerated and further calcified. The calcified lesions are referred to as psammoma bodies (blue arrows).

Ⅳ. Clinical pathological discussion

Case

A 5-year-old girl was admitted to the hospital with persistent headache and high fever for 24 hours. On physical examination, her temperature was 38.4℃, her pulse was 85/min, her respiratory rate was 18/min, and the blood pressure was 125/85 mmHg. CT scan of the head shows no mass and midline shift. A lumbar puncture was subsequently performed. The CSF results showed that the cerebrospinal fluid was cloudy and purulent. The total number of white blood cells increased significantly with $1\,000 \times 10^6$/L, and the leukocytes are mainly neutrophils; The glucose and protein concentrations were 0.9 mmol/L (normal 2.5 ∼ 4.5 mmol/L) and 1.3 g/L (normal 0.2∼0.4 g/L), respectively.

(1) What disease is considered firstly according to the clinical manifestations and laboratory examination?

(2) What are the common pathogenic microorganisms for the patient? What can be done to identify them?

V. Questions

1. What are the clinical manifestations of epidemic suppurative meningitis?

2. What is the difference between epidemic suppurative meningitis and epidemic encephalitis B?

3. What are the common types of neurologic tumors?

4. An adult has a spherical space-occupying lesion in the white matter of the frontal lobe of the brain, what lesions should be considered? What pathological changes can be used to diagnose the lesion?

5. Terms: Epidemic cerebrospinal meningitis, Satellitosis, Microglial nodules, Neuronophagia.

VI. 附图 (Figures)

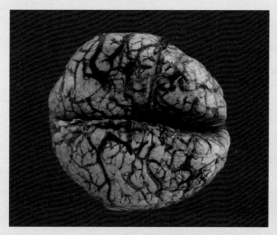

图 12-1　流行性脑脊髓膜炎
Fig.12-1　Epidemic cerebrospinal meningitis

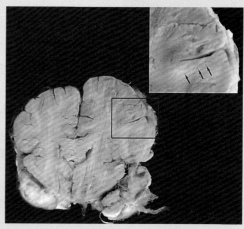

图 12-2　流行性乙型脑炎
Fig.12-2　Epidemic encephalitis B

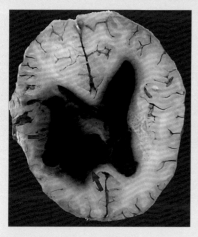

图 12-3　脑出血
Fig.12-3　Cerebral hemorrhage

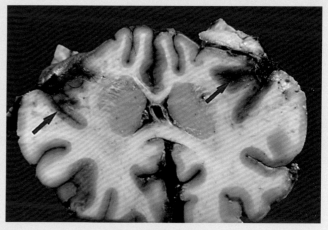

图 12-4　蛛网膜下腔出血
Fig.12-4　Subarachnoid hemorrhage

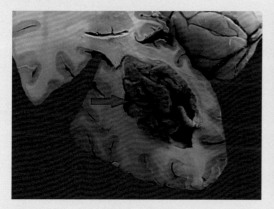

图 12-5　室管膜瘤
Fig.12-5　Ependymoma

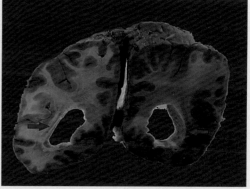

图 12-6　脑积水
Fig.12-6　Hydrocephalus

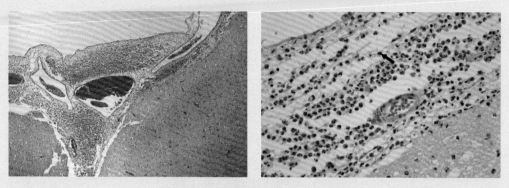

图 12-7 流行性脑脊髓膜炎(×40；×400)
Fig.12-7 Epidemic cerebrospinal meningitis(×40；×400)

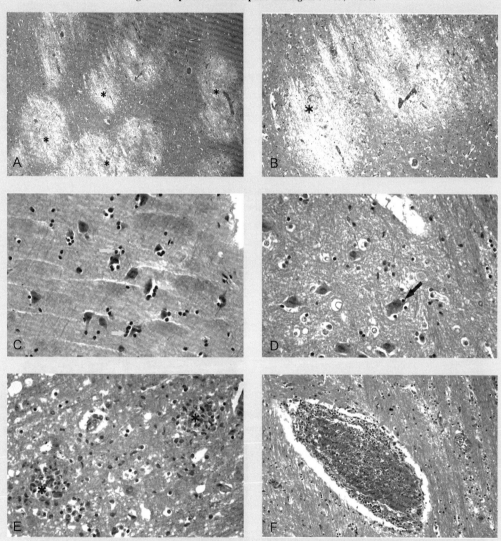

图 12-8 流行性乙型脑炎(A：×40；B：00；C～E：×400；F：×200)
Fig.12-8 Epidemic encephalitis B(A：×40；B：100；C～E：×400；F：×200)

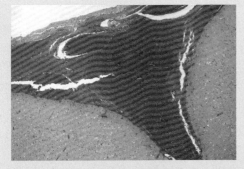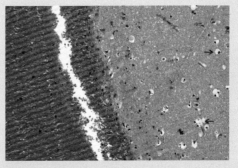

图 12-9　蛛网膜下腔出血（×40；×200）
Fig.12-9　Subarachnoid hemorrhage（×40；×200）

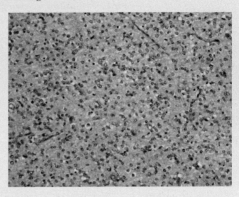

图 12-10　弥漫性星形细胞瘤（×100；×200）
Fig.12-10　Diffuse astrocytoma（×100；×200）

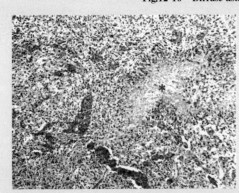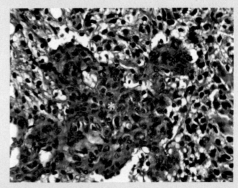

图 12-11　胶质母细胞瘤（×100；×400）
Fig.12-11　Glioblastoma（×100；×400）

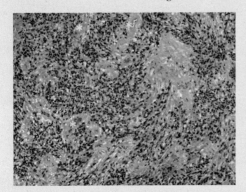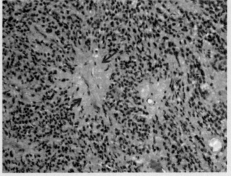

图 12-12　室管膜瘤（×100；×200）
Fig.12-12　Ependymoma（×100；×200）

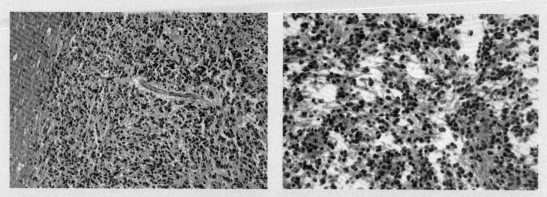

图 12-13　髓母细胞瘤（×200；×400）
Fig.12-13　Medulloblastoma（×200；×400）

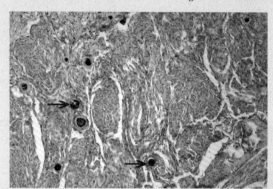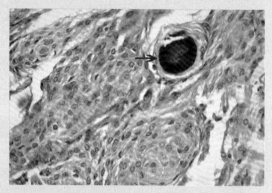

图 12-14　脑膜瘤（×100；×400）
Fig.12-14　Meningioma（×100；×400）

徐月霜,张爱凤（Yueshuang Xu，Aifeng Zhang）

第十三章

骨关节疾病

一、目的要求

1. 掌握骨软骨瘤、软骨肉瘤、骨肉瘤、骨巨细胞瘤、尤因肉瘤的基本病理特征。
2. 了解骨髓炎、佝偻病、痛风性关节炎、腱鞘巨细胞瘤的形态特点。

导学

肿瘤名称	好发年龄	好发部位	形态特征	生物学行为
骨软骨瘤	10～30 岁	股骨、胫骨、肱骨	软骨膜、软骨帽和基底部骨质三层结构	良性
软骨肉瘤	30～60 岁	骨盆、肋骨、股骨	可由髓腔发生（中心型）或骨表面发生（外周型），可有软骨黏液样基质产生或者不同程度的分化	恶性
骨肉瘤	10～25 岁	股骨、胫骨、肱骨	肿瘤细胞直接产生不成熟骨或骨样基质	恶性
骨巨细胞瘤	20～40 岁	股骨、胫骨、桡骨	溶骨性病变，出血、坏死常见，由肿瘤性的单核基质细胞和类似破骨细胞的巨细胞构成	潜在恶性（50％复发）
尤因肉瘤	5～20 岁	股骨、骨盆、胫骨	通常呈"小圆细胞肿瘤"形态，纤维间隔将小而一致的肿瘤细胞分割成巢片状	高度恶性

二、大体标本

1. 骨非肿瘤性疾病

佝偻病肋骨（图 13-1）

由于软骨和骨样组织的堆积，肋骨和肋软骨结合部位呈结节状隆起（蓝箭），多条肋骨同时受累之后，结节状隆起成行排列，类似串珠样改变，称为佝偻病串珠。

2. 骨肿瘤

2.1　骨软骨瘤（图 13-2）

结节状之不整形肿块，切面见肿物大部分由海绵状松质骨（绿星）构成，骨质上方有一层灰白色半透明软骨帽覆盖（蓝星），最外层有薄层纤维组织包绕（黑星），纤维组织部分已撕脱。

2.2　软骨肉瘤（图 13-3）

股骨上段瘤体主要位于骨外，呈现外围型生长，大部分肿瘤组织切面呈半透明、胶冻样（蓝星），股骨皮质部分破坏，肿瘤已侵入髓腔及周围软组织。

2.3　骨肉瘤（图 13-4）

股骨下段干骺端灰红色、均匀致密的肿瘤组织已充满髓腔（蓝星），骨皮质被广泛破坏，肿瘤组织与正常组织界限不清，且向外侵入周围组织形成肿块（黑星）。

2.4　骨巨细胞瘤（图 13-5）

胫骨上段干骺端充满灰红色肿瘤组织，受累部位的骨皮质变为薄壳样，部分区域出血、坏死及囊性变（蓝星）。请思考：该肿瘤的生物学行为。

三、组织切片

1. 骨非肿瘤性疾病

1.1　亚急性骨髓炎（图 13-6）

骨髓腔内小血管扩张充血，可见大量的炎性渗出物，渗出物中所含中性粒细胞较少，以淋巴细胞和浆细胞为主，可见炎细胞小灶状聚集（蓝圈）。

1.2　慢性骨髓炎（图 13-7）

骨髓腔内可见大量的慢性炎细胞和成纤维细胞混杂（黑圈），部分区域已明显纤维化（蓝圈）。

2. 骨肿瘤

2.1　骨软骨瘤（图 13-8）

肿瘤表面被覆薄层纤维结缔组织（黑星），与骨膜延续，其下方可见由透明软骨构成的软骨帽（蓝星），厚薄不一，细胞增生活跃，但缺乏明显的异型性，肿瘤基底部为骨质成分（绿星）。

2.2　骨肉瘤（图 13-9）

肿瘤组织在髓腔内弥漫分布（蓝星），或呈小巢状聚集，破坏周围骨质，瘤细胞（蓝箭）大小不一，核不规则，异型性明显，可见肿瘤组织产生的骨样基质（黑箭）。

2.3　骨巨细胞瘤（图 13-10）

肿瘤主要由两种细胞构成，单核基质细胞（黑箭）和多核巨细胞（蓝箭），多核巨细胞均匀分布在圆形或梭形的单核基质细胞背景之中，两种细胞的核形态基本类似，可见核仁。

2.4　尤因肉瘤（图 13-11）

肿瘤细胞被纤维性间隔（黑箭）分割为不规则的巢片状（蓝星），瘤细胞小而一致，核染色质呈粉尘状，有时可见瘤细胞围绕血管呈假菊形团样排列（蓝圈），具有原始神经外胚层分化的形态。

3. 关节疾病

3.1　痛风石（图 13-12）

纤维结缔组织内可见多灶分布的淡伊红染、大小不等的无定形物质（蓝星），周围有巨噬细胞、成纤维细胞、淋巴细胞等包绕（黑星），偏振光显微镜下可显示淡伊红染区域中沉积的尿酸盐晶体呈针状结构。

3.2　腱鞘巨细胞瘤（图 13-13）

腱鞘巨细胞瘤主要由致密纤维组织背景中混杂的单核基质细胞（黑箭）、多核巨细胞（蓝箭）和泡沫样组织细胞（绿箭）构成。注意：低倍镜下观察分叶状的肿瘤组织结构以及分布不均匀的多核巨细胞。

四、临床病理讨论

案例　患者，男，46 岁，因"双侧臀部、双下肢疼痛麻木 20 余天"入院。胸部 CT 示右肺门占位性病变，腰椎 MRI 示 S1－S2 椎体异常信号。图 13-14 中可见经支气管镜肺活检术（A）以及骶骨病灶切除术（B）后送检组织的镜下病理形态。

（1）该患者肺和骶骨内病变最可能的病理诊断是什么？
（2）请思考骶骨内病变的发生发展过程。

五、思考题

1. 引起化脓性骨髓炎的感染途径主要有哪些？
2. 骨软骨瘤的病理特征中可见哪三层结构？
3. 影像学中诊断骨肉瘤的特征性表现主要有哪些？
4. 尤因肉瘤主要的分子遗传学特征是什么？
5. 痛风的发病机制主要涉及哪些因素？
6. 名词解释：Codman 三角，纤维结构不良，动脉瘤样骨囊肿，痛风石。

Chapter 13

Bone and Joint Diseases

Ⅰ. Aims

1. To grasp the pathological characteristics of osteochondroma, chondrosarcoma, osteosarcoma, giant cell tumor of bone and Ewing sarcoma.

2. To understand the morphological characteristics of osteomyelitis, rickets, gout arthritis and tenosynovial giant cell tumor.

Guidance to study

Tumor	Age (years)	Bones most commonly affected	Morphological characteristics	Behavior
Osteochondroma	10~30	Femur, tibia, humerus	Show three layers of fibrous tissue, hyaline cartilage cap and underlying cortical and cancellous bone.	Benign
Chondrosarcoma	30~60	Pelvis, rib, femur	Locate into central (in the medullary cavity) or peripheral area (on the surface of bones), produce cartilaginous myxoid stroma, and show a remarkably wide range of differentiation.	Malignant
Osteosarcoma	10~25	Femur, tibia, humerus	Show direct production of immature bone or osteoid produced by neoplastic cells.	Malignant
Giant cell tumor of bone	20~40	Femur, tibia, radius	A radiolucent lesion involving the epiphysis and metaphysis. Hemorrhage and necrosis may be prominent. The two main components are the mononuclear stromal cells and giant cells.	Potentially malignant (50% for recurrence)
Ewing sarcoma	5~20	Femur, pelvis, tibia	Usually show small round cell tumor in morphology, present solid sheets or irregular nests of tumor cells divided by fibrovascular septa.	Highly malignant

II．Gross specimens

1．Non neoplastic diseases of bone

Rachitic ribs（Fig.13-1）

Due to the accumulation of cartilaginous and osteoid tissue, the junction of rib and costal cartilage presents nodular swelling（blue arrows）. When several ribs are involved at the same time, the nodules arrange in rows, which is called rachitic rosary.

2．Neoplasms of bone

2．1　Osteochondroma（Fig.13-2）

There is a nodular, irregular mass on the section. Most of it is composed of spongy cancellous bone（green asterisk）, covered by a layer of translucent cartilage cap（blue asterisk）. The outer layer of tumor is surrounded by a thin fibrous tissue（black asterisk）, and part of the fibrous tissue has been torn off.

2．2　Chondrosarcoma（Fig.13-3）

The tumor of the upper femur is mainly located outside the bone, showing peripheral growth pattern. Most of the tumor section is translucent and gelatinous（blue asterisks）. Part of the cortex has been destroyed, and the tumor has invaded both the medullary cavity and adjacent soft tissues.

2．3　Osteosarcoma（Fig.13-4）

The tumor tissue at the metaphysis of the lower femur has filled the medullary cavity （blue asterisk）, which shows a gray-red, uniform and dense appearance. The tumor causes destruction of bone cortex, and the boundary between the tumor and the normal tissue is unclear. The tumor tissue has spread outside the periosteum and into adjacent soft tissue, forming a peripheral mass（black asterisk）.

2．4　Giant cell tumor of bone（Fig.13-5）

The metaphysis of the upper tibia is filled with tumor tissue, and the cut surface is solid or friable and has a variegated red-brown and yellow appearance. The involved bone cortex has thin shell-like appearance, and hemorrhagic or necrotic cysts（blue asterisks）are prominent in the tumor. Please think about biological behaviors of the giant cell tumor of bone.

III．Tissue sections

1．Non neoplastic diseases of bone

1．1　Subacute osteomyelitis（Fig.13-6）

The small blood vessels in the marrow are dilated and congested with inflammatory exudate. In subacute osteomyelitis, the inflammatory infiltrate contains more lymphocytes and plasma cells, less neutrophils. Small focal aggregation of inflammatory cells (blue circle) can be observed.

1. 2   Chronic osteomyelitis (Fig.13-7)

A large number of chronic inflammatory cells and fibroblasts (black circle) are in the marrow, and some areas have obvious fibrosis (blue circle).

2.   Neoplasms of bone

2. 1   Osteochondroma (Fig.13-8)

The surface of the tumor is covered with a thin layer of fibrous connective tissue (black asterisk), which continues with the periosteum. Below the fibrous tissue, there is a hyaline cartilage cap (blue asterisks) with different thickness. The cells in the cap of osteochondroma actively proliferate, but they lack obvious atypia. The base of the tumor is composed of cancellous bone (green asterisks).

2. 2   Osteosarcoma (Fig.13-9)

The tumor tissue is diffusely distributed or nest-like gathered in the medullary cavity (blue asterisks), destroying the surrounding bone trabeculae. The tumor cells (blue arrows) are of different sizes, and obvious atypia with irregular nuclei. The immature bone or osteoid (black arrows) produced by the tumor cells can be observed.

2. 3   Giant cell tumor of bone (Fig.13-10)

The two main components of giant cell tumor are mononuclear stromal cells (black arrows) and multinucleate giant cells (blue arrows). The giant cells are evenly dispersed among a population of round and oval mononuclear stromal cells. The nuclei of the two components are similar in morphology, and nucleoli are visible.

2. 4   Ewing sarcoma (Fig.13-11)

The tumor cells are partitioned into irregular nests (blue asterisks) by fibrovascular septa (black arrows). The tumor cells are primitive, small, and uniform with a typically fine granular ("dusty") chromatin. Sometimes, they surround the vessels in a pseudorosette fashion (blue circle), providing morphological evidence for neuroectodermal differentiation.

3.   Joint diseases

3. 1   Gouty tophi (Fig.13-12)

There are lightly eosin-stained and amorphous substances (blue asterisks) of different sizes in the fibrous soft tissue, and the substances are surrounded by macrophages, fibroblasts and lymphocytes (black asterisks). The monosodium urate crystals appear as needle-like structures under polarized light microscope.

3. 2   Tenosynovial giant cell tumor (Fig.13-13)

The tenosynovial giant cell tumor is composed of mononuclear stromal cells (black arrow), multinucleated giant cells (blue arrows), and foamy histiocytes (green arrows) in dense fibrous tissue. Note the lobulated morphology and unevenly distributed multinucleated giant cells under low power microscope.

Ⅳ. Clinical pathological discussion

Case

A 46-year-old male was hospitalized with "pain and numbness of bilateral buttocks and lower limbs for more than 20 days". Chest CT revealed an occupying lesion at the right hilum, and lumbar MRI showed abnormal signals of S1-S2 vertebral bodies. Fig.13-14 shows the microscopic pathological morphology of the tissue from bronchoscopic lung biopsy (A) and sacral lesion resection (B).

(1) What is the most likely pathological diagnosis of pulmonary and sacral lesions in this patient?

(2) Please think about the occurrence and development of sacral lesions.

Ⅴ. Questions

1. What are the main ways of infection causing suppurative osteomyelitis?

2. Which three layers can be visible in the morphological characteristics of osteochondroma?

3. What are the main radiographic features of osteosarcoma?

4. What are the main molecular genetic features of Ewing sarcoma?

5. What factors are involved in the pathogenesis of gout?

6. Terms: Codman triangle, Fibrous dysplasia, Aneurysmal bone cyst, Gouty tophi.

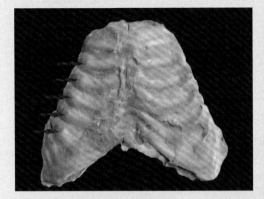

图 13-1　佝偻病肋骨
Fig.13-1　Rachitic ribs

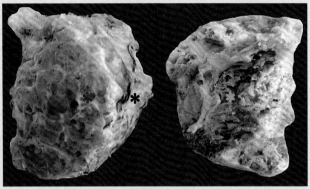

图 13-2　骨软骨瘤
Fig.13-2　Osteochondroma

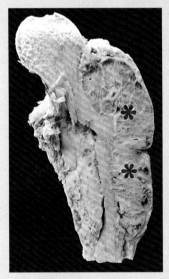

图 13-3　软骨肉瘤
Fig.5-3　Chondrosarcoma

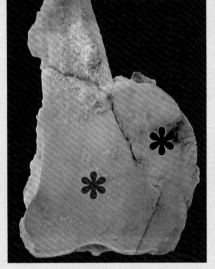

图 13-4　骨肉瘤
Fig.13-4　Osteosarcoma

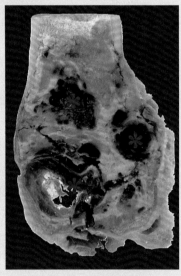

图 13-5　骨巨细胞瘤
Fig.13-5　Giant cell tumor of bone

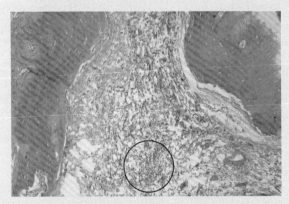

图 13-6　亚急性骨髓炎（×100）
Fig.13-6　Subacute osteomyelitis（×100）

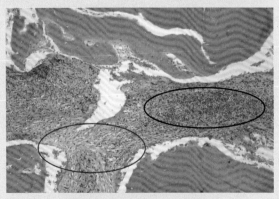

图 13-7　慢性骨髓炎（×100）
Fig.13-7　Chronic osteomyelitis（×100）

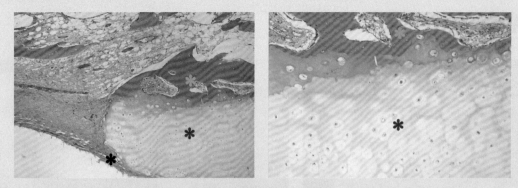

图 13-8　骨软骨瘤（×40；×100）
Fig.13-8　Osteochondroma（×40；×100）

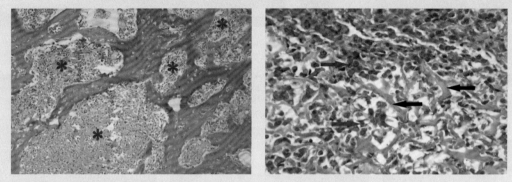

图 13-9　骨肉瘤（×100；×400）
Fig.13-9　Osteosarcoma（×100；×400）

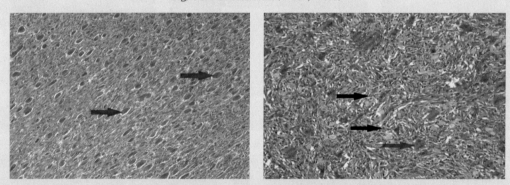

图 13-10　骨巨细胞瘤（×100；×200）
Fig.13-10　Giant cell tumor of bone（×100；×200）

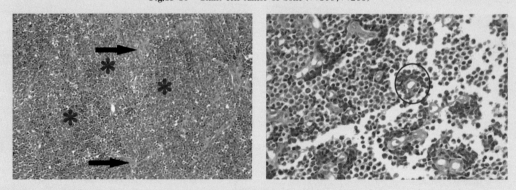

图 13-11　尤因肉瘤（×200；×400）
Fig.13-11　Ewing sarcoma（×200；×400）

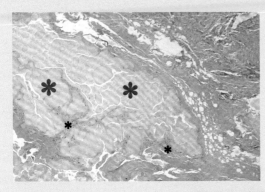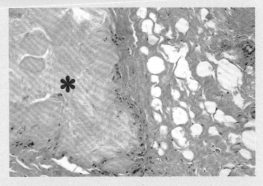

图 13-12　痛风石（×40；×200）
Fig.13-12　Gouty tophi（×40；×200）

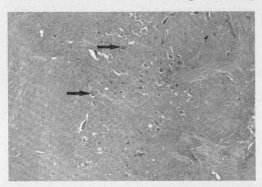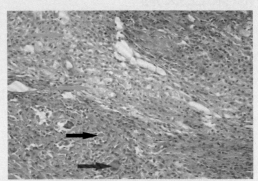

图 13-13　腱鞘巨细胞瘤（×40；×200）
Fig.13-13　Tenosynovial giant cell tumor（×40；×200）

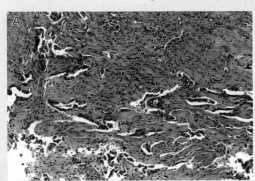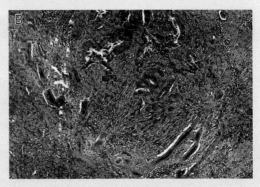

图 13-14　案例（×200；×100）
Fig.13-14　Case（×200；×100）

卜晓东（Xiaodong Bu）

第十四章

感染性疾病

一、目的要求

1. 掌握结核病的基本病变及主要传播途径。
2. 掌握肺结核的主要类型、各型的形态特点及转归。
3. 掌握伤寒的分期和各期的形态学特征。
4. 掌握细菌性痢疾的病理形态特征。
5. 熟悉肺外器官结核的形态特点。
6. 熟悉尖锐湿疣、梅毒的基本病变。

导学

1. 感染性疾病的主要类型及主要特征可参考下表。

感染性疾病	致病微生物	炎症类型	病变特征
结核病	结核杆菌	肉芽肿性炎	结核结节,干酪样坏死(最常累及肺)
伤寒	伤寒杆菌	肉芽肿性炎	伤寒结节(回肠下段)
细菌性痢疾	痢疾杆菌	纤维素性炎	假膜和浅表小溃疡(乙状结肠和直肠)
尖锐湿疣	人乳头瘤病毒	增生性炎	凹空细胞(生殖器官皮肤黏膜交界部位)
梅毒	梅毒螺旋体	肉芽肿性炎	浆细胞恒定出现于基本病变(树胶肿、闭塞性动脉内膜炎和小血管周围炎)。三期梅毒常累及内脏、心血管和中枢神经系统

2. 结核病的主要类型可参考下图。

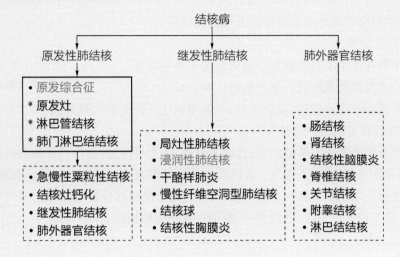

二、大体标本

1. 结核病

1.1 肺结核

1.1.1 原发性肺结核（图 14-1）

小儿肺脏切面可见的病变包括三部分：① 原发病灶（黄箭）：位于肺膜下，中央为干酪样坏死，蚕豆大小；② 结核性淋巴管炎（绿箭）：因切面上不一定正好切到，故标本一般很难见到；③ 淋巴结结核（蓝箭）：肺门淋巴结以及气管旁淋巴结明显肿大并互相融合，切面可见干酪样坏死。

1.1.2 原发性肺结核的结局（图 14-2～图 14-4）

① 急性粟粒性肺结核

两肺切面散在分布均匀、大小一致的灰黄色结节，结节弥漫分布、粟粒大小、边界清楚，切面可观察到结节微隆起（图 14-2）。

② 急性粟粒性脾结核

脾切面散在分布均匀、大小一致的灰黄色粟粒结节，结节切面略隆起（图 14-3）。

③ 慢性粟粒性脾结核

脾切面散在分布不均匀、大小不一致的灰黄色结节（绿箭）（图 14-4），这与急性粟粒结节形态特征上有何不同？为什么？

1.1.3 继发性肺结核（图 14-5～图 14-9）

① 局灶型肺结核

肺尖部有多个边缘清楚，绿豆或黄豆大小病灶（绿箭），病灶中央干燥，呈灰黄色，周围有明显纤维组织包绕（图 14-5）。

② 浸润型肺结核

肺上叶尖段见一灰黄色病灶（黄箭），切面呈干酪样坏死形态，边界模糊（图 14-6）。请思考：该类型临床多见的主要原因及可能的结局。

③ 干酪样肺炎

肺切面散在大小不等灰黄色不规则形的干酪样坏死灶（绿箭）、边界不清，多为浸润型肺结核沿支气管播散所致。部分区域已融合成片（图 14-7）。如果病变累及的范围和大叶性肺炎或小叶性肺炎相仿，请思考：如何鉴别这三种类型的肺炎。

④ 慢性纤维空洞型肺结核

肺上叶有两个紧邻的厚壁空洞，边缘不整齐，但边界清楚，腔内可见残存干酪样坏死物（黄星），空洞壁较厚，分为数层，最内层为干酪样坏死层，周围为结核性肉芽组织，最外围为纤维组织（绿箭）（图 14-8）。空洞内液化的干酪样坏死物可持续向支气管输送细菌，引起双肺出现大小不等、性质不一、新旧程度不同的病灶。

⑤ 肺结核球

肺组织标本，可见一孤立的圆形、灰白色干酪样坏死灶（绿箭），周围境界清楚，外有薄层纤维组织包裹（图 14-9）。

1.2　肺外器官结核

1.2.1　肠结核（图 14-10）

回肠一段，黏膜面见多个环形溃疡（绿圈）。溃疡长径与肠管长轴垂直，边缘不整齐如鼠咬状，底部不平坦，可见坏死。

1.2.2　肠和肠系膜淋巴结结核（图 14-11）

该段组织包括一段肠管及肠系膜淋巴结。肠管可见多个长径与肠管长轴垂直的溃疡（绿箭），肠管周围的肠系膜淋巴结肿大粘连，切面见干酪样坏死（绿圈）。

1.2.3　肾结核（图 14-12）

肾脏肿大，肾实质内有多个干酪样坏死病灶（绿箭）。右图的肾组织切面可见多个空洞，空洞壁粗糙、内有干酪样坏死物。请思考：空洞是怎么形成的以及对毗邻组织的影响。

1.2.4　结核性脑膜炎（图 14-13）

脑膜血管充血，脑回变宽，脑沟变窄。脑顶部蛛网膜下腔内可见灰白色、半透明、略呈胶冻状的渗出物（绿箭）。

1.2.5　脊椎结核（图 14-14）

标本为椎骨的纵切面，其中两个椎骨（绿箭）大部分结构破坏消失，其内为黄白色干酪样坏死组织，造成脊椎骨成角畸形，临床可表现为驼背，也可因压迫脊神经引起病变部位以下神经功能受损。

1.2.6　关节结核（图 14-15）

肘关节切面见骨质广泛破坏，为干酪坏死物质及结核性肉芽组织取代，并已向软组织及皮肤穿破，形成窦道（绿圈）。

1.2.7　附睾结核（图 14-16）

附睾切面可见干酪样坏死灶（绿箭），睾丸未被累及。基于附睾的功能，请思考该病变对病人最主要的影响是什么。

2. 肠伤寒（图 14-17）

左侧图为髓样肿胀期，回肠黏膜孤立淋巴小结（绿箭）和集合淋巴小结（绿圈）高度肿胀，呈圆形或椭圆形向表面突出，其表面高低不平形似脑的沟回，灰红、质软。

中间图为坏死期，肿胀的淋巴滤泡及其表面覆盖的黏膜发生坏死（绿星），因而表面粗糙，失去光泽。部分区域坏死组织已开始脱落。

右侧图为溃疡期，由于坏死组织全部脱落，形成肠伤寒典型的纵形溃疡（绿圈），其长轴与肠长轴平行，溃疡一般波及黏膜下层，严重时可波及深部组织，甚至发生穿孔。请思考该溃疡与肠结核在大体形态上的主要区别。

3. 肠细菌性痢疾（图 14-18）

细菌性痢疾主要累及大肠，以乙状结肠和直肠病变最为严重。该标本为一段结肠，肠壁增厚，黏膜面皱襞消失，覆盖以灰白色糠皮样膜状物（假膜，蓝箭），部分已脱落，形成不规则地图状溃疡（绿箭），溃疡一般较小且浅表。

4. 性传播疾病

肝树胶肿（图 14-19）

肝组织来源于三期梅毒患者，切面见多个灰白色的不规则结节（绿箭），大小不一，质韧富有弹性，边界相对清楚。

三、组织切片

1. 结核病

1.1　粟粒性肺结核（图 14-20）

肺组织充血、散在分布多个圆形、卵圆形结核结节（蓝圈），中央可有干酪样坏死，外周是大量的上皮样细胞夹杂少量朗汉斯巨细胞（蓝箭）。上皮样细胞形态多样，排列常较紧密，边界不清，体积较大，胞浆丰富，轻度嗜酸性，胞核为圆形或卵圆形，染色浅。朗汉斯巨细胞体积较大，卵圆形或不规则形，胞浆丰富、嗜酸性，核圆形或卵圆形，一般数个到数十个，细胞核多排列在细胞膜的边缘呈马蹄形或环形排列。

1.2　干酪样肺炎（图 14-21）

所示肺组织大部分为干酪样坏死灶（蓝星）取代，与周围组织无明显分界。坏死区不整形、片状，周边有大量的核碎片。附近未坏死的肺组织中，肺泡腔内见大量巨噬细胞（蓝箭）及少量中性粒细胞，并混有多少不等的浆液和纤维素（绿箭）。左图的右上插图为抗酸染色，紫红色弧形结构为结核杆菌。

1.3　肺结核球（图 14-22）

绿星示结核球内大片的干酪样坏死，周围为炎性纤维结缔组织包膜（蓝星），主要为大量增生的纤维组织和慢性炎细胞。棕星示邻近肺组织。

1.4　肠结核（图 14-23）

一段回肠组织，黏膜下层和肌层均可见结核结节（蓝圈）。这些结节主要由上皮样细胞构成，可见少数朗汉斯巨细胞，周围为多量淋巴细胞。绿星和蓝星分别示结肠壁的黏膜层和黏膜下层。

1.5　肾结核（图 14-24）

肾组织大部分结构被大小不等的结核结节（蓝星）所取代，部分结节中心可见干酪样坏死（红箭），结核结节内有大量上皮样细胞（黑箭）和少量朗汉斯巨细胞（黄箭）。间质有多量炎细胞浸润，蓝箭示肾小球。

1.6　输尿管结核（图 14-25）

输尿管上皮细胞脱落（蓝箭），其下为大片干酪样坏死（蓝星），输尿管壁各层均可见炎细胞浸润和结核结节（蓝圈）形成，肌层尤为明显。结核结节中央主要为上皮样细胞，间杂有朗汉斯巨细胞（绿箭），外围是淋巴细胞和成纤维细胞。

1.7　附睾结核（图 14-26）

附睾管（蓝箭，黑箭）之间可见边界清楚的结核结节（蓝星），内有朗汉斯巨细胞（绿箭），部分附睾管结构被结核结节破坏（黑箭），上皮细胞变性坏死脱落入管腔。

1.8　结核性脑炎（图 14-27）

脑组织灶性破坏，原有结构被结核结节（蓝圈）取代。其内可见朗汉斯巨细胞（红圈），未被结核结节累及的区域可见神经元（蓝箭）、神经胶质细胞和神经纤维等脑组织成分。

1.9　胸椎结核（图 14-28）

切片取自胸椎，绿箭示椎骨组织。骨组织间查见结核结节，其内有朗汉斯巨细胞（蓝箭）。

1.10　淋巴结结核（图 14-29）

淋巴结部分区域淡伊红色，为干酪样坏死区（绿星），坏死彻底，失去正常组织结构，呈红染无结构的颗粒状物。周边残存淋巴组织（黄星）中散在大小不等的结核结节（蓝星），有的结节内有朗汉斯巨细胞（蓝箭）。

2. 肠伤寒（图 14-30）

切片取自回肠末段肿胀的淋巴小结。大部分区域黏膜组织已脱落形成溃疡，左侧可见少量残存的上皮组织（蓝箭）。淋巴小结肿大明显，部分区域坏死，结构模糊（蓝圈）。该区域淋巴小结原有结构消失，被大量增生的巨噬细胞取代。这些细胞体积较大、圆或卵圆形，胞浆丰富，核圆形或肾形，多数细胞内可见吞噬的淋巴细胞、红细胞及一些坏死细胞碎片，即伤寒细胞（黑箭）。伤寒细胞常聚集在一起，形成结节，称伤寒结节。

3. 肠细菌性痢疾（图 14-31）

肠壁各层结构尚清楚，黏膜浅层大部分区域坏死、脱落，仅见少许残存的黏膜上皮（蓝箭），其表面为一层较厚的膜状物（蓝圈），由坏死的黏膜组织、渗出的纤维素（蓝箭头）、中性粒细胞及核碎片混合构成,该结构称为假膜。固有层、黏膜下层、肌层和浆膜层充血水肿,有多量炎细胞浸润。

4. 性传播疾病

4.1 尖锐湿疣(图 14-32)

表皮角质层轻度增厚,棘层肥厚,基底膜完整。表皮钉突增粗延长、浅层(绿星)可见凹空细胞(HPV 感染的特征细胞)。凹空细胞(绿箭)体积较正常细胞大,核大居中,圆形、椭圆形或不规则形,核周胞浆有空晕,核仁清楚。真皮层毛细血管和淋巴管扩张,伴间质水肿和炎细胞浸润。

4.2 梅毒性主动脉炎(图 14-33)

切片为主动脉管壁,A 图中央可见大量炎细胞浸润和纤维结缔组织增生。B 图炎性区可见炎细胞主要为淋巴细胞(蓝箭)和浆细胞(绿箭),小血管内皮细胞增生(黑箭),致管壁增厚、管腔狭窄,周围环绕有淋巴细胞和浆细胞。C 和 D 图为 Weigert's 弹力纤维染色,示中膜弹力纤维断裂(绿星),损伤部位被瘢痕组织所取代。

四、 临床病理讨论

案例 1 患者,女性,38 岁,体检时胸部 X 线发现右肺有一直径 22 mm、边缘清晰的结节;患者自诉无任何不适症状,进一步检查提示:血常规无异常,结核菌素实验阳性,痰涂片抗酸染色阴性。后行病灶切除,并送检病理科,典型图片见图 14-34。

(1)请给出该病人的病理诊断,并说明理由。

(2)患者为何无任何不适症状?

(3)如果对该结节不做任何处理,会对患者有哪些影响?

案例 2 患者,32 岁,男性,工人。午饭后大约 2 小时开始出现下腹部疼痛,伴恶心,无呕吐。后又腹泻多次,黏液脓血便,伴恶心呕吐、发热,急诊就医。体格检查结果为,体温 38.7℃,中下腹有压痛,肠鸣音亢进。其余无异常。血常规和粪便检查结果如下。

血常规:白细胞总数为 11.6×10^9/L,中性粒细胞比例 82%。

粪便检查:查见红细胞 10~15 个/高倍视野,大量中性粒细胞 20~30 个/高倍视野、脓细胞(偶见成堆脓细胞聚集),伴黏液及片状膜样物。

(1)请给出该患者最可能的病理诊断为下列疾病中的哪一个:肠结核、肠细菌性痢疾、肠伤寒? 给出诊断要点以及不选其他两种疾病的理由。

(2)根据诊断,描述病人肠道可能出现的形态学变化。

(3)根据形态学变化分析患者为何会发热、粪便为何会出现片状膜样物?

五、 思考题

1. 结核病具有诊断价值的形态学病变是什么?

2. 干酪样坏死与其他坏死有何不同?

3. 原发性肺结核与继发性肺结核在形态学变化和播散时的特点各是什么?

4. 一位伤寒病人突然发生肠穿孔,因抢救不及时不幸死亡。在尸检时,哪些器官或组织可能会发现与伤寒相关的病理改变?

5. 请说明结核病、伤寒和细菌性痢疾三者肠道病变的炎症性质及特征性的形态学改变。

6. 名词解释:结核结节,原发综合征,原发性肺结核,结核瘤,冷脓肿,伤寒细胞,伤寒结节,凹空细胞,硬性下疳,树胶样肿。

Chapter 14

Infectious Diseases

Ⅰ. Aims

1. To grasp the basic pathological characteristics and infectious routes of tuberculosis.

2. To grasp the types, pathological characteristics, and outcomes of pulmonary tuberculosis.

3. To grasp the main stages and corresponding morphological features of typhoid fever.

4. To grasp the pathological features of bacillary dysentery.

5. To familiarize with the pathological characteristics of extrapulmonary tuberculosis.

6. To familiarize with the basic pathological features of condyloma acuminatum and syphilis.

Guidance to study

1. The main features of infectious diseases can be referred in the following table.

Infectious disease	*Pathogenic microorganism*	Type of inflammation	Pathologic characteristics
Tuberculosis	Mycobacterium tuberculosis	Granulomatous inflammation	Tubercle and caseous necrosis (mostly involving lungs)
Typhoid fever	Typhoid bacillus	Granulomatous inflammation	Typhoid nodule (lower part of ileum)
Bacillary dysentery	Shigella dysenteriae	Fibrinous inflammation	Pseudomembrane and superficial small ulcers (sigmoid flexture and rectum)
Condyloma acuminatum	Human papillomavirus	Proliferative inflammation	Koilocytes (the junction between skin and mucosa of genital tissues)
Syphilis	Treponema pallidum	Granulomatous inflammation	Plasma cells are invariably present in the basic pathological changes (gumma, occlusive endoarteritis and periarteritis). Visceral organs, cardiovascular system and central nervous system are commonly involved for the patients with tertiary syphilis

2. The main types of tuberculosis are shown in the following figure.

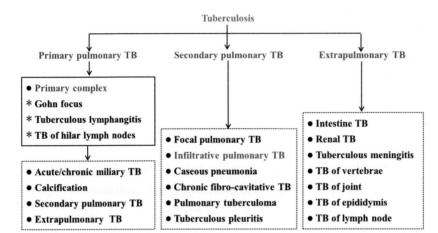

Abbreviation：TB, tuberculosis

Ⅱ. Gross specimens

1. Tuberculosis

1.1　Pulmonary tuberculosis

1.1.1　Primary pulmonary tuberculosis（Fig. 14-1）

Three lesions are observed in the child's lung: ① Primary tuberculous focus (Ghon focus, yellow arrow): The gray-white parenchymal focus with caseous necrosis is visualized under the pleura. ② Tuberculous lymphangitis (green arrow): It is a disseminated lesion linking Ghon focus with tuberculous lymphadenitis. ③ Tuberculosis of lymph nodes (blue arrow): The homolateral hilar lymph nodes as well as parabronchial lymph nodes become swollen and coalesced, and the cut surface is yellow-white caseous necrosis.

1.1.2　Outcomes of primary pulmonary tuberculosis（Fig. 14-2～14-4）

① Acute miliary tuberculosis of lung

Many gray-yellow tubercles diffusely distribute on the surface and cut surface of lung, and the tubercles are round millet-sized with clear borders (Fig.14-2).

② Acute miliary tuberculosis of spleen

Numerous miliary tubercles uniformly distribute on the surface and cut surface of spleen. The tubercles are gray-yellow and round with clear margin (Fig.14-3).

③ Chronic miliary tuberculosis of spleen

The gray-yellow tubercles (green arrows) distribute nonuniformly on the surface and cut surface of the spleen. The tubercles are different in both pathological nature and size of the lesions (Fig. 14-4). Pay attention to the difference between acute and chronic miliary tuberculosis in morphology.

1. 1. 3   Secondary pulmonary tuberculosis (Fig. 14-5～14-9)

① Focal pulmonary tuberculosis

Some round, gray-yellow, soybean-sized foci (green arrows) are at the apex of the lung. The boundary between the foci and the surrounding fibrotic tissue is clear (Fig.14-5).

② Infiltrative pulmonary tuberculosis

The focus presents caseous necrosis with undefined edge (yellow arrow). It is the most common type of secondary pulmonary tuberculosis in clinic (Fig.14-6). Please think about the reasons and possible outcomes.

③ Caseous pneumonia

The yellow-white lesions containing caseous necroses (green arrows) scatter on the cut surface of the lung. Among them, some foci are enlarged and coalesced (Fig.14-7). If the whole lobe is involved, how do you distinguish it from lobar pneumonia? If only the lobules are affected, how do you differentiate it from lobular pneumonia?

④ Chronic fibro-cavitative pulmonary tuberculosis

Two closely contiguous thick-wall cavities are observed in the upper lobe. The cavities have necrotic, ragged walls, with adherent yellow-white cheesy debris (yellow star). The thick wall of the cavity is divided into three layers: caseous necrosis, granulation tissue and fibrous tissue from inner to outer (green arrow) (Fig.14-8). The cavities may continuously spread mycobacteria tuberculosis by bronchi and cause more lesions in the lung. The lesions are different in both morphology and size.

⑤ Pulmonary tuberculoma

A nodular, conglomerate area (green arrow) is observed at the apex of the lung. This nodule shows caseous necrosis circumscribed by well-defined fibrous capsule (Fig.14-9).

1. 2   Extrapulmonary tuberculosis

1. 2. 1   Intestinal tuberculosis (Fig. 14-10)

This is a segment of ileum. Several transverse ulcers (green circles) are noticeable, which are slightly bulge with rough edges on the mucosa. The bases of ulcers are uneven with necroses.

1. 2. 2   Tuberculosis of intestine and mesenteric lymph nodes (Fig. 14-11)

A segment of ileum is firmly adhered to the surrounding mesenteric tissue. A few enlarged lymph nodes (green circle) are coalesced each other. Yellow-white cheesy necrotic material and several transverse ulcers (green arrows) are observed on the cut surface in the ileum.

1. 2. 3   Renal tuberculosis (Fig. 14-12)

Both kidneys are enlarged, and some caseous necroses (green arrows) are obviously observed on the section. The kidney in the right picture presents several cavities lined by yellowish white caseous necrosis.

1. 2. 4　Tuberculous meningitis（Fig. 14-13）

Gray-white, turbid, gelatinous exudate（green arrows）is obvious within subarachnoid space at the top of the brain, especially around the blood vessels. The blood vessels are easily observed due to congestion. The gyri become widened, and the sulci are narrowed.

1. 2. 5　Tuberculosis of vertebrae（Fig. 14-14）

This is the sagittal section of vertebrae. Among them, two vertebrae（green arrows）are destroyed and replaced by caseous necroses. The vertebrae are deformed by a certain angle. In clinic, the patient must be humpbacked.

1. 2. 6　Tuberculosis of joint（Fig. 14-15）

The osseous area near the elbow joint is extensively destroyed. The surrounding tissue is involved, and a sinus（green circles）is noticeable on the skin.

1. 2. 7　Tuberculosis of epididymis（Fig. 14-16）

The cut surface of the epididymis shows caseous necrosis（green arrows）. The testis is not affected. Consider the main effect of the lesion on the patient based on the function of epididymis.

2. Typhoid fever

Typhoid fever of intestine（Fig.14-17）

The images shows the intestine with typhoid fever. The left image is for hyperplasia stage, the middle one for necrosis stage, and the right one for ulceration stage.

Hyperplasia stage: This is one segment of ileum opened longitudinally. Note the enlarged solidary（green arrows）and aggregated lymphoid nodules（Peyer's patches, green circles）. The surfaces of Peyer's patches are convoluted and swollen, which resembles the gyri of the brain （sharply delineated, plateau-like elevations）.

Necrosis stage: The necrotic areas（green stars）are pronounced on the surface of the enlarged Peyer's patches.

Ulceration stage: The longitudinal ulcers（green circle）usually destroy submucosa layer. Severe lesions may involve the deep tissue, even penetrate the serosa and lead to perforation. The longitudinal ulcers with typhoid fever are different from the transverse ulcers with tuberculosis.

3. Bacillary dysentery

Bacillary dysentery of colon（Fig.14-18）

The colonic mucosa becomes thickened, and shows the gray-white pseudomembrane（blue arrow）with small and superficial ulcers（green arrows）.

4. Sexual transmitted diseases

Gumma of liver（Fig.14-19）

The liver sample is from a patient with tertiary syphilis. On cut section, there are some irregular gray-white nodules with relatively clear borders (green arrows),and the nodular changes are resilient with different sizes.

Ⅲ. Tissue sections

1. Tuberculosis

1. 1　Miliary tuberculosis of lung（Fig.14-20）

There are many well-defined and equal sized tubercles with clear margins(blue circles)in the lung, and some tubercles contain Langhans' giant cells (blue arrows). The giant cell distributes among epithelioid cells, and displays abundant red-stained cytoplasm and multiple nuclei. The nuclei arrange in garland or horse's hoof form. The epithelioid cell looks like epithelial cell with unclear margin, and presents round or oval nucleus, and light staining cytoplasm with unclear margin.

1. 2　Caseous pneumonia（Fig.14-21）

Most of the lung tissue is replaced by irregular caseous necroses(blue stars), and there is no distinct boundary between the necrotic and normal tissue. The peripheral zones are full of exudate containing abundant fluid, fibrins (green arrows), many macrophages (blue arrows) and a few neutrophils.

The upper-right small micrograph in the left image displays mycobacteria tuberculosis labelled by acid-fast staining.

1. 3　Pulmonary tuberculoma（Fig.14-22）

The green star indicates caseous necrosis surrounded by an intact capsule. The capsule (blue star)is composed of plentiful fibrous tissue and chronic inflammatory cells. The brown star shows the adjacent lung tissue.

1. 4　Intestinal tuberculosis（Fig.14-23）

The histological section is from the intestinal wall. Some tubercles(blue circles)exist in the submucosal layer and muscle layer. The dominant cells of tubercles are epithelioid cells. A few Langhans' giant cells and numerous lymphocytes are also seen in the tubercles. The green and blue stars indicate mucosa and submucosal layer, respectively.

1. 5　Renal tuberculosis（Fig.14-24）

Some areas are replaced by tuberculous granulomas(blue stars)and caseous necroses(red arrows)in the kidney. Epithelioid cells (black arrows), Langhans' giant cells (yellow arrows), and mass of inflammatory cells are observed in the granulomas. The blue arrows indicate glomeruli.

1. 6　Ureter tuberculosis（Fig.14-25）

The epithelial cells detach from the wall of ureter (blue arrows) and replaced by caseous necrosis (blue star). Tubercles (blue circle) and inflammatory cells can be observed in the all layers of the ureter, especially muscular layer. Two contiguous granulomas appear in the muscular layer of the magnified right image. The granulomas display that epithelioid cells and Langhans' giant cells (green arrow) are surrounded by lots of lymphocytes and fibroblasts.

1. 7　Tuberculosis of epididymis（Fig.14-26）

Some tubercles (blue star) are seen among the epididymal ducts (blue arrows, black arrow). Some granulomas show Langhans' giant cells (green arrows). An epididymal ducts is damaged by the granuloma (black arrow), and some epithelial cells fall off into the lumen due to necrosis.

1. 8　Tuberculous encephalitis（Fig.14-27）

Some regions are injured and replaced by tubercles (blue circles) including Langhans' giant cells (red circles). The uninvolved areas present alterative neurons (blue arrows), glia cells, and nerve fibers.

1. 9　Tuberculosis of thoracic vertebra（Fig.14-28）

The tissue is taken from the thoracic vertebrae. Among the osseous tissue (green arrows), tubercles with Langhans' giant cells (blue arrows) are visible.

1. 10　Tuberculosis of lymph node（Fig.14-29）

The pink areas lose original tissue structure of lymph node and replaced by caseous necroses (green stars). The surrounding tissue presents residual lymphatic tissue (yellow stars), tubercles (blue stars), and a few Langhans' giant cells (blue arrows).

2. Typhoid fever of intestine（Fig.14-30）

The tissue is from the swollen lymphoid follicles in the lower segment of ileum. Most of the mucosal tissue has dropped off and developed an ulcer, and only small amount of epithelia are visible in the surrounding tissue (blue arrows). Lymph follicle (blue circle) presents necrotic tissue and large macrophages. The proliferative macrophages display phagocytized erythrocytes, lymphocytes, and nuclei debris in the cytoplasm, which are the marker cells of typhoid fever and defined as typhoid cells (black arrows). The typhoid cells aggregate into typhoid granuloma/nodule.

3. Bacillary dysentery of colon（Fig.14-31）

The layers of intestinal wall are still clear, and show inflammatory response such as congestion, edema, and leukocytes infiltration. However, the superficial part of mucosal layer is necrotic with a few residual epithelial cells (blue arrows). The necrotic mucosa is covered by the pseudo-membrane (blue circle), which is composed of fibrins (blue arrowheads), neutrophils, cell debris, and erythrocytes.

4. Sexual transmitted diseases

4. 1   Condyloma acuminatum (Fig.14-32)

The epidermal cuticle and prickle cell layer become thickened, and the basal membrane is intact. Epidermis are thickened and prolonged. The superficial layer (green star) presents some koilocytes with perinuclear haloes (indicative cells for HPV infection). The koilocytes (green arrows) are larger than normal prick cells, and the nuclei are big and centered around pronounced nucleoli. The dermis shows dilated capillaries and lymphatic vessels with interstitial edema and inflammatory cells infiltration.

4. 2   Syphilitic aortitis (Fig.14-33)

In the aortic wall, mass of inflammatory cells and fibrous tissue are apparent (Fig.14-33A). The inflammatory cells are mainly located in the inflamed area, especially around the small blood vessels. The dominant infiltrating cells are lymphocytes (blue arrow) and plasma cells (green arrows). The blood vessels are lined with proliferating endothelial cells (black arrows) with narrow lumens (Fig.14-33B). The Weigert's staining for elastic fibers shows the broken elastic fibers (green stars) in the media, and the destroyed part is replaced by scar tissue (Fig.14-33C, D).

Ⅳ. Clincal pathological discussion

Case 1

A female aged 38 has been told to have a well-circumscribed nodule in her right lung. The nodule is 22 mm in diameter. The patient had no any discomfort, and the results from further clinical examination were as follows.

(1) Blood routine test: Normal;

(2) Tuberculin test: Positive;

(3) Acid-fast staining of her sputum smear: Negative;

The patient took a surgery to remove the nodule, and the nodule was detected by pathological doctors. The typical pictures are shown as Fig.14-34.

(1) Please make a diagnosis of the nodule.

(2) The patient has a large nodule in her lung, but she hasn't complained any discomfort, why?

(3) If no medical intervention is done against the nodule, what will possibly happen on the patient in future?

Case 2

A male worker complained that he had been suffering lower abdominal pain, nausea after lunch for about 2 hours.

Physical examination: Acute appearance, body temperature 38.7℃, tenderness in his middle-lower abdomen, and hyperactive bowel sounds.

Routine blood test: Leukocytes count is 11.6×10^9/L, and neutrophils percentage is 82%.

Stool test: Red blood cells 10～15/HPF (high power field), neutrophils 20～30/HPF, pus cells (occasionally aggregate), mucus fluid, and laminar membrane-like substance.

(1) Which is the most likely pathological diagnosis for his intestinal tissue, tuberculosis, bacillary dysentery, or typhoid fever? Why?

(2) Describe morphological changes which are possibly observed in his intestine.

(3) Why did the patient suffer fever? Why did laminar membrane-like tissues appear in his stool?

Ⅴ. Questions

1. What morphological changes are diagnostic for tuberculosis?

2. Compare caseous necrosis with other types of necroses.

3. Compare primary type with secondary type of pulmonary tuberculosis in both morphology and transmission routes.

4. A patient died of intestinal typhoid fever due to the complication of intestinal perforation, and sent to autopsy. Please list the tissues possibly presenting morphological changes related to typhoid fever.

5. Please explain the nature of inflammation and characteristics of pathological changes in the intestine with tuberculosis, typhoid fever, and bacillary dysentery.

6. Terms: Tubercle, Primary complex, Primary pulmonary tuberculosis, Tuberculoma, Cold abscess, Typhoid cell, Typhoid nodule, Koilocyte, Hard chancre, Gumma.

VI. 附图 (Figures)

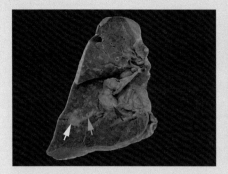

图 14-1　原发性肺结核
Fig.14-1　Primary pulmonary tuberculosis

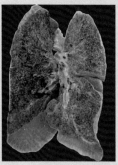

图 14-2　急性粟粒性肺结核
Fig.14-2　Acute miliary
tuberculosis of lung

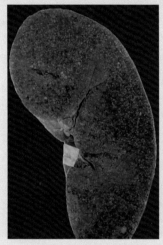

图 14-3　急性粟粒性脾结核
Fig.14-3　Acute miliary
tuberculosis of spleen

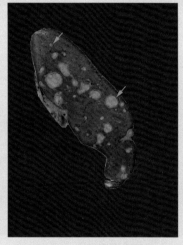

图 14-4　慢性粟粒性脾结核
Fig.14-4　Chronic miliary
tuberculosis of spleen

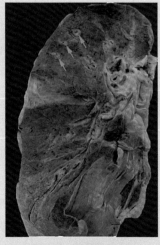

图 14-5　局灶型肺结核
Fig.14-5　Focal pulmonary
tuberculosis

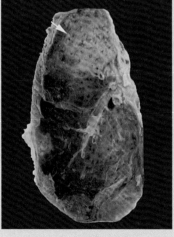

图 14-6　浸润型肺结核
Fig.14-6　Infiltrative pulmonary
tuberculosis

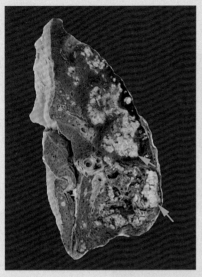

图 14-7 干酪样肺炎
Fig.14-7 Caseous pneumonia

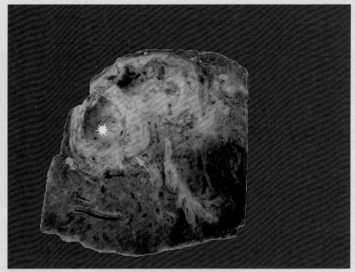

图 14-8 慢性纤维空洞型肺结核
Fig.14-8 Chronic fibro-cavitative pulmonary tuberculosis

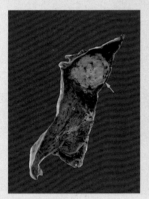

图 14-9 肺结核球
Fig.14-9 Pulmonary
tuberculoma

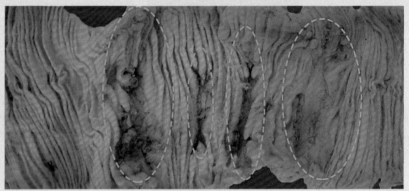

图 14-10 肠结核
Fig.14-10 Intestinal tuberculosis

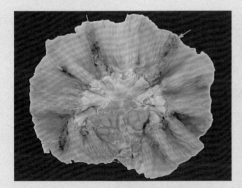

图 14-11 肠和肠系膜淋巴结结核
Fig.14-11 Tuberculosis of
intestine and mesenteric lymph nodes

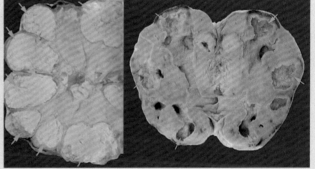

图 14-12 肾结核
Fig.14-12 Renal tuberculosis

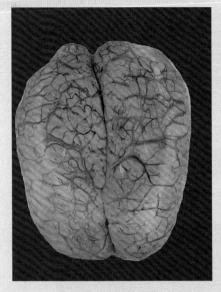
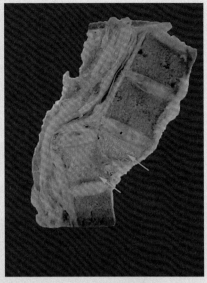

图 14-13　结核性脑膜炎
Fig.14-13　Tuberculous meningitis

图 14-14　脊椎结核
Fig.14-14　Tuberculosis of vertebrae

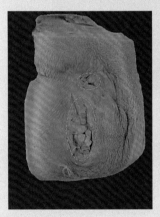
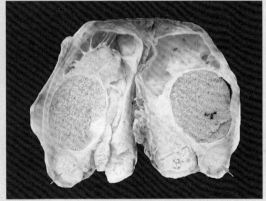

图 14-15　关节结核
Fig.14-15　Tuberculosis of joint

图 14-16　附睾结核
Fig.14-16　Tuberculosis of epididymis

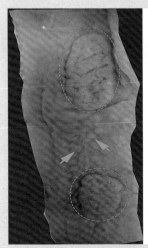
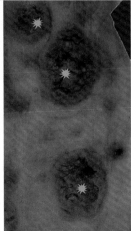
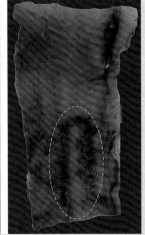

图 14-17　肠伤寒
Fig.14-17　Typhoid fever of intestine

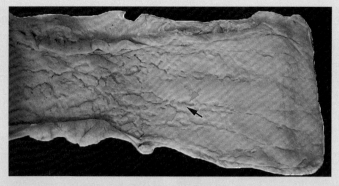

图 14-18　肠细菌性痢疾

Fig.14-18　Bacillary dysentery of colon

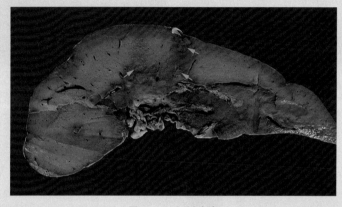

图 14-19　肝树胶肿

Fig.14-19　Gumma of liver

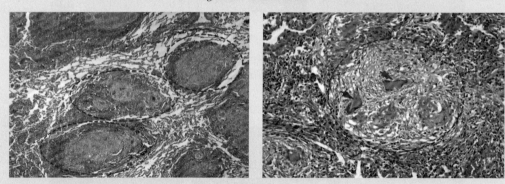

图 14-20　粟粒性肺结核（×40；×200）

Fig.14-20　Miliary tuberculosis of lung（×40；×200）

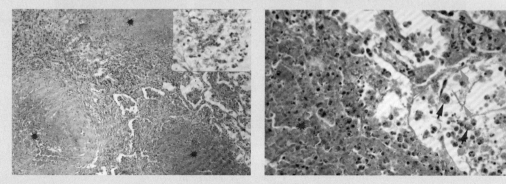

图 14-21　干酪样肺炎（×100；×400）

Fig.14-21　Caseous pneumonia（×100；×400）

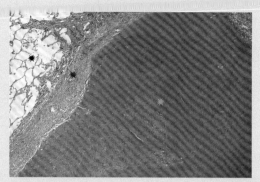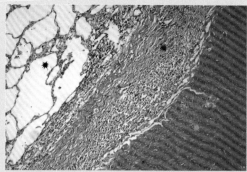

图 14-22　肺结核球（×40；×100）

Fig.14-22　Pulmonary tuberculoma（×40；×100）

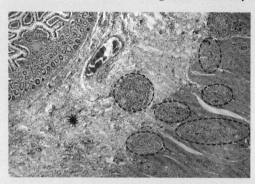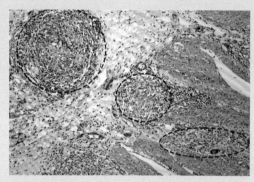

图 14-23　肠结核（×40；×100）

Fig.14-23　Intestinal tuberculosis（×40；×100）

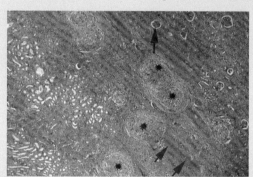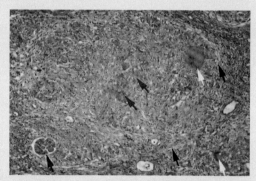

图 14-24　肾结核（×40；×100）

Fig.14-24　Renal tuberculosis（×40；×100）

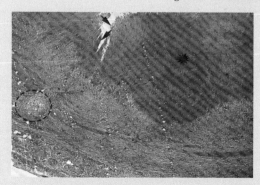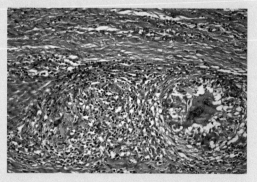

图 14-25　输尿管结核（×40；×200）

Fig.14-25　Ureter tuberculosis（×40；×200）

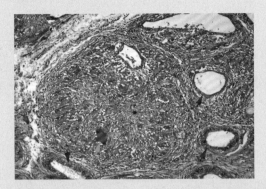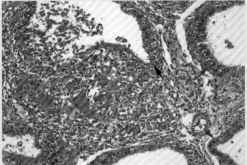

图 14-26　附睾结核（×100；×200）
Fig.14-26　Tuberculosis of epididymis（×100；×200）

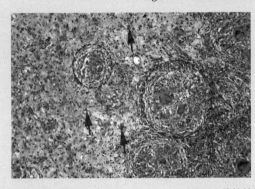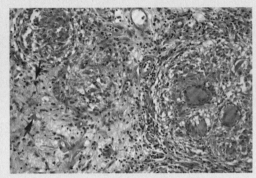

图 14-27　结核性脑炎（×100；×200）
Fig.14-27　Tuberculous encephalitis（×100；×200）

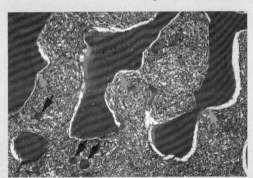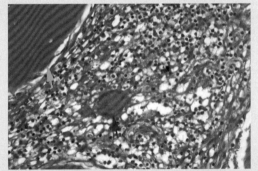

图 14-28　胸椎结核（×100；×400）
Fig.14-28　Tuberculosis of thoracic vertebra（×100；×400）

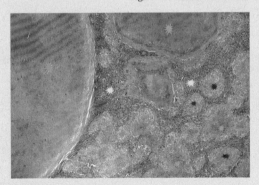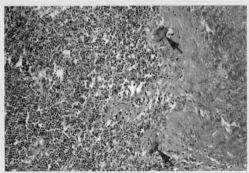

图 14-29　淋巴结结核（×40；×200）
Fig.14-29　Tuberculosis of lymph node（×40；×200）

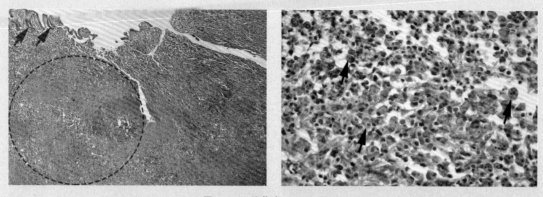

图 14-30 肠伤寒（×40；×400）

Fig.14-30 Typhoid fever of intestine（×40；×400）

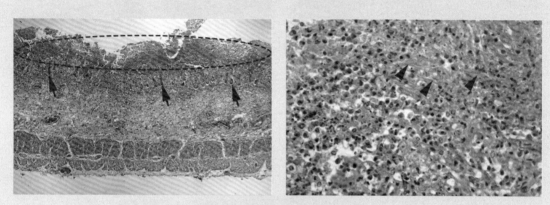

图 14-31 肠细菌性痢疾（×40；×400）

Fig.14-31 Bacillary dysentery of colon（×40；×400）

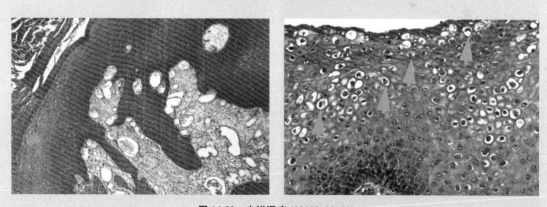

图 14-32 尖锐湿疣（×100；×400）

Fig.14-32 Condyloma acuminatum（×100；×400）

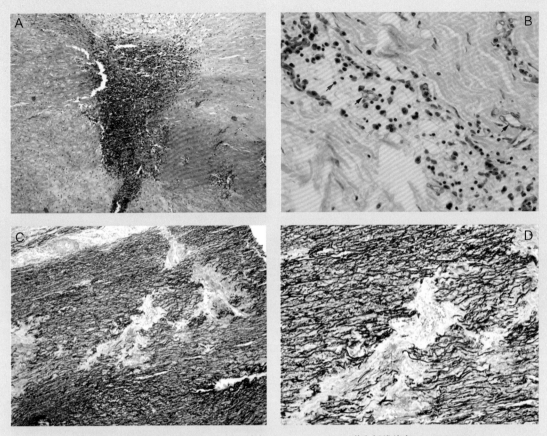

图 14-33　梅毒性主动脉炎（A,B:H.E. 染色×40；×400；C,D:弹力纤维染色×40；×400 ）
Fig.14-33　Syphilitic aortitis（A,B:H.E. ×40；×400；C,D:Weigert's staining×40；×400）

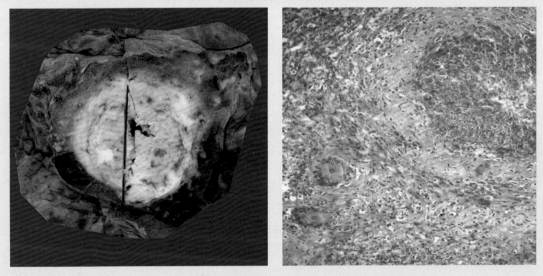

图 14-34　案例 1:肺结节（手术切除标本、H.E. 染色×200）
Fig.14-34　Case 1:Pulmonary node（Specimen from surgical operation，H. E. staining×200）

李懿萍（Yiping Li）

第十五章

寄生虫病

一、目的要求

1. 掌握阿米巴病、血吸虫病主要累及的器官及其病理形态特征。
2. 熟悉丝虫病主要累及的器官及其病理形态特征。

导学

　　理解病变组织中寄生虫的存在是诊断寄生虫病最直接、最可靠的证据,体会不同种类的寄生虫在不同的发育阶段主要侵犯的组织以及损伤的形态学特征并不相同,而且病变在急性期和慢性期的呈现也各具特点。

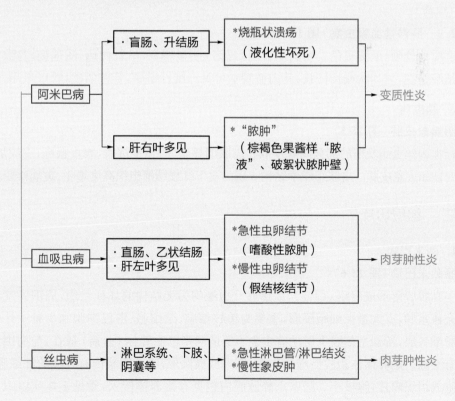

二、 大体标本

1. 阿米巴病

1.1　肠阿米巴病（图 15-1）

溶组织阿米巴通常寄生于结肠，以盲肠、升结肠最多见，标本见结肠黏膜表面散在有大量大小不等，圆形或不整形的溃疡，溃疡边缘肿胀且潜行，致溃疡呈口小底大烧瓶状（绿箭）。溃疡底部和边缘有灰黄色絮状物附着，溃疡之间肠黏膜尚正常。相邻溃疡还可观察到在黏膜下层相互融合，形成较大的不规则形溃疡（绿圈）。

1.2　阿米巴肝脓肿（图 15-2）

肝组织切面上见两个较大"脓肿"（绿圈），脓肿壁上附着破絮状尚未完全坏死液化的肝组织，脓肿内容物为液化的棕褐色果酱样坏死组织，在标本切开时已流失。此类病人行肝穿刺可抽出特征性的棕褐色果酱样内容物，可为临床诊断提供重要线索。这种内容物由坏死液化的肝组织混杂溶解的红细胞组成，不同于真正的脓肿。

2. 血吸虫病

2.1　结肠慢性血吸虫病（图 15-3）

肠黏膜表面粗糙不平，黏膜皱襞消失、萎缩、增生和坏死区域并存。黏膜表面区域或散在小溃疡，或不同程度萎缩致皱襞变平坦（黄箭），或颗粒状隆起似砂粒、或增生呈息肉状（绿箭）。

2.2　肝慢性血吸虫病（图 15-4）

肝质地变硬，呈黄褐色。切面汇管区（绿箭）明显增宽，呈灰白色、质地韧，为致密的纤维结缔组织，呈片状或长杆状，其内血管壁可见纤维性增厚，管壁僵硬，管口哆开。

3. 丝虫病

阴囊象皮肿（图 15-5）

标本为丝虫病晚期的部分阴囊皮肤。皮肤明显增厚，色素沉着，表皮粗糙，皮纹加深，质地变韧如大象皮肤。皮肤组织学结构表现为皮下纤维结缔组织高度增生、玻璃样变。

三、 组织切片

1. 阿米巴病

肠阿米巴病（图 15-6）

肠黏膜脱落形成溃疡（绿箭），溃疡底及边缘均为无结构的坏死组织，周围肠壁各层轻度充血水肿，有大量炎细胞浸润，主要为单核细胞、浆细胞、淋巴细胞和少量中性粒细胞。肠壁各层，特别是黏膜下层见有多少不等的阿米巴滋养体（蓝箭）散在，与周围组织之间有空隙。滋养体体积较巨噬细胞大，圆形或椭圆形，有的胞浆内有吞噬的红细胞、淋巴细胞或组织碎片，胞核小。肠壁小静脉腔内也见有滋养体侵入，常见于坏死组织与正常组织的交界处。黑箭示病灶周围肠黏膜腺上皮。

2. 血吸虫病

2.1 结肠慢性血吸虫病（图 15-7）

肠壁各层尤其黏膜下层可见大小不一的多个结节（蓝星），其内有许多不同形态的血吸虫虫卵成堆或散在沉积。虫卵结节内可观察到：① 中央的虫卵（蓝箭），有的已钙化，有的可见紫蓝色密集小圆点（成熟虫卵）；② 嗜酸性粒细胞（黑箭）、淋巴细胞、巨噬细胞、浆细胞等炎细胞；③ 上皮样细胞和多核异物巨细胞（绿箭）。

2.2 肝急性血吸虫病（图 15-8）

A 图黑星所示区域为扩大的汇管区，其内可见小叶间血管和小叶间胆管，大量炎细胞浸润（绿星）。绿圈所示区域为汇管区内的急性虫卵结节，邻近肝小叶结构基本正常，界板区肝细胞受压萎缩、小灶性变性坏死。B 图虫卵结节内可见位于中央的残留虫卵（蓝箭）、周围的坏死组织（蓝星）以及炎细胞。炎细胞（绿星）主要为嗜酸性粒细胞，伴上皮样细胞和成纤维细胞增生。C 图虫卵结节结构与左侧基本一致，可观察到数个多核巨细胞（绿箭）。

2.3 肝慢性血吸虫病（图 15-9）

肝小叶结构尚完好，无假小叶形成，汇管区扩大明显，挤压肝小叶导致小叶界板周围肝细胞萎缩、小灶性变性坏死。汇管区内见扩张淤血的血管（蓝箭）、增生的纤维组织、再生的胆管（黑箭）、浸润的炎细胞，其间查见数量不等的虫卵结节（蓝星），有的已钙化（黄箭），周围可见多核异物巨细胞（绿箭）和嗜酸性粒细胞（红箭）。

3. 丝虫病

丝虫性肉芽肿（图 15-10）

纤维结缔组织内可见围绕数段虫体断面（蓝箭）形成的肉芽肿性病变，其内可见密集微丝蚴、坏死组织（蓝星）。坏死组织及虫体周围有多量嗜酸性粒细胞和少量淋巴细胞及浆细胞浸润，并可见数量不等上皮样细胞和多核异物巨细胞（绿箭）。

四、临床病理讨论

案例 患者，男性，42 岁，2 个月前曾和朋友一同去户外游泳。当时感觉小腿皮肤有些刺痛瘙痒，出现几个红色丘疹，患者以为是皮肤过敏，未做处理。但一天前开始出现左下腹痛、腹泻、脓血便，且有发热。体格检查显示：体温 39.0℃，血压 120/80 mmHg，呼吸 18 次/分，脉搏 86 次/分。心肺无异常。左下腹压痛明显、无反跳痛，肝肋下 0.5 cm，脾未触及。余无异常。患者粪便检查为白细胞和红细胞计数增加，且查见虫卵（图 15-11）。

（1）患者罹患的疾病可能是什么？诊断依据是什么？

（2）试分析患者腹痛、腹泻、脓血便、发热和肝肿大的可能病理学基础。

五、 思考题

1. 阿米巴肝脓肿是真的脓肿吗？为什么？
2. 血吸虫病的慢性虫卵结节为何称为假结核结节，其与结核结节形态学有何不同？
3. 请比较嗜酸性脓肿、脓肿和冷脓肿。
4. 请比较阿米巴病、血吸虫病、细菌性痢疾、伤寒和结核时肠道的病理学变化。
5. 名词解释：嗜酸性脓肿，假结核结节，阿米巴肝脓肿，血吸虫病肝。

Chapter 15

Parasitosis

Ⅰ. Aims

1. To grasp the commonly involved tissues and morphological characteristics in amoebiasis and schistosomiasis.

2. To familiarize with the commonly involved tissues and morphological characteristics in filariasis.

Guidance to study

First clarify that the direct proof of parasites existence in the samples is the most convincing evidence, then understand that morphological changes and involved tissues are different considering various species and developing stages of pathogenic parasites. Furthermore, pathological characteristics are inconsistent at acute and chronic stage of infection.

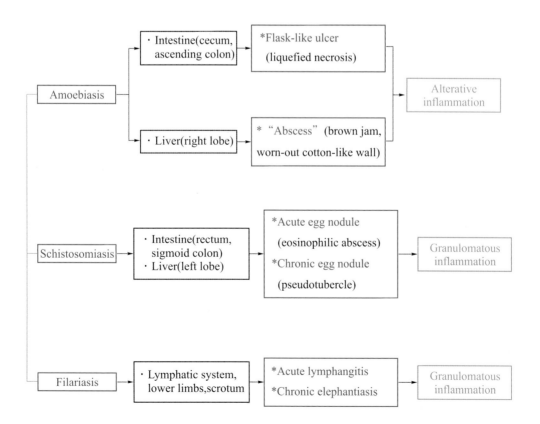

Ⅱ. Gross specimens

1. Amoebiasis

1.1　Amoebiasis of intestine (Fig.15-1)

This is a segment of colon. There are multiple ulcers, and some ulcers coalesce into a big ulcer in the submucosal layer (green circle). The ulcers are flask-shaped (a narrow neck and a broad base, green arrows), and the mucosal tissue between ulcers is relatively normal.

1.2　Amoebic abscess of liver (Fig.15-2)

The liver presents two "abscesses" (green circles) with irregular margins. The abscesses are brown jam-like materials composed of liquefied necroses as well as old hemorrhage. On cut section, most of the contents have flowed away, and the incompletely liquefied necroses have attached to the wall, therefore, the abscesses present worn-out cotton-like appearance. Are amoebic abscesses true abscesses?

2. Schistosomiasis

2.1　Chronic schistosomiasis of colon (Fig.15-3)

This is a segment of the colon. The mucosal surface is rough with the lesions of proliferation, atrophy and necrosis. On the cut section, small ulcers, necrotic areas (yellow arrow) coarse granules, and small polyps (green arrow) are observed.

2.2　Chronic schistosomiasis of liver (Fig.15-4)

The liver is yellow-brown, small and hard. On the cut surface, portal areas (green arrows) becomes broad with gray-white dense connective tissue that is flake-like or rod-like in shape.

3. Filariasis

Elephantitis of scrotum (Fig.15-5)

The specimen is from the scrotum skin with late-stage filariasis. The tissue is visibly thick, hard, and rough, with marked pigment deposit and deep dermatoglyph. The pathological skin tissue has the same appearance as an elephant's skin, which is referred to as elephantitis.

Ⅲ. Tissue sections

1. Amoebiasis

Amoebiasis of intestine (Fig.15-6)

The green arrows point to an ulcer, and the bottom and margin of the ulcer are necrotic. The intestinal wall presents mild congestion and edema. Mass of leukocytes (macrophages, lymphocytes, and plasma cells) and some amoebic trophozoites (blue arrows) are observed. The trophozoites are large and round with an irregular outline, basophilic cytoplasm, and round nuclei. The typical trophozoites contain phagocytosed erythrocytes, lymphocytes and cell debris in the cytoplasm. Around the trophozoites, empty spaces commonly exist because the surrounding tissues have been dissolved. The black arrows indicate the surrounding mucosal epithelia.

2.　Schistosomiasis

2. 1　Chronic schistosomiasis of colon（Fig.15-7）

Multiple nodules（blue stars）of varying sizes are visible in the intestinal wall, and the schistosoma eggs deposit in aggregated or scattered pattern. The egg nodules contain the components, ① Eggs of schistosoma（blue arrows）, some are dead and calcified, and others are mature with purple-blue dense dots, ② Inflammatory cells including eosinophils（black arrows）, lymphocytes, macrophages, and plasma cells, ③ Multinucleated foreign body giant cells（green arrow）and epithelioid cells.

2. 2　Acute schistosomiasis of liver（Fig.15-8）

Figure A shows a widened portal area（black star）, where interlobular blood vessels, bile ducts, and a large number of inflammatory cells（green star）can be examined. The green circle indicates acute egg nodule, and the adjacent hepatic lobule is normal, but the hepatocytes in the margin of lobules display atrophic or alterative changes. Both figure B and C display magnified egg nodules composed of necrotic tissue（blue star）, remained eggs（blue arrow）, inflammatory cells, fibroblasts, and multinucleated giant cells（green arrow）. The infiltrating cells are mainly eosinophils and epithelioid cells.

2. 3　Chronic schistosomiasis of liver（Fig.15-9）

The structure of hepatic lobules is almost intact, while some portal areas are broadened with proliferative fibrotic tissues, regenerative bile ducts（black arrow）, dilated and congested blood vessels（blue arrows）, and infiltrating inflammatory cells. There are some schistosoma egg nodules in portal areas（blue stars）. Among them, eggs are surrounded with multinucleated foreign giant cells（green arrows）, eosinophils（red arrows）, and fibrous tissue. Some eggs are calcified（yellow arrows）.

3.　Filariasis

Filaria granulomas（Fig.15-10）

Some filarial granulomas distribute in the fibrous connective tissue. The granulomas present some sections of worms with numerous microfilaria（blue arrows）, necrotic tissue（blue stars）, epithelioid cells, and multinucleated giant cells（green arrow）.

Ⅳ. Clincal pathological discussion

Case

A male aged 42 went swimming outdoors together with his friends two month before. At that time, he felt tingling and itching in the skin of his lower legs and found some red papules, which was thought to be allergic, and ignored. However, he has got abdominal pain and diarrhea with bloody purulent stool, and fever since yesterday. Physical examination showed his body temperature was 39. 0 ℃, blood pressure(BP)was 120/80 mmHg, respiratory rate was 18 beats per minute(bpm), and heart rate was 86 bpm. Tenderness, but no rebounding pain was examined at the left-lower abdomen. The liver was 5 mm below the costal margin, and the spleen was not touched. Stool routine test revealed that leukocytes and erythrocytes counts increased, and abnormal eggs were detected. The morphology of microbes are shown as Fig.15-11.

(1) What should be diagnosed for the patient? Why?

(2) Try to explain the clinical manifestations (abdominal pain, diarrhea, bloody purulent stool, and hepatomegaly) based on pathological changes.

Ⅴ. Questions

1. Is the amoebic liver abscess a true abscess? Why?

2. Chronic egg nodules of schistosomiasis are termed as pseudotubercles, why? What is the difference between pseudotubercle and tubercle?

3. Please distinguish eosinophilic abscess from abscess and cold abscess.

4. Please differentiate the pathological changes of intestines with amoebiasis, schistosomiasis, bacillary dysentry, typhoid fever, and tuberculosis.

5. Terms: Eosinophilic abscess, Pseudotubercle, Amoebic liver abscess, Chronic hepatic schistosomiasis.

VI. 附图 (Figures)

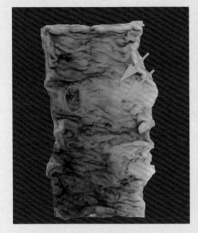

图 15-1 肠阿米巴病
Fig.15-1 Amoebiasis of intestine

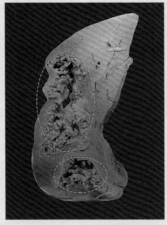

图 15-2 阿米巴肝脓肿
Fig.15-2 Amoebic abscess
of liver

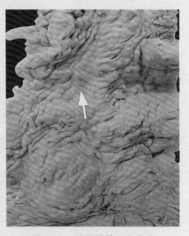

图 15-3 结肠慢性血吸虫病
Fig.15-3 Chronic schistosomiasis
of colon

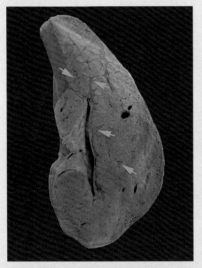

图 15-4 肝慢性血吸虫性病
Fig.15-4 Chronic schistosomiasis
of liver

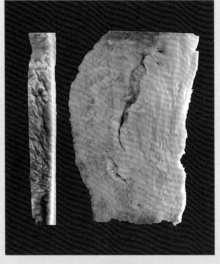

图 15-5 阴囊象皮肿
Fig.15-5 Elephantitis of scrotum

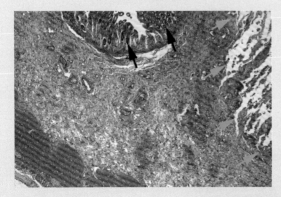

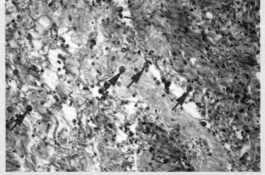

图 15-6 肠阿米巴病（×40；×400）
Fig.15-6 Amoebiasis of intestine（×40；×400）

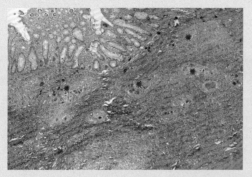
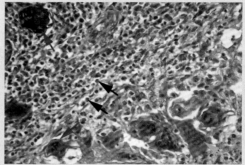

图 15-7　结肠慢性血吸虫病（×40；×400）
Fig.15-7　Chronic schistosomiasis of colon（×40；×400）

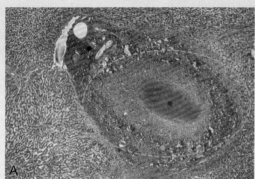
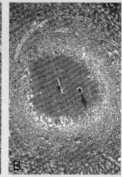
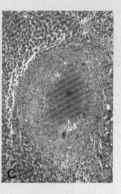

图 15-8　肝急性血吸虫病（×40；×100；×100）
Fig.15-8　Acute schistosomiasis of liver（×40；×100；×100）

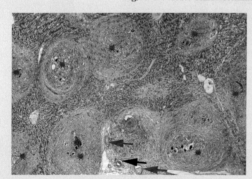
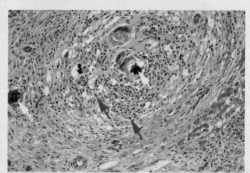

图 15-9　肝慢性血吸虫病（×40；×200）
Fig.15-9　Chronic schistosomiasis of liver（×40；×200）

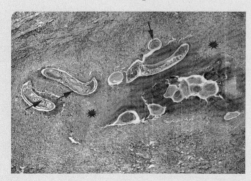
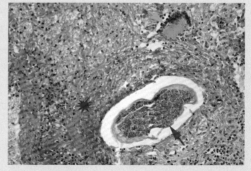

图 15-10　丝虫性肉芽肿（×40；×200）
Fig.15-10　Filaria granulomas（×40；×200）

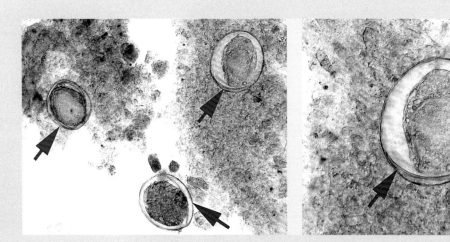

图 15-11　案例（×200；×400）
Fig.15-11　Case（×200；×400）

李懿萍（Yiping Li）

参考文献

［1］步宏,李一雷. 病理学［M］. 9 版. 北京：人民卫生出版社,2018.

［2］陈杰,周桥. 病理学［M］. 3 版. 北京：人民卫生出版社,2015.

［3］Vinay Kumar，Jon Aster，Abul Abbas. Robbins Basic Pathology［M］. 10th ed. Elsevier publisher，2017.

［4］病理与健康［EB/OL］. https：//www. icourse163. org/course/SEU-1001755397.

［5］病理形态实验学［EB/OL］. https：//www. icourse163. org/course/SEU-1206290801.

［6］普通病理学［EB/OL］. https：//www. icourse163. org/course/SEU-1463109174.

［7］系统病理学［EB/OL］. https：//www. icourse163. org/course/SEU-1206526803.

References

［1］ Hong Bu, Yilei Li. Pathology［M］. 9th ed. Beijing: People's medical publishing house, 2018.

［2］ Jie Chen, Qiao Zhou. Pathology［M］. 3rd ed. Beijing: People's medical publishing house, 2015.

［3］ Vinay Kumar, Jon Aster, Abul Abbas. Robbins Basic Pathology［M］. 10th ed. Elsevier publisher, 2017.

［4］ Pathology and health［EB/OL］. https://www.icourse163.org/course/SEU-1001755397.

［5］ Experimental pathology［EB/OL］. https://www.icourse163.org/course/SEU-1206290801.

［6］ General pathology［EB/OL］. https://www.icourse163.org/course/SEU-1463109174.

［7］ Systemic pathology［EB/OL］. https://www.icourse163.org/course/SEU-1206526803.